Pharmacokinetics

A MODERN VIEW

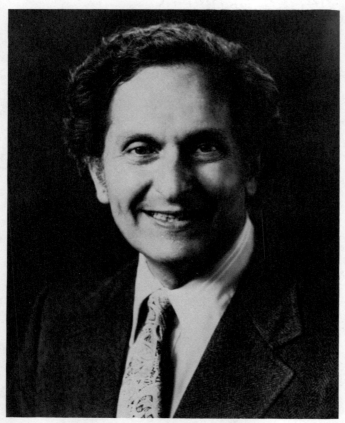

Professor Sidney Riegelman

Pharmacokinetics

A MODERN VIEW

Edited by

Leslie Z. Benet
University of California School of Pharmacy
San Francisco, California

Gerhard Levy
School of Pharmacy
State University of New York
Buffalo, New York

and

Bobbe L. Ferraiolo
University of California School of Pharmacy
San Francisco, California

Plenum Press • New York and London

Library of Congress Cataloging in Publication Data

Sidney Riegelman Memorial Symposium (1982: University of California, San Francisco)
  Pharmacokinetics, a modern view.

"Proceedings of the Sidney Riegelman Memorial Symposium, held April 22–24, 1982, at the
University of California, San Francisco, California"—T.p. verso.
  Bibliography: p.
  Includes index.
  1. Pharmacokinetics—Congresses. I. Benet, Leslie Z. II. Levy, Gerhard. III. Ferraiolo,
Bobbe L. IV. Riegelman, Sidney, 1921–1981. V. Title. [DNML: 1. Biopharmaceutics—
congresses. 2. Drugs—administration and dosage—congresses. 3. Drugs—metabolism—
congresses. 4. Kinetics—congresses. QV 38 S569p 1982]
  RM301.5.S53 1982   615'.7   84-15011
  ISBN 0-306-41810-X

Proceedings of the Sidney Riegelman Memorial Symposium, held April 22–24, 1982,
at the University of California, San Francisco, California

© 1984 Plenum Press, New York
A Division of Plenum Publishing Corporation
233 Spring Street, New York, N.Y. 10013

Printed in the United States of America

DEDICATION

This book and the symposium upon which it is based are intended as a tribute and memorial to our colleague, teacher and friend, Sidney Riegelman, Professor of Pharmacy and Pharmaceutical Chemistry at the University of California, San Francisco, School of Pharmacy. It is also intended to serve as a record of his accomplishments and a history of his outstanding service to his profession and his scientific discipline. Moreover we hope that this book will be an inspiration to present and future graduate students in the pharmaceutical sciences so that they may pursue their studies with the same vigor, commitment and enthusiasm that characterized Sid Riegelman's career.

There have been very significant and exciting advances in the young discipline of pharmacokinetics in recent years. Important concepts such as nonlinear pharmacokinetics, physiologically based models, presystemic biotransformation, effects of age and disease on drug disposition, relationship between plasma protein binding and drug distribution and elimination, kinetics of pharmacologic effects and population pharmacokinetics have been introduced, explored and applied in research and drug therapy. The late Professor Sidney Riegelman played a leading role in these developments and it is appropriate that this book in his memory be devoted to a comprehensive survey of the current status of pharmacokinetics and to a consideration of the likely future directions of research and practice in this discipline.

SIDNEY RIEGELMAN – 1921–1981

Sidney Riegelman was born July 19, 1921 in Milwaukee, Wisconsin. He attended the University of Wisconsin, graduating with a Bachelor of Science degree in Pharmacy in 1944. Since these were the war years, Sid went into the armed services, serving as a lieutenant in communications in the U.S. Navy. At the end of the war, he returned to Madison to enter graduate school receiving a Ph.D. in Pharmacy in 1948. Following his graduate work, Sid and his new wife of two years, Milli, came West to join the faculty of the School of Pharmacy at the University of California at San Francisco. Their children, Nancy, Mark and Carole, were born in the following years. At UCSF, Sid rose through the academic ranks holding the positions of instructor, 1948-50; assistant professor, 1950-56, and associate professor, 1956-62.

In 1958, Sid published a series of papers with graduate student Wilfred Crowell, which appeared in the scientific edition of the Journal of the American Pharmaceutical Association under the major heading of "The Kinetics of Rectal Absorption". For these studies Sid was awarded the Ebert Prize in 1959 which recognized Sid's publications as the best work published in journals of the American Pharmaceutical Association during the year 1958.

Sid was promoted to Professor of Pharmacy in 1962 and held a joint appointment in the Department of Radiology beginning in 1964. The quality of the research published by Sid together with his graduate students and postdoctoral fellows was recognized when Sid was awarded the American Pharmaceutical Association Research Achievement Award in Physical Pharmacy in 1968, followed by the Association's Award in Pharmacodynamics in 1970. In 1970, Sid was chosen Alumnus of the Year by the University of Wisconsin School of Pharmacy and was elected a Fellow of the Academy of Pharmaceutical Sciences.

In the early 1970s, Sid carried out two significant research-related tasks in addition to his own work. In 1972, he was the primary author for a pamphlet published by the Academy of Pharmaceutical Sciences entitled "Guidelines for Bioavailability Studies in Man." In 1973, Sid founded and became the Editor of the Journal of Pharmacokinetics and Biopharmaceutics, the first journal pub-

lished in this discipline. Sid was a visiting lecturer in Australia, Japan, Israel and South Africa and repeatedly was invited to
lecture in Europe, particularly in the Scandinavian countries. In
1978, he was selected to deliver the Karl Wilhelm Scheele Lecture
at the meeting of the Pharmaceutical Society of Sweden.

Sid always gave willingly of his time and energy. At the
time of his death he was a member of the Executive Committee of the
Academy of Pharmaceutical Sciences and Chairman of the Academy's
Task Force on Dissolution Methodology. Sid was also a leader in
pharmacy education. He developed the first courses related to
biology and pharmacy under the title of Biopharmaceutics. He was
Chairman of the Department of Pharmacy from 1967–78, a time when
the department grew in stature to assume an important leadership
position. He was instrumental in the development of Clinical Pharmacy at UCSF. Throughout much of the 1950s, with this discipline
in its infancy and with many doubters, he was a major and tireless
force in initiating and developing Clinical Pharmacy at UCSF. Even
in 1981, as a full Professor and Associate Dean for Research Services, Sid was Chairman of the school's Curriculum Committee.
Although Sid's interests and research were multifarious, he considered himself a pharmacist and a pharmaceutical scientist. All his
energy went into making his profession and scientific discipline
succeed.

Twenty-two graduate students received their Ph.D.'s under
Sid's direction, including three of the six students working with
Sid at the time of his death. An approximately equal number of
postdoctoral scholars and M.D. fellows have worked in Sid's laboratory. These young men and women collaborated with Sid in his 176
publications. Thirty-two of these Riegelman trained scientists are
contributing authors in this volume. A complete listing of Sid's
scientific publications may be found as an Appendix beginning on
page 519. The first six chapters of this volume describe in more
detail and from the perspective of his personal friends an overview
of Sidney Riegelman, the man, his work and his impact.

On April 4, 1981, Sid drowned while scuba diving with his wife
at Salt Point, California, a coastal area just north of San Francisco. It seems most appropriate to close this brief biographical
sketch by recounting the text of a memorial plaque located outside
the office of the Department of Pharmacy at UCSF. The plaque is
dedicated to Sid "by his graduate students, who honor his scientific achievements and excellence, his inspiration and contagious
enthusiasm in research and teaching. We shall always remember Sid
as our mentor, scientific father and most importantly, as our
beloved friend and confidant."

Leslie Z. Benet

ACKNOWLEDGMENT

The Editors gratefully acknowledge the efforts of the individuals whose expertise, dedication and loyalty made the publication of this tribute to Sidney Riegelman possible: Trinity Ordona, Linda Roman, Jude Thilman, Martha Barba, Maria Rosen and Joan Apodaca.

CONTENTS

xi

PHARMACOKINETICS – CONCEPTS, THEORY AND APPLICATION

PHARMACOKINETICS AND DRUG METABOLISM

APPENDIX AND INDEX

Chapter 1

SIDNEY RIEGELMAN - THE WISCONSIN YEARS

Louis W. Busse

School of Pharmacy
University of Wisconsin
Madison, Wisconsin

I am pleased to be able to participate in this Symposium in which we pay honor and respect to Sidney Riegelman, a friend and colleague to so many of us. His many contributions to pharmacy, pharmaceutics education and research will be outlined in the chapters to follow. It is my pleasure to recall for you events in Sid's preparative years which we call The Wisconsin Years.

Sid was born on July 19, 1921 in Milwaukee, Wisconsin, the second son of Marcus (Max) and Irma R. Riegelman. His brother Robert preceded him by about three years. It is quite clear that the Riegelman family was a "pharmacy" family and as the brothers grew into early adulthood they were initiated into the pharmacy environment by their father and worked with him diligently through their high school and college careers.

The development of Sid's pharmaceutical career must have been influenced by the example his father set for him. Max Riegelman's life was devoted entirely to pharmacy. He was a medical service representative for Eli Lilly & Co. for many years before he opened his pharmacy, at 12th and State Streets, across from Mt. Sinai Hospital in Milwaukee, in the year 1918. His early work with medical professionals proved helpful and he became the primary supplier of pharmaceutical services in the hospital. A friendly relationship was established between the medical personnel of the hospital and the pharmacy personnel and the pharmacy soon became the "hangout" for the doctors, interns and nurses.

It is interesting to note that out of this rather unique pharmacy environment Robert, Sid's brother, found and developed a strong attachment to the so-called "people" side of the profession

1

and opened his own community pharmacy in Milwaukee which he
operated for over 30 years. Sid, on the other hand, became very
interested in pharmacy as a profession, but was more attracted to
the why and what, or the science, of the chemicals and pharmaceuticals. He indicated to me that his early exposure to the hospital
setting and his contacts with the physicians and house staff had a
great influence upon the direction of his career.

Sid's elementary and secondary education was all in the
Milwaukee school system.   His brother Bob says Sid's academic
record in those years was good but nothing to get excited about; he
says it wasn't until Sid was stimulated in the fields he enjoyed
that his real abilities appeared. Of course, this is substantiated
by his marvelous academic performance in his professional and post-
graduate work.

Our first personal knowledge of Sidney came about in the form
of a letter to Dr. Uhl on May 22, 1940. In it, Sid stated that he
was enrolled in the first pre-pharmacy year at the Milwaukee Extension Center and that he was looking forward to finishing his
"ordinary course in Pharmacy" and then perhaps going on to get a
Master's Degree in Pharmaceutical Chemistry. He requested information on the other courses he would need, the mathematics courses in
particular. He wanted to get these out of the way through correspondence courses that summer.

You can imagine Dr. Uhl's delight at receiving a letter like
that.   Sid came to the Madison Campus in September 1940 and a
mutual admiration relationship soon arose between Sid and Dr. Uhl.
He couldn't wait to get Sid into graduate school.   Dr. Uhl did not
hesitate to maneuver Sid's professional requirements so that Sid
could take elective courses to prepare for graduate school. This
soon got Dr. Uhl into trouble with the Dean of the College of
Letters and Science (Pharmacy was not a separate school at that
time), who wrote:

> "Dear Professor Uhl: It seems to me in the case
> of Sidney Riegelman, and similar cases, where the
> student wishes to take the lecture portion of courses
> during the semester and the laboratory work during the
> vacation, you ought to send up a recommendation to that
> effect, since the procedure is irregular, although I
> have no doubt justifiable. Will you, therefore, please
> send me such a recommendation for Mr. Riegelman. Yours
> very truly, G.C. Sellery, Dean."

Needless to say, Dr. Uhl responded promptly to Dean Sellery's
request.   Dr. Uhl had apparently learned his lesson, for on
December 16, 1942 we have a request to the Dean as follows:

"Mr. Sidney Riegelman is short one credit of Pharmacy 51 which is a required subject in the School of
Pharmacy. His program was arranged this semester to
include physical chemistry, a course I wanted him to
have as a prerequisite for work he expects to take later
on. I will be on the campus this Christmas recess and
will direct the work in Pharmacy 51. I recommend that
Mr. Riegelman be given permission to register for this
course during the Christmas recess."

Sid graduated with a B.S. degree in Pharmacy, became a regis-
tered pharmacist and, although continuing on into graduate school,
maintained a life-long interest in the profession and worked
consistently to improve its practice through better educational
programs.

My own personal contact with Sid came about through the
teacher/student relationship. This relationship was enhanced when,
in his senior year, he completed his thesis requirement under my
direction by doing a "Study of the Effect of Electrolytes on Acacia
Emulsions." Through this work we came to know quite a bit about
heterogenous and disperse systems which stimulated our interest in
surfaces, sizes, areas, and so forth, of liquid and solid pharmaceutical disperse systems. When Sid entered into graduate school
in January of 1943, we began to study ways and means of producing
solids with large surface areas and decided that spray drying would
be a process we might investigate.

We had very little money to work with at that time so we
designed and had the University shops build the chamber and the
atomizer spray nozzle. We conjured up a turbine fan and gas air
heater to go with the chamber. We were not sure about our abilities with an air cyclone (centrifuge) precipitator so we decided
to construct and attach a Cottrell precipitator system. Believe it
or not, it worked, and we were able to substantiate this procedure
as a method for achieving very small, uniformly sized particles and
for adsorbing mucilaginous and surface active agents on the
surfaces of these powders. As a result, we were able to receive
research support for these studies, and also to purchase a commercial laboratory spray dryer for future studies.

I mention this in some detail because it exemplifies a part of
Sid's nature. Those of us who knew Sid certainly would not
consider him to be adept or well-coordinated with his hands - not
the builder type. However, what he lacked in natural ability, he
made up for in tenacity. He was one of the most determined and
intense young men I knew in those days; and insofar as I know, this
tenacity continued throughout his career.

The war period began and, in the first two years of Sid's
graduate studies, we were constantly involved with registration and
deferment problems. By the spring of 1943, it was obvious that we
were not going to be able to maintain a deferment status for Sid so
he applied for a commission in the Navy and this was granted in
June of 1944. By September, I was in Washington D.C. with the War
Production Board.

During the next two years Dean Uhl and Sid were in continuous
communication. Sid would write and tell Dr. Uhl of his experiences
in the Navy and then ask about journals he should read, the school
and the staff. He told Dr. Uhl what he wanted to do when he
returned. Dean Uhl would reply to Sid's questions and tell Sid
about his plans for the school when the war was over. In the
spring of 1945, long before there was any sign that the war with
Japan would end, Dr. Uhl sent Sid an application for a research
assistantship to begin in September 1946. Sid, of course, complied
and, fortunately for me, we both were able to be back on the campus
in 1946.

The 1946-48 years were significant years for Sid for many
reasons. First, he was part of the school's effort to bring the
application of physical chemical principles to pharmaceutical
science and pharmaceutical systems, and to bring these subjects
into the pharmacy curriculum. Dr. Higuchi came to us also in 1947
and he, along with graduate student Joe Swintosky, gave strong
support to Sid's interest in physical chemistry and mathematics.

The first Pharmaceutical Education Seminar, sponsored by the
American Foundation for Pharmaceutical Education, was held on the
Wisconsin campus in the summer of 1949. This seminar was devoted
to discussing the need to explain pharmaceutical problems and techniques from a scientific standpoint, and the need for pharmacy
students to have adequate training in mathematics and physical
chemistry. Sid and Joe were strongly involved in this effort along
with Dr. Wurster, Dr. Higuchi and myself.

Publicity from seminars and presentations at national meetings
led some book publishers to initiate new textbooks which would
incorporate these new philosophies and apply them to the solution
of old problems. Lippincott sought contributions from Dr. Higuchi,
Dr. Wurster and myself. I discussed this with Sid and Joe and they
said they would like to participate in the writing of one of the
chapters on Colloids, Suspensions and Emulsions that I would be
responsible for; they did, and their names appeared as co-authors
with their titles as Research Assistants, University of Wisconsin
(1). Sid's participation in these efforts to modernize pharmaceutical science was a marvelous outlet for his energy and his
ambitions; it developed in him a maturity far beyond that of the
average graduate student. Someone once said "timing" is

all-important. It was certainly true in Sid's case. In one sense, we can say it was fortunate for Sid that the evolving changes in the School of Pharmacy were in motion when he came, and that these fitted his ideas and needs perfectly. The reverse was also true. It was extremely fortunate for the school to have had Sidney Riegelman as one of its first graduate students; a student who would test the new programs and who would contribute so much to the success of the School.

Sid's thesis work was done in the powder technology area. His research centered on the importance of the state and subdivision of powders as this would affect therapeutic performance. Sid used the spray dryer to prepare the powders and studied the gas permeation method for particle size analysis. The philosophy behind both Sid's and Joe's work was that "particle size" was a poorly controlled factor in pharmaceutical systems. The USP did not have sub-sieve specifications for powders and there was evidence that size distribution could play an important part in the release of drug substances from pharmaceutical systems, thereby influencing the absorption of the drug in the biological system. Sid's thesis work substantiated this and that concept became the central part of his studies in his later career, eventually leading him into biopharmaceutics and pharmacokinetics.

If I have written too much about Wisconsin, I apologize. I must state, however, that for the period 1942-48 Sid was so intimately associated with our programs, and our hopes and dreams for the School, the profession and its science, that we would be doing Sid an injustice if we did not talk about it.

In this world we seem to be categorized as givers or takers. For me, there is no question that Sid gave back to the University, the profession, and its science much, much more than he took. To me, Sid was a giver, a contributor always willing to give more than he received. I was enriched by having Sidney Riegelman as a student in the professional and doctoral programs. He contributed significantly to my career as a teacher and researcher. Wisconsin pharmacy was enriched as well, through Sidney Riegelman's contributions as a student, teacher and researcher. We miss him as a friend and a colleague.

REFERENCE

1. S. Riegelman, J.V. Swintosky and L.W. Busse, Colloids, emulsions and suspensions, in: "American Pharmacy," (Vol. II), R.A. Lyman, ed., J.B. Lippincott Co., Philadelphia (1947), ch. 3.

Chapter 2

SIDNEY RIEGELMAN - FRIEND AND COLLEAGUE

Arnold D. Marcus

Research and Development Laboratories
Bristol-Myers Products
1350 Liberty Avenue
Hillside, New Jersey

To be asked to present some reminiscences about the distinguished scientist whose contributions we recognize here is an honor
which I, like all of us, would prefer to forego. Yet another giant
has fallen in the midst of a magnificent career. Why, I keep
asking, do we fail to acknowledge the living and wait to confer
posthumous honor? This gathering includes many whose work has been
at the cutting edge; those who have received medals, scrolls,
honorary degrees and the plaudits of scientists throughout the
world. They, too, face the menace of the years. What greater
tribute to Sid Riegelman than to have this symposium serve as a
spur to do honor to those who deserve honor inter vivos rather than
posthumously.

My own years with Sid as a friend and colleague resulted from
a letter I wrote to him shortly after Thanksgiving of 1950. I
wrote to ask him for his candid opinion about the University of
Wisconsin. Louis Busse, Joe Swintosky and Sid had written a
chapter for a recently published volume of **American Pharmacy.** That
chapter, along with one written by a then "unknown" Takeru Higuchi,
fascinated me. Since Louis, Joe and Tak were members of the
Wisconsin faculty, I thought that Sid, safely away in California,
would be the most candid, especially after two years away from
Madison. We had never met or communicated in any way; we were
unknown to each other. Yet, I received as long, detailed, thorough
and encouraging a response as if the inquiry had been made by a
close relative or life-long friend.

Although we were not then "friends" by any definition of that
word, Sid's letter was an act of friendship which I recalled

happily many times. Our friendship matured slowly but continuously
over a period of more than thirty years. Without question, in the
decade or so before April 1981, our friendship was firm. We sought
each other out, we could speak freely of personal matters, we could
seek advice and receive it. Even though the jet age reduced the
effect of great distance, and we both overcame depression-born
reluctance to make long-distance telephone calls, we realized that
a great deal had to be packed into the times we were together
physically. Unfortunately, we never developed a long and continuing correspondence and I don't know why. Neither of us regarded
words as things to be hoarded or used sparingly. Perhaps the fact
that we did use the phone and saw each other four or five times a
year inhibited a written correspondence.

    The bond between Sid and me developed more easily and was
surely stronger because of the close relationship between Milli and
Judy. Our wives enjoyed each other's companionship, looked forward
to being together, and were also able to share and confide; to lend
an understanding ear and a sympathetic response. Thus our friendship embraced our families and not the two of us alone.

    To return to my subject and to be fair to Sid's preference, I
must even now use words and conjure ideas with that meticulous
precision which marked Sid's scientific and professional contributions. I want to preserve a "cognitive accuracy."

    In a dictionary, which is quite old, yet treasured by me above
all others, the word "friend" has several definitions. The first -
paramour - can be dismissed immediately. The second - one who is
passive, contemplative without passion, seeking only inner light
and abhoring any violence - is also inappropriate. Sid's mission
was, and ours should be, to be active, not pacific; to be emotion-
ally involved; to strive, often at fever pitch; to introduce change
in scientific thought, professional practice and educational
policy. Sid intended to do violence to the status quo and intended
to shatter stale ideas in order to stand on the debris and thereby
surmount complacency and inaction. Sid thought things through
carefully and with attention to detail, but mere contemplation was
not his way. His mind was a maelstrom for ideas as well as a
processor for separating the worthy from the illogical. Those of
us who struggled to read his slides realized that the power of his
mental vortices was never quite equaled by the striving to make
sense or produce order. Those of us who heard his rising crescendo
of condemnation of the USP and NF - just after having served with
the U.S. Office of Technological Assessment, as discussed in Dr.
Kaplan's chapter - may have squirmed a bit, perhaps a good deal,
but we were made well aware that pacifism was not Sid's route to
progress.

The definition of friend which most closely fit our friendship is "one attached to another by affection and esteem." Our affection permitted serious differences over scientific matters, educational policy and social institutions to persist, without rancor, to the very end. We looked forward to serious exchanges, no matter how intense or violent, precisely because of our esteem for each other's intellectual rigor. During an Academy of Pharmaceutical Sciences business meeting, only a few days before Sid's death, I stated my annoyance about a report Sid's committee was about to issue. Our "discussion" continued at one of the hospitality suites and even during a harrowing cab ride with Judy and Stan Kaplan. It ceased for a few moments at the restaurant but didn't really end until we started eating. As I remember the occasion, it really only stopped after Stan tried to mediate and Judy told us to "shut up." That woman has winning ways!

A further example of this mutual esteem and affection is one which occurred during one of my brief visits to the University. Naturally, I stopped by Sid's office just to say hello. He was immersed in a sea of paper with sheets covering every space. He looked up and said, with rising irritation and increasing decibels, ceasing only a moment from the furious pace of writing, "Arnold, I don't have the time to talk to you. I have a grant application to finish and the deadline is here." He started another sentence and then stopped in mid-syllable as I started to leave while muttering my regards to Milli. "The hell with the application. Let's talk; we always have so many things to go over," were Sid's next words. About an hour later, after we had ranged over a wide spectrum of concerns and were in the middle of a heated debate over the predictive value of dissolution rates, Les Benet came by to remind me that the students were waiting for me. The "debate" ended, we shook hands and exchanged good wishes. Each of us had had a wonderful hour while remaining true to his nature. We parted, as always, firm friends.

I made brief mention earlier in these remarks of the close relationship enjoyed by Milli and Judy. Their views of Sid and me also served to cement the friendship I held so dear. In truth, they regarded us as not totally in the world of reality. One evening, after dinner and theater in New York, the four of us were walking north on Fifth or Sixth Avenue. Sid and I were deep into a discussion of nuclear arms, the need to provide more or less clinical education and the efforts to unionize the faculty at the University of California. We may have been slightly preoccupied; autos blew their horns, cab drivers their stacks, brakes screeched, and assorted philistines waved fists at us. We paid little heed but kept walking, past our destination, until Judy ran over to us and exclaimed, "You two would fall off Manhattan if we weren't here." In the face of such slander, our friendship could only thrive!

Our relationship as colleagues was somewhat different from the usual. We were not part of the same department, school, college, university or even a group working closely together dealing collegially with mutual problems, concerns and differences. Our arena was unlike the academic; in academia, I'm certain, conflicts are resolved dispassionately, rancor plays no role, ideology seldom intrudes, and the territorial imperative, "turf," is virtually unknown. In those groves, the only passions are those of logic and reason. Sid and I often arrived at our consensus-of-two tumultuously, if at all. It may be more than metaphor to say that our differences were hammered out.

At least one derivation of the word colleague suggests that such persons were originally part of a union formed or permitted by law. The law currently glorifies, or at least emphasizes, the adversary process as the way to the truth. Sid and I enjoyed that system. Sometimes we stood together, adversaries to all who espoused the conventional wisdom. Other times we were adversarial to each other, in public, on issues of educational philosophy, drug product selection, the vitality of the Academy of Pharmaceutical Sciences and many others. Our discussions were not dispassionate; they were loud and vehement; sometimes, even discourteous. Yet, not once did our disputes and disagreements mar our friendship or attenuate our desire to renew the battle.

My conclusion to this tribute to Sid Riegelman would be incomplete and inadequate if I failed to emphasize that his scientific skills ranged far beyond pharmacokinetics. This discipline was but the most recent into which he plunged with vigor and from which he emerged with great success. I must note that Sid achieved prominence in almost every area of pharmaceutical science. His reputation was built on and anchored to a thorough knowledge of the physical sciences and mathematics. Only because of his basic education in and mastery of the physical sciences was Sid able to contribute so much to the area which is the focus of this symposium.

Chapter 3

SIDNEY RIEGELMAN — THE EDUCATOR

Jere E. Goyan

School of Pharmacy
University of California
San Francisco, California

Of the many people I have known, few have been as complex as Sidney Riegelman. Since I have been given the task of discussing Sid, the complex educator, it is imperative that I lay out the credentials that enable me to comment in this regard. First of all, I was a student of his — a relationship that began when I was an undergraduate at the University of California at San Francisco and ended on the day he withdrew from the company of man. I attended the first pharmaceutics lecture he gave at UCSF in 1951. Later, he taught in the senior dispensing course, and I was there too. And even later, as a graduate student sharing problems with his first two graduate students, I had the opportunity to observe him as a graduate mentor.

I left, went off into the world, returned in 1963, and had the pleasure of working with him in a number of capacities. Eventually, I became the Chairman of the Department of Pharmacy, (can anyone imagine what it is like to be a chairman of a department with Sid Riegelman in it?), and later, I sat in the dean's chair. Yes, I have had the pleasure of observing Sid, the educator, for more than 30 years, during which I counted myself as his friend, colleague and admirer.

An audience listening to someone describe an exceptional educator perhaps expects to be told about the person's talents as a superb lecturer. Now, let us be totally truthful: Sid was a perfectly dreadful lecturer, difficult to follow, and from whom it was impossible to take notes. But all who ever had him as an instructor forgave him his shortcomings in this regard. We knew that his thoughts traveled so fast that he was always five steps ahead of us and we were dazzled by the bewildering stream of

11

stunning concepts with which he inundated us. We did not dare try
to slow him down, for that would be a tacit admission that we did
not understand, and none of us could bring ourselves to do that.
Instead, we studied, so as not to disappoint him, and so that the
gap would not increase to six steps. And we learned. Furthermore,
his habitual enthusiasm was infectious. He would become so excited
that he would stutter, and he would excite us, and we would study
all the more. Few teachers, regardless of their eloquence, succeed
in stimulating such a response in their students. I say that now
as a mature, former student of his who can look back and appreciate
the impact he had upon me and others.

Sid was a man of many interests, to each of which he was
totally committed. Among the many things he was dedicated to was
the profession of pharmacy and the education of pharmacists. He
made this clear in the opening paragraphs of a presentation
entitled, "One Man's Biased View of Pharmacy Education" (1):

> "The following is an extremely biased exposition
> of the views of one educator ... and somewhat overempha-
> tic in tone in a desire to make the message heard.
> Having grown up with and been involved with pharmacy
> throughout my life, it is a view through these jaundiced
> eyes of mine. Finally, since this message is primarily
> directed to the pharmacy educator, which I have
> professed to be for nearly thirty years ... it is in
> some ways an act of self-flagellation."

He went on to speak of the many errors that had been made in
pharmacy education, and did not hesitate to list his own role in
what he called its "trials and tragedies." He was unfair to
himself in many ways in that presentation, and I would like to set
the record straight by elaborating on the magnitude of his contributions to pharmacy education at UCSF, most of which, as history
has demonstrated, have had national repercussions.

Early in his teaching career, Sid made a number of original
contributions to the fledgling area of pharmaceutics, particularly
as it related to ophthalmologics, suppositories and dermatologi-
cals. Furthermore, with each dosage form, he addressed the issue
of the effect of formulation on the pharmacologic availability of
the active agent, something which much later became known as
biopharmaceutics. His chapter on suppositories in **American
Pharmacy** (2) is excellent reading even today and his syllabi on
ophthalmologic and dermatologic drugs were widely admired.

When Eino Nelson joined the UCSF faculty in the mid-'50s, he
and Sid accepted the responsibility for developing a course in
biopharmaceutics for the then emerging Doctor of Pharmacy program.
It was Sid's ever alert pharmacist's eye, however, that first saw

this as a tool to extend the pharmacist's role beyond the distribution of drugs. Few people may recall that generic drugs were just emerging at that time and Sid felt that an understanding of product formulation, drug stability and bioavailability would enable the pharmacy practitioner to assume a role in drug product selection. Although this did not come to pass in the manner Sid had envisioned, it did represent a drastic departure from the traditional passive role of the pharmacist, which, once suggested, set him to thinking about other roles.

The first I heard about it was when he and Don Sorby came to see me, in November 1965, to discuss a new practice concept they had been mulling over. Their timing was perfect; I, too, had been seriously considering the need for alternative roles for the pharmacist. They quickly convinced me that we needed to do an experiment to test the pharmacist as an expert on drug therapy. As an initial step, we hired five young, enthusiastic, UCSF graduates to establish a seven-day-a-week, around-the-clock clinical pharmacy service on the surgical ward of Moffitt Hospital. From that modest beginning evolved the curriculum we have today, with its intense clinical clerkship experience. Before 1965, no school of pharmacy offered required clerkships; today, none are without them. In a very real sense, Sid Riegelman is their originator.

Today, the practitioner faculty at UCSF School of Pharmacy stands more than 300 strong. Sid is also responsible for this development. It was he who had looked around in 1961 and realized that none of our faculty were practicing pharmacists. He saw to it that Dick Penna and then Bob Day were appointed to the faculty, and later suggested that we recruit a volunteer faculty to teach in the area of non-prescription (OTC) drugs. Incidentally, few people realize Sid's indirect role in OTC education. As early as 1957, he taught a course that critically evaluated the OTC external products on the market - something that just wasn't done in those days - and in so doing planted the seed in the minds of two students, later to be faculty, that led to the development of the APhA **Handbook on Non-Prescription Medications.**

In the presentation I referred to earlier, Sid described his commitment to the clinical program in the following terms (1):

> "From 1967 to 1972, Don Sorby and I virtually immersed ourselves in implementing the clinical pharmacy program. Most of the credit should go to Don Sorby and to Bob Miller, who was initially in charge of the Clinical Pharmacy Service, and to Eric Owyang, who kept our hospital pharmacy administration chores to a minimum. I must admit, though, I had virtually to give up being a researcher and spend most of my 60 hours per week as an administrator."

Sid did not exaggerate. He <u>did</u> immerse himself in the program and, as was his nature, generated not only intense light but some heat as well. I remember the observation of a faculty member that no one ever left Sid's presence without some emotion, whether it be confusion, anger or elation. Indeed, shortly after he dedicated himself totally to the clinical pharmacy program, I could depend upon visits by one or two faculty members each month who were absolutely enraged over something Sid had asked of them or, worse yet, had done. My advice was always the same: cool off and see what happens. One of two things <u>always</u> happened: Sid realized that his zeal had carried him too far, apologized and was loved again, or those who felt offended quickly saw the wisdom of his ways. Either way the program improved and those involved could look back and see how they had been intimately involved in something that was important. He had his finger on every facet of our clinical program, and no other member of our faculty had as much impact on it as he during its neonatal period.

How about Sid, the graduate educator? During his career, he trained 22 graduate students. From his first, Naseem Allawala, to his last, Man-Wai Lo, he was a stimulating, demanding, maddening, supportive, but most of all, inspiring mentor. Herein, too, he was a complex, sometimes confusing instructor, and, from all external appearances, the stereotypical absent-minded professor. There are tales that have rumbled through the years - too many, in fact, to be ignored - about meetings with Sid in which his attention was divided between the graduate student and three or four other activities that were going on simultaneously. And sometimes the student came to the realization that, although Sid had looked at him or her and had nodded attentively, Sid had not heard a single thing he or she had said. But perhaps the most disconcerting form of his intense preoccupation surfaced at those times when, in the middle of a discussion, Sid would stand up and leave, and the student would sit there, assuming that he would return shortly. Where had Sid gone? Off to take care of something that had suddenly popped into his mind, fully intending to return, only to think of something else, and something else again, and finally forgetting that the student was waiting.

Graduate students quickly learned that if they wanted Sid's full attention, the only way to get it was to catch him on a weekend, or at some other time when he was not doing five hundred other things. But when his attention was finally gained the ideas, questions, answers and guidance came tumbling out lightning fast, and those who had endured his distractions realized that it was all worthwhile. Whatever the frustrations, the magic he was capable of conjuring worked, as can be measured by the many contributions his former students have made in wide and diverse areas of pharmaceutics research.

In the early '70s, Sid decided that it was time for our Department of Pharmacy to spell out the professional competencies a pharmacist should possess. Since our clinical program was still in its formative stages, his directive was resisted by the fairly unanimous defense that it was "too early to nail ourselves down." Although a few competencies dribbled in from some members of the faculty, this did not satisfy Sid. So one night when he couldn't sleep, he got up and wrote down what he thought the clinical pharmacist should be capable of doing: four pages of competencies. They were magnificently defined, so much so that only a little editing was necessary before we adopted them. But, as was so typical of Sid's global concern for the profession, he realized that what we had envisioned was a pharmacist of a type as yet unrecognized anywhere in the nation. So he decided to change that sorry state of affairs, beginning with California. He met with the California Board of Pharmacy, presented the list of competencies, and the Board members were impressed, to say the least. The Board had been grappling with the notion of defining pharmacist competencies for many years, but had never been able to get the project off the ground. Sid's four pages were a godsend. Nevertheless, the Board asked that he meet with the faculties of the other schools in the state to see if they agreed with the proposed competencies. What resulted was a tri-school endorsement of something only slightly different from the original. If you are interested, you need only obtain a copy of **California Pharmacy Law** (3) to read them. They serve as the foundation upon which the State Board of Pharmacy licensing examination is constructed.

Several events took place that would have given any scientist/educator, even one as committed as Sid, ample excuse to say, "I have paid my dues to pharmacy education, let others take on the burden." The first was the informal separation of the clinical program from the Department of Pharmacy at UCSF, a process in which he assisted. The second was his retirement as chairman of the Department of Pharmacy. No one would or could have criticized him for redirecting his attention entirely to his research. After all, he had done more than anyone could have expected of him. But he was not that kind of man; his love of education and pharmacy had no end. In 1978, I prevailed upon him to serve as chairman of the Curriculum Committee of the American Association of Colleges of Pharmacy. He was at the height of his research productivity then, yet he did not hesitate to accept. And at the time of his death, he was chairman of the Educational Policy (curriculum) Committee of our School, still pressing for change, still tilting with dragons, still stirring up emotions, and still a pharmacist for all seasons.

From the dawn of its history, our profession has been graced with dedicated teachers who have advanced the practice of pharmacy, and capable scientists who have pushed back the frontiers of its sciences. They are so many in number that they cannot be named.

However, we can count on one hand those who have made outstanding
contributions to both the practice and the science of pharmacy.
Sid Riegelman, complex scientist, educator and man, was a member of
that small, select fraternity. Few people like him come our way in
a lifetime, and when they do we seldom realize the immensity of
their presence until they are gone.

No man can die immediately; each leaves something behind, like
a pebble dropped into a placid pond, that sends forth ever-
diminishing ripples that long survive its passing. Sid was no
small pebble; the splash he made will never subside. He has left
an indelible mark on our sciences and our profession, and it will
never wash off. In this regard, he will live forever.

REFERENCES

1. Presentation to School of Pharmacy Faculty Conference, University of California, San Francisco, August 11 (1970).
2. S. Riegelman, Suppositories, in: "American Pharmacy, Textbook
   of Pharmaceutical Principles, Processes and Preparations,"
   (4th Edition), R.A. Lyman and J.B. Sprowls, eds., J.B.
   Lippincott Co., Philadelphia (1955), pp. 347-360.
3. "Business and Professions Code of the State of California,"
   Division 2, ch. 9, Section 4000 et seq.

Chapter 4

SIDNEY RIEGELMAN – THE SCIENTIST

Leslie Z. Benet

Department of Pharmacy
School of Pharmacy
University of California
San Francisco, California

Every winter quarter, I participate, together with Jack Cooper and John Shell, in teaching a course at the University of California at San Francisco (USCF) entitled "Pharmaceutical Chemistry 208, Survey of Pharmaceutics." At the beginning of the course, I usually give a history of the field. I particularly enjoy this because I have known all of the principals personally. I had always told the students what a unique opportunity they have since they can meet, listen to and consult with one of those principals, Professor Sidney Riegelman.

As detailed by Professor Busse, Sid began his scientific career early in his undergraduate training. After World War II, he returned to Madison, Wisconsin to re-enter graduate school, not in the usual areas of pharmacy research at that time, such as medicinal chemistry, pharmacognosy or pharmacology, but in an area related to the manufacture and properties of drug dosage forms that was designated physical pharmacy. Sid chose to work with Dr. Louis Busse who was investigating the physical properties of powders, and he worked closely with another graduate student, Joe Swintosky, and Swintosky's former roommate, Takeru Higuchi. The group published four papers (2-5)*; Sid's special research related to the application of spray drying techniques to pharmaceutical powders. This was 1946-1948, long before either the food or pharmaceutical industries began utilizing such techniques routinely.

---

*Reference numbers refer to the corresponding publications in Dr. Riegelman's biography as found in the Appendix.

In 1948, Troy Daniels, Dean of the UCSF School of Pharmacy, recruited Sid to the West to join the faculty. In this new setting, Sid carried out some early studies with more established faculty members: Robertson Pratt, Don Brodie, John Oneto, Steven Dean, Einar Brochmann-Hansen and Louis Strait (6,7,22,30).

Sid attracted his first graduate student, N.A. Allawala, and began some studies of his own related to solubilization with surface active agents (8,9,22,26), an area of interest he maintained throughout his career. At a lunch at the Faculty Club, about a month prior to Sid's death, I was speaking with a senior scientist from Shell Development Corporation. This scientist didn't know Sid but knew his work, as he had gone back to search out in the literature the origins for the use of surface active agents in solubilization.

In 1958, Sid published a series of papers (16-18) with graduate student Wilfred Crowell under the major heading "The Kinetics of Rectal Absorption" in the Scientific Edition of the Journal of the American Pharmaceutical Association. These papers were important for a number of reasons. First, the work was good. The studies were recognized with the awarding of the Ebert Prize to Sid in 1959. This Prize is awarded for the best work published in journals of the American Pharmaceutical Association during the previous year. Second, the papers indicated the direction of Sid's future work and where he would make his major contributions to science: the relationship between drugs and biological systems. And third, this work reflected the new pharmacy course which Sid had conceived at UCSF, and which he jointly taught with Eino Nelson, integrating physical measurements with measurements in the biological system. A few years later, Gerhard Levy coined the word "biopharmaceutics" to describe this course and the field in which Sid had become involved. At this time, Sid was also very interested in drugs used in ophthalmology (11-13,15,19-21,23,28,35,36, 39,74), radiology (40-42,52) and dermatology (54,76,80,94,95,101, 104,106,113). He continued to publish in these medical specialty areas throughout his life; particularly in dermatology with faculty colleague and good friend William L. Epstein. At about this time, Sid developed and patented the methodology to stabilize epinephrine solutions (32,33). I remember reading the patents when I worked in a pharmacy in Cincinnati where we were trying to compound such solutions.

Sid was promoted to Professor in 1962 and held a joint appointment in Radiology beginning in 1964. I first met Sid in 1963 when I came to UCSF as a graduate student. He then had a tremendously active research group carrying out the first pharmacokinetic studies. Pharmacokinetics is the study of absorption, distribution, metabolism and excretion of drugs and metabolites, and their correlations with pharmacological measurements in man and animals; a definition which Sid helped to write. Although the word pharmacokinetics was originated by Professor Dost of Giessen in the 1950s, Sid was generally considered as one of the founders and world leaders in this fledgling field.

In 1963, when I came to California, Larry Fischer, now Professor of Pharmacology and Toxicology at the University of Iowa; Stan Kaplan, now Director of the Department of Pharmacokinetics and Biopharmaceutics at Hoffmann-LaRoche; and Bill Barr, presently Professor and Chairman of the Department of Pharmaceutics at Medical College of Virginia, were working in Sid's laboratory. They were carrying out the first significant absorption, distribution and metabolism studies on griseofulvin (37,38,43,44) and salicylamide (63,64).

In 1964, Sid went to England for his first sabbatical. At that time, Sid recruited a graduate student from Arnold Beckett's laboratory to come back to the U.S. as his first postdoctoral fellow. Malcolm Rowland arrived in 1965. Sid, Malcolm and graduate students Jack Loo and Phil Harris published a series of fundamental papers on pharmacokinetics establishing Sid's laboratory as a major center in this discipline in the 1960s. Riegelman, Loo and Rowland published four papers in 1968 (50,51,53,55) describing the need to use multicompartment pharmacokinetic models to adequately describe drug distribution. The first paper in this series, "Shortcomings in Pharmacokinetic Analysis by Conceiving the Body to Exhibit the Properties of a Single Compartment" (50), should be listed as a "Citation Classic" having been referenced over 400 times since its appearance. The third paper in the series, "New Method for Calculating the Intrinsic Absorption Rate of Drugs" (53), reports a method of determining absorption rate profiles of drugs with multicompartment pharmacokinetic characteristics which is generally referred to in the literature as the Loo-Riegelman Method.

Also in the late '60s, Sid published a series of papers with Malcolm Rowland and graduate student Phil Harris, describing for the first time the quantitative nature of the first-pass effect on the metabolism of aspirin. These papers (47,56) emphasized the difference between the extent of availability of a drug to the systemic circulation versus the amount absorbed from the gastrointestinal tract. "Thus, during the absorption of ASA, appreciable hydrolysis to SA must occur across the gut wall or during the first passage of this drug through the liver" (47). Sid's contributions were recognized with the awarding of the prestigious American Pharmaceutical Association Research Achievement Award in Physical Pharmacy in 1968, followed by the Association's award in Pharmacodynamics in 1970. In 1970, Sid was chosen Alumnus of the Year by the University of Wisconsin School of Pharmacy and was elected a Fellow of the Academy of Pharmaceutical Sciences.

From 1969 through 1971, Sid and graduate student Win Chiou
published a series of papers concerning the application of solid
dispersion systems (61,67,71-73).   Sid and Win patented this
process. I was surprised to learn that Sid's two patents - stabilization of epinephrine and solid dispersion of drugs - still
generate a considerable fraction of the total royalties received by
the entire University of California (9% in 1979-1980 and 12.5% in
1980-1981). In the early 1970s, Sid carried out two significant
research-related tasks in addition to his own work.   In 1972, he
was the primary author of a pamphlet published by the Academy of
Pharmaceutical Sciences entitled "Guidelines for Bioavailability
Studies in Man."   As reviewed by Dr. Kaplan in the next chapter,
this was the first publication to specifically state the criteria
for and the directions that such studies should take.   In 1973, Sid
founded and became editor of the Journal of Pharmacokinetics and
Biopharmaceutics, the first journal published in this discipline.
The journal, now in its 11th year, has established a reputation for
excellence for which Sid was justifiably proud.   Sid published the
first of many of his scientific papers in the fourth issue of
journal (87).   In the following year, graduate student Harold
Boxenbaum, Sid and statistician Bob Elashoff published an often
cited paper describing the limitations of statistical estimation
when one is attempting to select the most appropriate pharmacokinetic model (91).

In the 1970s, Sid attracted a growing number of graduate
students and postdoctoral fellows.   Three of these postdoctoral
scholars are presently members of the Department of Pharmacy
faculty: Wolfgang Sadée, Bob Upton and Nick Holford.   They, along
with their many colleagues from Sid's lab, published work relating
to the pharmacokinetics of propylthiouracil (87), spironolactones
(77-79), acetazolamide (110,111), phenytoin (112), diethylstilbestrol (105,115), acebutolol (127), ketoprofen (133,144,153), naprox-
en (133,144), isoniazid (93,97,107), iodipamide (108,114) and
iopanoic acid (103,124,128).

At the time of his death, Sid's research work was in its most
active phase.   In 1980, Sid published 18 papers, more than he had
published in any previous year.   Research in his laboratory was
concentrated on three major drugs.   One of these was theophylline.
Ten postdoctoral research associates and two graduate students co-
authored papers related to Sid's theophylline work (109,116,117,
121,131,132,134,138,139,141,142,145,152,156-160,162-164,172).   This
intensive effort was begun at the request of the FDA for whom Sid
carried out substantial contract research work for about four
years.   Diane Tang-Liu was Sid's last graduate student working on
theophylline and appropriately presents "A Composite View on
Theophylline Disposition in Man" in this book.

The second major drug undergoing investigation in Sid's laboratory at the time of his death was quinidine (120,122,123,126, 129,136,140,151,168,169,171). Sid's research group made a major contribution to the understanding of quinidine pharmacokinetics and pharmacodynamics by identification of new quinidine metabolites, particularly the N-oxide, and the development of sensitive and specific analytical procedures for measurement of the drug and its metabolites in plasma and urine. Approximately six months following Sid's death, Ashok Rakhit finished his work on the effects of phenobarbital induced enzyme induction on quinidine binding and disposition, a presentation which appears in this text. Another of Sid's students, Kathy Maloney, is continuing to study the covalent binding of quinidine. Her preliminary results, which are presented in this book, suggest that quinidine binds covalently to tissue molecules following cytochrome P-450 activation via an epoxide.

The third major drug being studied in Sid's lab at the time of his death was propranolol (135,137,143,155,165,167,170,173). Man-Wai Lo was the last of Sid's students to have his major professor sign the thesis. Man-Wai investigated the nonlinear aspects of the first-pass metabolism of propranolol in dogs with a portacaval transposition. This allowed him, and faculty colleagues David Effeney and Susan Pond, to differentiate gutwall/intestinal metabolism from hepatic metabolism and thereby to determine that propranolol did not undergo gastrointestinal metabolism to any significant extent. The studies indicated that two of propranolol's metabolic pathways, side chain oxidation and aromatic ring hydroxylation, are saturable. Sid was very aware of the need to define the pharmacokinetics of racemic drug mixtures in terms of the active and nonactive species. Graduate student Bernie Silber developed a stereochemical assay for S (-) and R (+)-propranolol along with the corresponding glucuronide conjugates (143). These studies, also described in this book, demonstrated for the first time that propranolol undergoes stereoselective disposition in man.

Throughout his career, Sid approached scientific problems from both experimental and theoretical perspectives. While his laboratory was in one of its most productive phases, Sid was also very concerned with the development of mathematical methods. He was firmly committed to a population-based approach to clinical pharmacokinetics in conjunction with faculty colleagues Lew Sheiner and Stuart Beal and Clinical Pharmacology Fellows Sam Vozeh and Keith Muir. Sid supported the view that estimates of pharmacokinetic parameters could be obtained from the vast amounts of highly relevant, yet ostensibly free, data obtained during routine use of drugs in patients where only a few blood samples are available from each subject. He also investigated the use of statistical moment theory to evaluate in vivo dissolution and absorption times (146) in collaboration with Paul Collier, who spent his sabbatical year in Sid's laboratory.

Sid was most of all an enthusiastic and excited scientist. We who were close to him will not forget that quick smile, that bear hug arm that came around your shoulder as Sid greeted you, the excitement in his eyes and voice as he told of the latest magic to come out of his laboratory and his mind. I had said to others that whenever I ran out of research ideas, all that I needed to do was to follow Sid around for half an hour and collect all the projects he discarded. He was a fountainhead of ideas.

Sid was proud of his work and proud of the students, postdoctoral fellows and visiting scientists who worked in his laboratory. I know that he would be pleased that so many of his students and fellows are represented in this volume. He also would be pleased that his scientific colleagues and friends all chose to contribute to this book and to be members of the Symposium faculty. Unfortunately, Sid cannot be here to share his insights with us. As stimulating and rewarding as this volume may be, you and I know that we would willingly trade it for a short scientific discussion with Sid.

Chapter 5

SIDNEY RIEGELMAN – HIS CONTRIBUTIONS TO PUBLIC POLICY IN PHARMACY AND THE PHARMACEUTICAL SCIENCES

Stanley A. Kaplan

Department of Pharmacokinetics and Biopharmaceutics
Hoffmann–La Roche, Inc.
Nutley, New Jersey

Consider the professional, scientific and regulatory world that Sidney Riegelman found and, because of his efforts, the world he left. Consider Sid's role in our public policy. His impact with regard to so many aspects of our profession, be it academic, regulatory, or industrial, has been immense, and these contributions, their interrelationships and Sid's perseverance have resulted in a more reasonable, rational and creative environment in the pharmaceutical sciences.

Sid was very direct with people, yet he was a patient teacher and, because of this style, his insight and expertise, he was able to influence his students, fellow scientists and administrators at the FDA and international regulatory agencies, industrial researchers, and his colleagues on various panels in professional societies. His trend-setting research in bioanalytical chemistry, physical pharmacy, biopharmaceutics, pharmacokinetic modeling, clinical pharmacokinetics and pharmacodynamic interrelationships provided a solid base upon which his visions were able to materialize.

During the 1960s, Sid was concerned that the pharmacy curriculum was overtraining the majority of pharmacy practitioners. They were evolving into merchandisers of products, and this role required very little of their training. He also observed that in hospitals where pharmacists were involved with the manufacture and control of a large array of products, these pharmacists were working with staff and equipment insufficient for their tasks. In light of the therapeutic variables that could result from inappropriate product manufacture and control in large, well-equipped

23

industrial laboratories, he wondered how pharmacists in hospitals could manufacture safe and effective drugs with minimal equipment and no independent verification of quality. If, in fact, it was safer and cheaper to buy and dispense manufactured pharmaceutical products, rather than prepare them, what was there for future pharmacists to do and was their training geared to a new role?

At that time, Sid's involvement in both pharmacy education and research triggered visions that went beyond the generation of clinical pharmacokinetic data and quality drug products. Technological advances had virtually obliterated the compounding and analytical responsibilities of the practicing pharmacist, and the rate of change of these advances made it impossible for these pharmacists to even try to keep up. There were also significant advances in our knowledge of disease states and drugs, with the physician bearing newer burdens in the areas of selecting proper therapy and monitoring the care of the patient. Sid believed this information should be properly disseminated to health care professionals to improve patient care. In this regard, he was instrumental in creating a professional curriculum that would result in the development of clinical pharmacists.

The question was whether the pharmacy student was receiving the proper training to fulfill all of the roles he could effectively secure within the health care team, or whether his training allowed solely for the passive role of being a distributor of drugs. Although the pharmacy curriculum had continued to expand in the areas of physical pharmacy, biopharmaceutics, pharmacokinetics and pharmacodynamics, there was no concerted effort to train pharmacy students to utilize this conglomeration of isolated facts in their relationship with the physician and the patient. Sid pondered how best to teach pharmacy students to communicate information to the physician, and what information the physician really needed to know. Sid's goal was to develop a pharmacist trained to interact in the clinical scene as a therapeutician along with the physician-diagnostician.

Fortunately, the location of the UCSF School of Pharmacy on a teaching hospital campus provided the perfect environment for such a program to take shape, develop and grow. How should pharmacy training change? Sid discovered that students had to experience the language of disease states and therapeutics, not just the language of textbooks: they needed to translate the medical literature and isolated facts into clinically significant answers. He believed that pharmacy training was concentrated on the avoidance of side effects, rather than on the broad therapeutic requirements of the patient. Sid observed that because pharmacists had no direct clinical exposure, they lacked confidence in their ability to integrate available clinical data with their knowledge regarding therapy. He believed pharmacy students must see patients react to various drugs to gain this confidence, so that they could better understand the problems and questions of the physician and provide relevant answers.

The curriculum at UCSF changed to allow the pharmacists to become more patient-oriented in their pharmaceutical services. Sid preferred the term clinically trained pharmacist to clinical pharmacist. He believed that this individual was capable of practicing pharmacy in any setting, be it community, institutional, or industrial, and not just in a hospital practice. The curriculum that Sid espoused has become a successful model for pharmacy education. Clinical pharmacists today provide consultative services to the physician on proper drug selection and drug utilization problems, and monitor patients with respect to their current clinical status and drug-use profiles.

Sid also believed that the pharmaceutical researcher's solid scientific knowledge of chemistry, biology and pharmacokinetics constituted rigorous tools which needed focus. His instincts told him that the growth and contributions of the pharmaceutical scientist would be manifested by first understanding the patient and disease variables, and then looking back into the basic sciences for the concepts and tools to solve health problems. As with the clinically trained pharmacist, he envisioned a clinically trained pharmaceutical scientist as well as a scientifically trained clinician. In this regard, Sid also developed an innovative joint program with Ken Melmon in the Division of Clinical Pharmacology at UCSF which received support from the National Institutes of Health. The marriage of these disciplines with regard to patient care has resulted in well-trained scientists capable of successful research efforts at the most critical juncture of our disciplines: i.e., the therapeutic consequences of biopharmaceutic and pharmacokinetic variables.

Sid was a highly respected consultant in the scientific and administrative echelons at the FDA. His interactions with them began in the early '70s when he did extensive "missionary" work and some problem-solving through which he attempted to convince the FDA that this academic curiosity called "pharmacokinetics" had a variety of practical and therapeutic implications. Problems with theophylline, quinidine, digoxin, specificity of assays and pharmacokinetic interpretation of mean data versus data from individual subjects all highlighted the need for the sophisticated application of pharmacokinetics as a tool in clinical therapeutic evaluations.

Many of these discussions raised questions that the regulatory agencies could no longer ignore or avoid and, in November 1971, the Drug Research Board of the National Academy of Sciences - National Research Council, co-sponsored a conference on the "Bioavailability of Drugs" along with the APhA Academy of Pharmaceutical Sciences, FDA, PMA, USP, and NF. This was the first major national conference of its kind which included representative input from these concerned groups. The politics at the time tended to shift the focus of any problems to manufacturing variables per se; therapeutic concerns were ignored or downplayed. Sid's contributions at this NAS-NRC Conference highlighted the physiologic and pharmacokinetic variables associated with bioavailability testing and their therapeutic implications. Sid played a major role in defining bioavailability as an overall medical problem of concern to all health professionals.

During this time, Sid was a member of an Academy of Pharmaceutical Sciences Committee which developed the "Guidelines for Biopharmaceutical Studies in Man," issued in February, 1972. This was the first written document which not only discussed the importance of such studies in drug development and therapeutics, but dealt with methods to achieve the stated objectives. This Academy document became the basis for establishing generally acceptable standards for study design and interpretation of pharmacokinetic data. Many of the concepts contained in this document were incorporated into the FDA's Bioequivalency and Bioavailability Regulations. These include criteria and evidence for establishing a bioequivalence requirement based on physicochemical and pharmacokinetic data; various requirements for in vitro, in vivo animal and in vivo human studies; and bioavailability testing principles such as protocol design, assay methodology, control of physiological factors, and statistical evaluation.

In the early '70s, the consensus was that problems resulting from a lack of biopharmaceutical/pharmacokinetic data affected only a handful of drugs, and that due diligence in manufacturing and quality control would cause such concerns to disappear. However, only a few drugs had been studied at that time. Debate and controversy ensued in governmental circles about the generic equivalency issue and reimbursement for multisource drugs. The result was that the Office of Technology Assessment (OTA) authorized the formation of a Drug Bioequivalence Study Panel to examine the relationships between clinical and therapeutic equivalency of drug products (short of therapeutic trials), and to assess the capability of current technology to determine whether drug products with the same physical characteristics and chemical composition produce comparable therapeutic results.

Sid and Jim Doluisio were the two pharmaceutical scientists amongst the ten OTA panelists. The panel solicited data, primarily unpublished studies from industry, which revealed the nature and magnitude of biopharmaceutically related drug product quality problems. Sid's imprint on most of the conclusions and recommendations of the OTA report are obvious. For example, he believed that current standards and regulatory practices did not assure product bioequivalence or uniformity; that bioavailability variables can have therapeutic implications; that physico-chemical properties, potency and therapeutic index were important in determining biopharmaceutical concerns about drugs; that continuous "state of the art" updating of compendial standards and manufacturing practices were essential; that we needed to develop in vitro and animal models to predict bioavailability in man; that application of statistical methodology was necessary, and that the merging of FDA and USP information pertaining to testing and record keeping practices was fundamental to achieving uniform, relevant and enforceable standards for drug quality.

It was the publication of the OTA report in April 1974, subsequently submitted to Congress, that finally convinced the hierarchy at the Commissioner's level of the FDA that biopharmaceutics was a concern for drug products in general, and not just a generic equivalency question for a handful of problem compounds. The impact at the FDA caused the creation of a Division of Biopharmaceutics separate from the Division of Clinical Research; the allocation of budget for both internal and external biopharmaceutical research programs; employment of skilled pharmacokineticists, and the formulation of guidelines for bioavailability studies which were formally issued in the Federal Register on January 7, 1977. Probable additional fallout from the OTA report included revisions by the FDA or USP in the area of Current Good Manufacturing Practices, the establishment of the Quality Assurance Program, the expansion of drug related information such as specific assay and dissolution testing, and the improvement of compendial standards contained in the official monographs pertaining to raw materials, excipients and finished products. Subsequently, a good number of Sid's students have worked in the FDA Division of Biopharmaceutics, impacting on both FDA and industrial research. In addition, Sid was a consultant to the FDA for several years and active on FDA advisory boards.

Sid was deeply concerned about the many vagaries in the regulation of drug product quality and the possible therapeutic implications. He saw many inconsistencies in the application of so-called "state of the art" technology as perceived by the FDA, USP/NF, industrial GMP's and Quality Assurance programs. He was concerned about the conservative views expressed by the USP Committee of Revision. His criticisms could not be ignored because they always contained scientific detail as to the basis of a problem and possible approaches to its solution. He felt these interagency inconsistencies discouraged the development and/or application of adequate tests to guarantee purity, strength and quality of products. As a result of much in-depth evaluation, as part of his interactions with the FDA and USP, Sid observed a variety of weaknesses at these organizations and in the interactions between them.

Sid did much to foster dialogue between the FDA and USP. Although often heated, the dialogue resulted in considerable reflection and some progress.

Sid observed an ever increasing use and abuse of dissolution technology in our scientific community, and believed that it was time that the interpretation and application of in vitro dissolution testing be reevaluated. In general, his guiding principle was that every drug is unique and must be treated individually, such that no single set of rules or guidelines could apply to every drug or drug product. Sid took the task of forming and chairing the Academy of Pharmaceutical Sciences Dissolution Committee, consisting of scientists from academia, industry, the FDA, and USP.

During the week preceding his death, at the Academy meeting in St. Louis, Sid was actively involved as a scientist and diplomat with the In Vitro Dissolution White Paper Committee, of which I was a member, attempting to establish a foundation for the applicability of in vitro dissolution testing to drug product development, and quality control specifications, that would assure safety and reproducibility in a drug product. He hoped that the document would serve as a starting point from which meaningful investigations could be planned.

Although this task remains to be completed by others, his ability to command the respect of many diverse groups, his teacher's patience and perspective to lead all of us to the best answer and his groundwork, all guarantee a successful conclusion to this dissolution document, as well as the perpetuation of his many visions, which pharmaceutical scientists, health care personnel and patients take for granted.

Sid was a true pathfinder. He enjoyed the thrill of discovery, conquest and success. His goals, however, were not limited to pathfinding, but extended to fulfilling his visions for pharmacy and the pharmaceutical sciences. He believed that our manifest destiny was to impact directly on patient care. His efforts provided us with the philosophy to push ahead, the tools to achieve goals and the programs and experiences to properly integrate ourselves into the scientific and health care communities.

His career spanned our evolution from the early days of chemical synthesis to improve natural products, to his innovative contributions in physical pharmacy in the fifties, to biopharmaceutics and pharmacokinetics in the sixties, to pharmacodynamics and the practice of clinical pharmacy in the seventies. The variety of his involvements and the quality of his contributions continued to grow during his career which was at an all time peak at the time of his death.

Although his leadership will be sadly missed, the foundations he established and the driving force he instilled in so many of us to fulfill his many visions, will keep him at the forefront of the pharmacy and the pharmaceutical sciences for many years to come.

Chapter 6

SIDNEY RIEGELMAN – CONTRIBUTIONS AT THE CLINICAL INTERFACE

Kenneth L. Melmon

Department of Medicine
Stanford University Medical Center
Stanford, California

Although it may seem presumptuous to say, I think Sidney Riegelman would have been delighted to attend most of the Symposium upon which this book is based. It deals with his science and is representative of his life interests. He'd probably have been sitting toward the back of the room, a mass of papers on his lap – half scanning, half listening – using every minute to the fullest.

I think of Sid in terms of what has been said about Lewis Thomas. One critic appraising **The Medusa and the Snail** said that if Montaigne had possessed a deep knowledge of 20th century biology, he would have been called Lew Thomas. Similarly, Sid deserves that type of distinction. I believe that if Lew Thomas or others ever focus on the biology of pharmacokinetics and optimal therapeutic decision making, they will have to recall Riegelman's contributions. Sid's thinking evolved toward development of the interface between the pharmaceutical sciences and clinical pharmacology; by his work, he helped unify them.

He would have been proud of the prior five chapters in this book because they reflect how he used his life to accomplish fundamental tasks. It is my function here to identify his ideas on the clinical interface. Sid had a very broad perspective on biology and, I believe, he had more pride in his contributions in this area than in any of the others that have been discussed. He was a person who saw the big picture and, although he was shy and therefore not readily able to express himself eloquently, hearing substantive talk about the clinical interface would have made him raise his eyes from his papers, and moved him to enthusiastic outbursts of participation.

The arrangement of the chapters in this book more or less follows Sid's priorities. It links all of his unusual talents and reflects the flair he had for transferring new data in his sphere of knowledge to man. Sid wanted to make important contributions to the clinical interface and made no bones about it. He set about the task in a quiet, unassuming way and he went a long way toward accomplishing his goal.

Let me give you some idea of just how far Sid went with his clinical interest. Before our collaboration began, his clinical studies were of trivial importance to therapy but latent in his approach were significant contributions. At that point, one of my confreres, who was somewhat dubious about clinical pharmacology, approached me after hearing that I was going to try to interest Sid in a collaboration. Julius Comroe had read Sid's bibliography and, in his clipped and joking way, said he felt that Sid's interest in therapeutics was limited to the effects of drugs given by enemas and the pharmacokinetics of salicylates. "Where could we go in our collaboration?" he asked.

Sid had a deep understanding of the mathematics related to the kinetics of drug ingestion, distribution and elimination but he realized that the clinical subjects he had so far considered investigating were therapeutically minor. He was determined to pursue important clinical problems aggressively from a scientific point of view. As one might have predicted, his dedication was not dictated by the politics of pharmacy, nor was he diverted into analyses of the survival of pharmacy; he was moved by a sincere interest that was an integral part of his being.

Although he was in a discipline that I have in the past accused of sometimes being unjustly medically aggressive, Sid's interest was not simply to extend the field into clinical medicine in order for it to survive by giving medical advice. Rather, he wanted to use the talents of those in pharmacy to concentrate on a discipline that physicians had shunned. He sensed that physicians were generally deficient in the management of pharmacologic and pharmaceutic data at the bedside and, in consequence, made suboptimal therapeutic decisions. Sid recognized that the pharmacist was never likely to take the place of the physician who made therapeutic decisions, for the pharmacist's background was in pharmaceutics, pharmacognosy, pharmacokinetics and pharmacology, but inadequate in biology and medical disease processes. Sid wanted a true symbiosis and worked for it. He knew that if the two professions could work together, investigatively and clinically, therapeutic benefit would result. His was a wide-eyed interest, typical of him, that resulted in recognition of the need to identify important problems in therapeutics that could best be solved by a firmer understanding and more systematic application of pharmacokinetics.

Who would ever have suspected that a fateful 1965 conversation at my house on a redwood terrace overlooking the untouched hills, oaks, redwoods and madrones of Black Canyon in San Rafael, California would lead to a solid trio dedicated to the integration of biopharmaceutic sciences, pharmacokinetics and clinical medicine? Sid influenced Malcolm Rowland and me to commit ourselves to making clinical pharmacology in the United States cognizant of the contributions that could be made by the pharmacokineticist. This commitment led to the discovery of significant answers in a wide area of the therapeutic decision process then embryonic in the world of biological sciences and almost non-existent in the United States. That meeting led to changes at the University of California at San Francisco which will persist far into the future.

What did Sid commit himself to in 1965 at that meeting in Marin County across the Golden Gate Bridge from San Francisco? He said that we would develop important areas of collaboration between his entire department, the School of Pharmacy and the Department of Medicine. He said that we would recruit personnel sympathetic to this cause in pharmacy, even if they were physicians. He said we would develop a training and program project grant application that would clearly indicate to others our interests, our abilities and our direction. Skepticism is common at the inception of any innovative collaboration, and the outcome seemed more dubious to Malcolm Rowland and to me than to Sid. Yet Sid was not about to drive something through by force; rather, his interest was to stimulate cooperation by leadership. So, you may ask, what did he do to help create an interface then barely nascent between medicine and pharmacokinetics?

First and foremost, Sid helped create a new atmosphere in clinical pharmacology at the University of California. He believed in the discipline, committed his space and facilities to it, and began a recruitment process that was sure to augment it greatly. He helped solidify the commitment made by the school to Malcolm Rowland; he recruited Les Benet, Wolfgang Sadée and others, and he intrigued people such as Lew Sheiner by helping him to apply kinetics appropriately to individualize the therapeutic decision process. He involved himself in the recruitment, selection and development of approximately 100 trainees in clinical pharmacology from 1965 to 1978. His unwavering support of the program project and training grants was what helped us win them and use them with remarkable effectiveness. Both the training program initiated in 1966 and the program project initiated in 1967 are still thriving, no small feat in today's real world of bureaucracy and budget cuts. He helped develop weekly conferences, which he rarely missed, that linked the fundamental research interests of people who were in the Department of Medicine as well as those who were in his School of Pharmacy. He helped draw an everwidening group of people into those conferences and created the atmosphere in which initial tolerance to a host of different subjects eventually amalgamated diverse interests. The amalgamation greatly enhanced the effectiveness of all of us in investigation.

Sid helped establish the first therapeutic drug assay laboratory at UCSF and convinced Jere Goyan and others that this laboratory should be located in the School of Pharmacy. He persuaded the Geheimrat of Pathology to recognize the importance of this new laboratory discipline and he coped with the administrative details required to insure effective laboratory function. He and Jere Goyan, along with others, promoted the development of pharmacy stations in the hospital to allow pharmacists to understand the real clinical problems that existed, and to help them apply their knowledge in a collaboration with physicians making therapeutic decisions that involved actual patients. He underwrote the establishment of a drug study unit which employed physicians and which included key pharmacokinetic information in the work-up of new chemical entities. He listened as we discussed disease aspects likely to influence kinetics and helped design the protocols through which the kinetics of lidocaine, digoxin, clonidine and morphine were placed in the context of dynamic disease. This led to new principles of therapeutics in use today, though less widely than we would like. He was interested in helping us develop models of shock, congestive heart failure and liver disease in order to help determine the role that each of these diseases might play in fundamental alterations of the pharmacokinetics of commonly used drugs, even though they were not likely to be used in the management of such diseases.

It is difficult to isolate one man's input when his great strength lies in his ability to work in concert with others; when his drive is to achieve a mutual goal with little regard for personal aggrandizement. Many who knew Sid as I did believe that he helped to change the overall orientation of training in pharmacy as it related to medicine. The changes were substantial and these advances formed the basis of irrefutable arguments that elements of synthetic and analytical chemistry, applied mathematics, and quantitative measurements of drugs that could be correlated with quantifiable pharmacologic effects, had to be incorporated into research in biology and medical biology if drug therapeutics were ever to be optimal and individualized.

No doubt I am attributing more to Sid than he would have. He often was not an author on the papers that he inspired and he always carried on a very independent research program unrelated to the collaboration. He was responsible for involving others in an area in which he had faith even though he lacked the eloquence to define and defend that faith. What he was able to do was to pour vigor, curiosity, enthusiasm, imagination and insight into all these areas, without abrading anyone who had claimed parts of these investigations as private territory.

Sid died while he was doing his best work on both a personal and institutional level. In selfish terms, we lost him at a crucial period for clinical pharmacology and at a critical moment in his own work. I refuse to lose sight of the fact that he was not only responsible for his own work, but for a much more important endeavor that influenced a spectrum of people in biology. I, for one, will never be able to understand any justification for an untimely death, but what better compliment could he, or we, be paid than to have it said about us that we died too soon because we had not completed what was remarkably good. It might be easier to accept death if it arrives when an individual has reached a stage in his life when he feels that his major work is finished. If he had started to simply vegetate in quietness and retirement, as so many famous scientists do, we would not have had this morning's talks. Yet we must take these comments a step further. Despite our hurt at being left, we must realize that Sid did establish a living trust. What he helped to start is very likely to be perpetuated because it was socially and scientifically appealing and has now developed its own momentum for life and growth. Entropy is a word that cannot be applied to the disciplines of pharmacokinetics or clinical pharmacology. The perpetuation of the field will be traceable in part to the contributions of a quiet, self-effacing man with an enormous zest for life and understated enthusiasm for his science and the world around him, which he expressed by willingly and actively giving it his all to his last moment.

Sid and his attitudes are identified to me in the words of Lewis Thomas, the current chronicler of biology, who wrote: "We pass the word around; we ponder how the case is put by different people; we read the poetry; we meditate over the literature; we play the music; we change our minds; we reach an understanding. Society evolves this way, not by shouting each other down, but by the unique capacity of unique, individual human beings to comprehend each other."*

Had Sid simply done in his professional life what most of us do, focus his research and creative interests on a specific area (in his case pharmacy, where he felt most comfortable), pharmacokinetics and clinical pharmacology would not be as developed as they are today. Sid Riegelman did not survive to see the role both will occupy or their increasing importance in making health care decisions responsive to the therapeutic imperatives of heterogenous

---

*L. Thomas, "The Medusa and the Snail," Viking, New York, (1979), p. 120.

disease in individuals. Sid provided the impetus which led many of us into these fields and we take this occasion to render our appreciation.

Chapter 7

PERSONAL EXPERIENCES IN THE EARLY DAYS OF BIOPHARMACY
AND PHARMACOKINETICS

Joseph V. Swintosky

College of Pharmacy
University of Kentucky
Lexington, Kentucky

I am glad to be a participant in this symposium as a memorial
to Sidney Riegelman. I knew him and members of his family when we
were undergraduates in pharmacy. We worked together on research
and graduate courses under the same major professor when I was a
half-time instructor and he was a full-time graduate student.
Working across the hall from each other at the University of
Wisconsin School of Pharmacy, our paths crossed thousands of
times. I completed my Ph.D. thesis examination in August of 1948
and he completed his a month or two later. We were the first Ph.D.
physical pharmacists to emerge from the physical pharmacy graduate
studies program started at Wisconsin in the 1940s. In 1946-47,
together with our major professor Louis W. Busse, we shared the
responsibility for writing the chapter entitled "Colloids,
Emulsions and Suspensions" for the book **American Pharmacy.** We took
courses together from Takeru Higuchi and benefited immensely from
his teaching and research leadership at the College after he joined
the faculty in 1947. Louis Busse and Takeru Higuchi influenced our
professional attitudes and our scientific development more than I
can possibly articulate in this brief chapter. In the '40s at
Wisconsin, pharmacy graduate education for pharmaceutics majors
began to be compounded with the ingredients of mathematics,
physical chemistry, qualitative organic analysis, advanced organic
chemistry and analytical instrumentation. To my knowledge, Sid and
I were the first at the College of Pharmacy at Wisconsin to include
mathematics, physical chemistry and related physical pharmacy
courses in our graduate study programs to the degree that we did.
When Tak Higuchi joined the faculty, graduate students clearly got
the message that a physical-chemical course background would be
very important to their thesis research projects and to their

37

scientific careers in pharmaceutics. When I and others persuaded
Tak to join the College in 1947, it was with the expectation that
this astute physical organic chemist would become our leader in
this discipline as it would be applied to pharmacy. He brought
authoritativeness, vigor and rapid growth to physical pharmacy, set
standards for graduate education in this area, and influenced the
direction and progress of the physical pharmacy research projects
that both Sid and I were working on for our theses. Sid and I did
our research on related problems. We were co-authors, in 1949 and
1950, with Louis W. Busse and Takeru Higuchi on the first four
scientific publications coming out of Wisconsin that bore the
physical pharmacy imprint. We became full-time faculty members in
1948, he at the University of California, and I at the University
of Wisconsin. We remained good friends throughout Sid's life.

I left academia to join Smith Kline and French Laboratories
(SK&F) in July of 1953. At that time, I started work on some pharmaceutical research and development problems to which I could apply
the breadth of biologic and physical science knowledge, and drug
knowledge, that one acquires in becoming a pharmacist, a Ph.D.
physical pharmacist, and a pharmaceutical educator. The organizers
of this Symposium have recommended that I dwell on some of my
biopharmaceutical research and development activities in that era,
comment on the status of pharmacy research then, make some
comparisons with the present, and point to opportunities for
research and innovation in this area for the future.

My first assignment as a "bench" scientist at SK&F was to make
oral sustained release tablets of aminophylline and theophylline,
on a project called Aminophylline Spansule®* Tablet. Heretofore I
have not described this project publicly, yet this is the one that
originally pointed me in the direction of biopharmaceutical study,
and generated for me a great deal of interest in research and
development at SK&F. I viewed my new job primarily as one in
applied physical pharmacy and pharmaceutical technology. The term
biopharmaceutics had not yet been coined. The expression "drug
biologic half-life" had not been a part of my educational experience and, to my knowledge in 1953, the concept it represents was
not taught in pharmacy schools. How, where, and at what rates
drugs were absorbed in the gastrointestinal tract were not well
understood. The classic studies of Brodie, Schanker, Hogben and
others on drug absorption, using the in situ rat gut technique,
came several years later. The technology of oral sustained drug
release from capsules and tablets was just emerging, and the first
successfully marketed Spansule® capsule had just been developed in

---

*Spansule® is the SK&F trademark name for their brand of sustained
 release products.

1952. No blood or urine data on this first capsule product had been published that I was aware of, and the FDA did not demand such data. In 1953, if preliminary results in humans looked promising, one could make a decision to develop a product, and within two years have the product ready and on the market. Good products, such as chlorpromazine tablets, developed in the Pharmaceutical Chemistry Section at SK&F, were introduced to the market within a two-year development time frame, and in my estimation the work was done carefully and well.

In 1953 scientists in pharmacy did not have a foothold yet in research areas dealing with absorption, distribution, metabolism and excretion. Passive and active absorption processes were foggy ideas and not a part of our research experience. Adrien Albert had written fascinatingly about prodrugs in the 1950s, but the concept was not yet being widely used by pharmacists in the pharmaceutical industry to mask taste, influence absorption, reduce toxicity, prolong drug action, or improve compounding of a drug entity.

I had become a close friend of Tak Higuchi in 1939, when I was an undergraduate in pharmacy and he a graduate student in chemistry. As a pharmacy undergraduate I benefited from Tak's thinking about the mathematical and physical sciences in research, and he learned a little about pharmacy from me. My teachers and friends had heard about Tak, but organized pharmacy didn't begin to know him until he accepted a position in academic pharmacy at Wisconsin in 1947. His Ph.D. graduates began entering the pharmaceutical industry and academia in about 1951, so very little physical pharmacy science was being applied to industrial pharmaceutical practice before that time. The Arrhenius equation for shelf-life study and drug stability prediction was not yet being used routinely, however, rule of thumb exaggerated temperature and handling conditions were being followed to forecast stability. The concepts pertaining to polymorphic forms of drugs and their relationship to drug absorption efficiency, bioavailability and stability were unknown in pharmaceutical science. The importance of particle size to dissolution and absorption rates of poorly soluble drugs was just being uncovered. Also just being recognized was the importance of the crystal forms of the fatty-waxy (lipid) materials that were being used to coat or imbed drugs in order to achieve controlled drug release. Drug interactions that occurred upon simultaneous administration of several drugs were hardly recognized, and the reduction in the excretion rate of penicillin upon probenecid administration was puzzling. High pressure liquid chromatography and mass spectrometry instrumentation were not yet available commercially to detect and measure drug concentrations in body fluids. Penicillins G and V were the only significant penicillins on the market. Analytical methods available for measuring organic nitrate in body fluids and assessing the worth of organic nitrate products were unsatisfactory, and brought about the

demise of a development project on oral sustained action organic
nitrate to which I was assigned.

In the early 1950s very few pharmacists employed in the research and development laboratories of the pharmaceutical industry
had doctoral degrees. They perceived themselves less as scientists
than as technical collaborators with scientists; at SK&F, however,
Rudolph Blythe was promoting the idea that pharmacists could be
innovators, research leaders and reformers of product development.
Only a handful of pharmacists in the industry were viewed as prominent pharmaceutical scientists at that time. Almost none were
publishing scientific data in refereed scientific journals because
most perceived themselves as development people rather than research and development people. Mostly, the research done by the
pharmacists in industry was incomplete and unpublishable. Development pharmacists did very little, if anything, to use animals and
humans as subjects to compare dosage forms of drugs, to study drug
absorption and excretion rates to help them understand dosage form
design or to help them establish dosage regimens. Pharmacy people
worried that work with animals and humans might be an intrusion on
the turf of the physician, pharmacologist or biochemist and, therefore, little research along these lines was initiated and published
by pharmacists.

When I undertook my first assignments at SK&F I began asking
questions such as how rapidly are these drugs absorbed orally, are
they absorbed in various portions of the gastrointestinal tract,
what is the purpose of ethylene diamine in the aminophylline
complex, how is theophylline eliminated from the body and at what
rate, in what kind of matrix can we disperse these drugs, how
stable are these compounds in lipid "melts," how easily can the
dispersions be granulated, how do the granulations flow in tablet
machine hoppers, how do the granulations compress, what unit dose
weight variability does one encounter in such tablets, and so on.
I kept a thorough notebook and insisted that data of sufficient
quality and completeness be generated such that, in due time, we
could publish at least some of our basic findings. At that time I
was not encouraged to do work in such a way that it could lead to
publication. In fact, the idea of publication was foreign to most
industrial research and development people schooled in pharmacy,
and to some its motivation was suspect.

At the time my work began various glyceryl stearates and
palmitates, along with the usual pharmaceutical waxes, were being
used as lipid matrices for effecting sustained release. In my
search for a food grade triglyceride that would be a more
granulateable, compressible and stable matrix for sustained action
tablets than the glyceryl stearates, I came upon hydrogenated
castor oil, a fairly waxy substance that melted at a somewhat
higher temperature than the commercial stearates. For quite a few

months I worked intensively on developing hundreds of granulations and tablets, utilizing lipid matrices from which drug release was protracted in vitro and in vivo, and we studied their in vitro and in vivo release profiles. Ultimately I concluded that we would have much better control of the drug release profile if we could make double layered tablets, one a quick release layer and the other sustained release (1). With the help of the R.J. Stokes Machine Co. and some very mechanically adept shop workers at SK&F, a tableting machine was devised to manufacture multilayered tablets. The idea was to formulate one layer as a typical quick release dose, and the other as a thin layer with wide cylindrical dimensions, so that dissolution of the remaining drug would approach zero-order release kinetics. The dose and release rate over a period of hours should approach the rate of theophylline loss from the body at therapeutic blood concentrations, thus requiring the patient to take only one tablet, morning and night. We succeeded in making a functional sustained release tablet, learned a lot about sustained release drug technology, but, as sometimes happens in product development, this product idea was shelved after a decision by company management not to market. It is ironic that sustained release theophylline products began to be marketed 30 years later and that the market for them is fairly large. In the process of developing the technology for making certain kinds of sustained release granules, coatings and tablets, we probably made the first use of hydrogenated castor oil, with or without ethylcellulose dissolved in it, as a plasticizer and as a matrix substance for effecting sustained drug release. A number of pharmaceutical companies since that time have adopted hydrogenated castor oil for use in their sustained release products.

An equally exciting part of my first product development experience was concerned with determining the appropriate dose and release characteristics of theophylline from the sustained release tablet. We made the assumption that therapeutic response to theophylline would be related to blood or tissue concentrations. Therefore, any sustained action oral dosage form should release drug and be absorbed at a rate that compensated for loss from the bloodstream and body tissues. I began searching the literature for plasma concentraton data for theophylline disappearance in humans. There was published data, but they were plotted on cartesian coordinate paper. They were in the form of the typical fall-away plasma concentration curve after peak plasma concentrations were obtained following a single dose. When these data were plotted on semilogarithmic paper, they yielded approximately straight lines during the fall-away phase of drug elimination. It was easy to compute the rate of disappearance of theophylline from the human body at a given plasma concentration and body content of theophylline, as well as the amount of theophylline that would have to be released and absorbed per hour from a tablet to just compensate for the theophylline disappearance rate. In the course of this work, I learned much technology and pharmaceutical science that would be applicable to the next development project that was to come along in 1954. That project dealt with a sustained release dosage form of sulfaethylthiadiazole (sulfaethidole or SETD), and lent itself to various biopharmaceutical studies.

After discovering for myself, in 1953, the exponential disappearance of theophylline from the body, I began to plot blood or plasma concentration data for "sulfas," which were being screened as possible candidates for sustained release, and similar data for other drugs. It was of great interest to me that the family of sulfa drugs had such a large range of biologic half-lives and that many other drugs seemed to be eliminated from the body by a process that approximated first-order kinetics. Working intensively in this field, in 1953 and 1954 I began to find some key literature references, such as articles by Dominguez (2), Boxer (3) and Axelrod (4). Later, I encountered the classic work of Teorell (5) and several other researchers, and this revealed that others outside the pharmacy field had explored the mathematics of drug absorption, distribution, metabolism and excretion. I turned up an old book from the turn of the century that contained data of Arrhenius, showing plots of exponential disappearance of antibodies from the blood. So these concepts were not new. Elementary pharmacokinetics reaches back to the 19th century, but these concepts were not being taught in pharmacy schools and they were not being applied in the pharmaceutical industry to any extent prior to the 1950s. They were new to pharmaceutical science, and to people like myself, in the pharmaceutical industry, who were trying to develop dosage forms and regimens based on sound science. I realized that the ability to describe blood or tissue drug concentrations and elimination rates in terms of biologic constants such as k and $t_{1/2}$ would be a major step forward since these constants are scalar quantities which lend themselves to comparison and tabulation.

By 1954, knowledge of some of the details of our work could not be contained. Consultants and other visitors learned about it. However, until a product was marketed, I was not free to submit for publication any of the experimental data that we generated. Therefore, I gave several lectures entitled, "Illustrations and Pharmaceutical Interpretations of First-Order Drug Elimination Rate from the Bloodstream," at colleges of pharmacy around the country. I submitted a paper for publication (6) under that title in 1955, anticipating the publication of our SETD studies in 1956. This paper, plus those published in 1956 through 1958 (7-12), which consisted mainly of our very extensive investigations with SETD in humans during 1954-56, stirred the interest of a lot of pharmaceutical scientists and educators. Within a few years hundreds of pharmacy-oriented people were undertaking research in the kinetics of drug absorption, distribution, metabolism and excretion.

In 1954, a plot I made of penicillin G concentration data illustrating a biologic half-life of 30 minutes had a profound effect
on my thinking about this drug. We attempted to prolong the oral
absorption of penicillin G by formulating it into an oral sustained
release product, but quickly discovered that it was not well
absorbed beyond the duodenum. Additionally, penicillin in oral
sustained release form was maintained in the adverse acidic
environment of the gastrointestinal tract for too long a time, and
the efficiency of absorption was dreadfully low. Further thought
about the short half-life of this drug prompted me to advise
management in 1954 that there would be new marketable products
possible among the penicillins and that we should begin looking for
some with longer biologic half-lives and/or a different antibacterial spectrum. After bringing in a respected consultant and
authority on penicillin development and production, who was also of
the opinion that this was possible, management's decision was that
the practice of medicine did not need another penicillin. When
management reversed its decision about three or four years later,
the development effort was too late. The new penicillin that SK&F
had begun to develop was already covered by a competitor's patent
application. The company lost its opportunity to become strong in
the marketplace with new penicillins; however, it was very successful in finding new marketable drugs in the mental health field and
other therapeutic areas.

As I look back now at my own scientific career and the
evolution of biopharmaceutics and pharmacokinetics in American
pharmacy, I see that they were closely linked to SK&F's decision in
the early '50s to use the principle of sustained drug release from
oral dosage forms as a means of developing and marketing new and
better products. The expectation was that numerous oral products
could be made for once-in-the-morning and once-in-the-evening
administration, and that this was a convenience factor for the
patient that would result in better patient compliance. In
addition, there would be less peak and valley variation in blood
and tissue drug concentrations, presumably leading to fewer side
effects, and there would be a uniqueness about such multipelletted
capsule products that would make oral sustained release products
credible in the eyes of the physician and pharmacist. Such
products, representing new drug delivery systems, would be a
marketing man's dream. Finally, at a stage in the company's
history when it was small, had only $50 million in annual sales and
was in need of new products, here were a number of products
available for development that didn't require the discovery of new
drugs. All that was needed was to put previously marketed drugs
into a new, more acceptable, dosage delivery form. History has
shown that this was sound scientific and management strategy, and
that a number of useful and acceptable drug products were developed
and marketed that could meet the therapeutic needs of patients.
The ideas pertaining to sustained drug release from oral and other

dosage forms remain viable and useful today, and many companies are currently pursuing such development work because better products are possible, development times for these products are much shorter, and costs of development are much lower than those associated with developing new chemical entities. SK&F slowed its efforts in this direction in the mid-'60s, but still retains a large share of the oral sustained release drug market.

The history of the development and design of oral sustained release medications at SK&F has been published (13) and will not be dealt with further in this chapter; however, I will attempt to relate some interesting episodes and present some further experimental data illustrative of what we were generating, mostly in the '50s, when I had the privilege of being the Program Team Director on research programs of Time Delay Principles, Formulation Principles, Drug Absorption and Prodrugs consecutively.

Some of the SETD data generated in 1954 and 1955 were interesting and instructive, especially at a time when blood concentrations of drugs were not being portrayed as exponential plots. The exponential plots of four different doses of SETD, shown in Figure 1, clearly indicate that, in the blood concentration range studied, the biologic half-life of SETD was independent of dose. Figure 2 depicts maximum and minimum limits of blood concentrations predicted for human subjects who exhibited a half-life of 8 hours for SETD and who received the drug according to a fixed protocol. The experimental data agreed with the predictions. The role which $t_{1/2}$ and k (the velocity constant for drug elimination) played in the scientific approach to establishing dosage regimens and formulas in product development was illustrated. This same concept is now widely used in clinical pharmacokinetic monitoring of hospitalized patients to change doses or dosage regimens when patients require such individualized attention. In recent years, we have helped pioneer this concept at our University Hospital in Kentucky and hope to extend its application to community pharmacy practice. Figure 3 illustrates the results of our attempt to determine how much human subjects might vary in their biologic half-lives with respect to a specific drug. The study showed a distribution of half-lives from 5 to 14 hours, with most subjects in the range from 7 to 10 hours. Figure 4 shows that, for drugs whose elimination is affected by urine pH, one can determine the half-life change as a function of urine pH (15,16). In this instance, at pH 5 SETD was eliminated with a half-life of about 11 hours, while at pH 8 the half-life was about 4 hours. We, and our associates at Temple University, were able to demonstrate for the first time the precise quantitative effect of urine pH on the biologic half-life when there is a pH sensitive excretion process. These kinds of data were important not only in the design of the sustained release SETD product, but also provided some perception of factors that might influence the performance of other drugs for

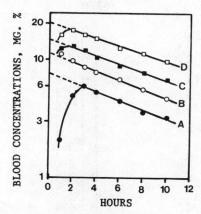

Figure 1. Sulfaethylthiadiazole concentrations in the blood of a single subject following oral doses of 1.0, 2.0, 3.0 and 4.0 g. Reprinted from (9), with permission of the copyright owner.

which we were developing sustained action delivery systems and for which we needed to recommend dosage regimens.

   Though some of our emphasis was given to evaluating drugs and their products in terms of blood concentrations, we also were interested in quantitating pharmacologic responses, understanding

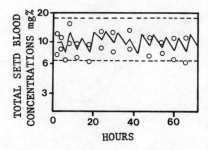

Figure 2. Total SETD blood concentration data for four adult human subjects receiving 2 g initial doses followed by a 1 g dose every six hours for 72 hours. Steady-state blood concentrations calculated from appropriate equations utilizing k or $t_{1/2}$ predict maximum and minimum limits shown by the broken lines. Actual data lie within the predicted limits. Reprinted from (12), with permission of the copyright owner.

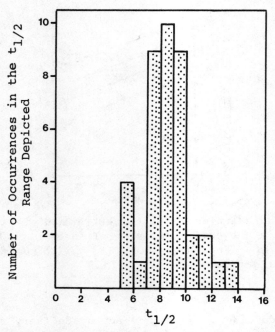

Figure 3. Histogram of the half-lives in hours observed from blood concentration data following oral or intravenous administration of 39 individual SETD doses ranging from 0.5 to 4.0 g in 13 normal human adult subjects (14).

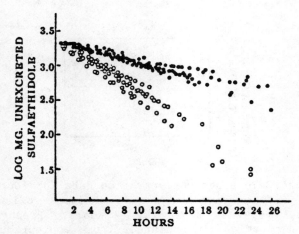

Figure 4. Illustration of first-order elimination of SETD after a 2 g oral dose in humans when urine was maintained at pH 5 (closed circles) and pH 8 (open circles). Reprinted from (15), with permission of the copyright owner.

and innovating drug delivery systems for sustained drug action, understanding factors that affected the stability of sustained release drug delivery systems, studying factors that influenced absorbability of drugs and their metabolism, making prodrugs to overcome some of the deficiencies of parent drugs, and understanding how coated pellets functioned as sustained release vectors for drugs.

Figure 5 is an example of an effort to quantitate the anti-sialogogue effect of the belladonna alkaloids which were important in the sustained release product area (17). The salivary suppression response could be quantitated, showing a pharmacologic half-life on the order of 1-1.5 hours in humans. Similarly, for some drugs we could quantitate pharmacologic response as a function of pupil dilation or reduction in pupil size versus time, or body temperature in excess of normal as a function of time (17). We felt it was important for the company to furnish data that would provide a basis for product claims. The company also needed to be able to make claims demonstrating its products' differences from and superiority to competitors' products or dosage regimens.

In making sustained action oral products that were marketable, much effort went into technology development by several SK&F pharmacists. Lipid material selection, coating solvents and techniques, storage techniques, stability evaluation systems and pellet blending techniques were all areas that were deemed important for developing and marketing a series of products and also for product improvement. The results of many of these experimental studies remain confidential; however, some of the extensive studies on

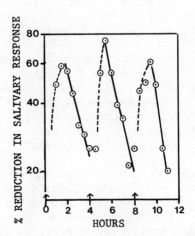

Figure 5. Mean salivary response by two human subjects given 2.4 ml of tincture of belladonna at zero, four and eight hours. Reprinted from (17), with permission.

physical properties of lipids used in these and related pharmaceutical processes were published (18-20). The pharmaceutical use of lipids (as matrices, coatings and additives in dosage forms) often demands a high degree of physical and chemical stability. To maintain the stability, moisture permeability, acceptability of appearance and use, and efficacy in lipid-containing products, such lipid properties as crystal size, refractive index, density, hardness and film integrity must not change sufficiently during the life time of the product to impair its utility.

Glyceryl esters and waxes, used in some sustained release products, are polymorphic and they are also complex chemical mixtures. This polymorphism means that the lipids can exist in various crystal forms that are subject to transition. Since their transition rates vary with temperature, the species that exist after creation of the final dosage form depend on the heating-cooling-processing that occurs during manufacture, and the polymorphs that are most stable will depend upon the storage conditions to which the product is exposed. Investigations of such mixtures are challenging. We studied these complex lipids, not so much to determine the transition states of every molecular species of these complex substances, but the way an engineer would study a material. We wanted to discover the temperatures at which major transitions would occur in the storage temperature range of pharmaceutical products, which storage conditions would hasten the attainment of stable forms, and which temperatures would cause transitions to virtually cease. We used heating-cooling curves as one approach to studying the characteristics of numerous lipid blends. The reading and studying that accompanied this experimental technique were perhaps as important in understanding how to use lipids as sustained drug release regulators as the complex series of connecting lines of different slopes derived from plots of log temperature difference (bath temperature minus sample temperature) versus time.

Heating-cooling curves were useful for detecting the propensity of various lipid substances to undergo polymorphic change, determining the temperatures of rapid polymorphic change, evaluating the effects of time-temperature history on the polymorphic forms which a lipid coating material may assume, and establishing what manufacturing and handling procedures result in the unstable or the relatively stable crystalline forms.

The great effort and time that went into trying to develop various coating agents and techniques for making each new sustained release product recalls another type of study we undertook. This involved screening of lipid materials by photomicrography for information about their storage sensitivities and physical integrity. This procedure was designed to detect lipids which were likely to undergo sufficient physical change to alter the appearance and efficacy of dosage forms made from them. The basic assumption of the test procedure was that the nature and degree of physical change in thin lipid films could be used to predict the physical changes these same lipids might undergo in dosage forms. In this procedure lipid films were cast from the molten state onto microscope slides. Photomicrographs were taken before and after storing the thin lipid films at different temperatures. Comparisons of identical fields on the photomicrographs revealed if there were crystal transformations, crystal growth or the development of minute cracks. In many respects the study of film stability by this technique, as a function of time and temperature of storage, mimicked stability studies on experimental lots of tablets or other dosage forms. The cast slides were stored at −15°C, room temperature, 37°C and 45°C for 24 months with a regular schedule of observations, and this proved to be a useful study method.

Understanding how coated pellets released their drug and sugar excipient was an interesting and challenging study because SK&F's Spansule® capsule contains many hundreds of pellets, some uncoated, but most coated with varying thicknesses of a water immiscible film. A simple single mechanism for drug release appeared unlikely, however, after numerous experimental studies including observations of pellets under the microscope after various periods of exposure to turbulence in digestive fluids. One could observe hairline cracks in some pellets, and some of these pellets were devoid or partially devoid of their solid contents. Some pellets had single holes in them as though a piece of the film had been blasted off, while others ended up as half shells with little or no other solids attached. An osmotic process by which water enters the pellet, begins to dissolve the contents and further attracts water until the pellet cleaves slightly or snaps apart at its weakest point, seems to be the way most of the pellets release their contents. Since coat thickness of the hundreds of pellets per capsule is variable, this results in a variable rate of in-flow of water into each coated pellet. Cleavage of the pellets at various times after exposure to digestive fluids, along with some physical attrition, adequately explains the observed drug release profile which covers a number of hours with the Spansule® capsule.

Another program from the '50s that deserves some mention because it is so closely identified today with biopharmaceutics, drug delivery systems and drug product improvement, is the program of prodrugs and the subject of drug latentiation. A prodrug has certain features that may confer upon it some distinctly advantageous properties; at the appropriate time and place in the body it converts to an active form of the drug. Following the presentation of the prodrug concept to SK&F management in 1959, we got that program underway. We made several hundred compounds that we thought were prodrugs, but I will only describe one that was studied in the '60s. One of our goals was to make a compound that was as good as aspirin (acetylsalicylic acid), but which lacked

aspirin's gastrointestinal tract irritant properties when administered over the long term.   In proceeding in this direction we
assumed that aspirin itself is a kind of transport form of salicylate; the acetyl portion is cleaved and disposed of when the
aspirin molecule is transported to the appropriate receptor site.

It was difficult to prove that aspirin is a prodrug, or that
it is or is not active when the molecule is intact. Thinking of it
as a prodrug, however, pointed out the possibility of making new
compounds with modified physical-chemical properties which could be
viewed as salicylate transport forms.   These could be made to have
less gastrointestinal tract irritancy but could retain the same
capability of cleaving as aspirin, thus leaving the therapeutic end
of the molecule at the receptor site.   We made the n-hexyl
carbonate of salicylic acid (compound SK&F 26070) and it had the
predicted properties (21-23).   On a molar basis, when it was
administered to small animals, the drug was virtually indistinguishable from aspirin both pharmacologically and in its acute
toxicity except that comparison studies in rats and dogs showed
that animals dosed with aspirin showed marked gastric bleeding
whereas those treated with SK&F 26070 showed virtually none (23).
Although the compound never reached development, we have recently
received IND status for it at the University of Kentucky. We have
determined recently that after oral doses to humans, one obtains
blood concentrations of salicylate comparable to those produced by
aspirin.

I never was able to generate much interest at SK&F in specific
prodrugs, but as noted in the chapters by Professors Higuchi and
Sezaki, the use of prodrugs as drug delivery systems is a concept
that is generating considerable new interest today.   In part this
is related to economics because even before we start development
work on the compound, we already have much scientific information
on the active moiety of the prodrug.   The investment of time and
money, up to the time of marketing, should be much less than that
required for developing a totally new therapeutic entity. Although
people knew almost as much in the '50s as they know now about how
and when to make prodrugs, the breadth of interest was not as great
as that which exists presently.

Since the advent of biopharmaceutics and pharmacokinetics on
the American scene, one sees an extraordinary emphasis on pharmacokinetics and related biopharmaceutic studies.   Thousands of
research articles and numerous books on this subject have been
written by pharmaceutical scientists since the 1950s.   This
reflects some of the drama and real importance of such research as
it relates to certain aspects of dosage form design, drug delivery
rate, and human and animal utilization and disposition of a drug.
In the '50s biopharmaceutics removed pharmaceutics from the
restraints of the beaker, test tube and pharmacy manufacturing

laboratory.   Research in biopharmaceutics resulted in many more
bridges and pathways that now increase the linkages of pharmaceutical analysis, nuclear pharmacy, pharmacognosy, microbiology,
molecular biology, pharmacology, physiology, biochemistry, toxicology, engineering and clinical drug product evaluation.   More of the
research in these disciplines of pharmaceutical science now focuses
on understanding dosage forms, drug delivery systems, dosage
regimens and their importance in optimizing therapy and discovering
new marketable drug products.   The concepts of biopharmacy have
given pharmaceutical scientists, educators and practitioners more
opportunity for interaction with biomedical scientists and physicians at the teaching, research, development and clinical services
levels.

Today I regard pharmaceutics and biopharmaceutics as essentially similar disciplines with a physical pharmacy basis, the
latter so named because of its biologic or clinical component.
Biopharmaceutics is essentially biophysical pharmacy which I
consider to be a mutant that grew from the seed of the physical
pharmacy tree. The biophysical pharmacy tree grew several more
branches than the parent and one of them was pharmacokinetics. The
volume of research and development originally being done in
physical pharmacy increased significantly when the biologic mutant
developed.   This development has made room for many more pharmacists and pharmaceutical scientists in the total health care
industry including the areas of traditional drug distribution,
services on interdisciplinary patient care teams, research in
federal research institutes, regulation in agencies for drug
product standards and control, research, development and services
in the pharmaceutical industry, and work in academic centers.
This new tree in pharmacy has been adorned with the fruits of
research and development since the 1950s, and many of these fruits
have come from pharmacokinetics. We need to give more attention to
the other branches and to harvest the other fruits of physical and
biophysical pharmacy that relate more to the creation and evaluation of new or improved drug delivery systems.   This means re-
examining all possible drug delivery routes and understanding
better the physical chemistry and physiology of the site as it
influences drug delivery.   We need further studies to understand
materials selection and materials science as various old and new
materials are selected as vehicles to carry drugs and control drug
delivery.   We need to understand better the absorption of drugs and
interactions between drugs and these vehicles, along with interactions of drugs with the body tissues they must traverse during
transport to receptor sites. We need to invent new dosage forms
from new materials. We need to research factors affecting the
stability and integrity of the dosage form per se, in addition to
the drug, as these relate to predicting and controlling drug
delivery.   We need to better understand the physical-chemical
structures and processes in the gastrointestinal tract that make

drugs more absorbable in one portion of the tract than in another. We need to study more thoroughly the rates of drug absorption from various parts of the gastrointestinal tract and other absorbing surfaces. We need to understand why some drugs exhibit one biologic half-life in one species and an entirely different biologic half-life in another, and how drug structural change influences this half-life and bears on drug product development. We need to get a better handle on how drugs are metabolized, and how this metabolism can be influenced for the benefit of the patient. We need to understand factors pertaining to drug and dosage form design that enable one to target a specific organ or tissue for drug delivery. We need more input from analytical scientists, pharmaceutical and natural product chemists, and from the new breeds of nuclear pharmacists and pharmaceutical biochemists, to not only make new or better therapeutic entities through advanced biotechnology, but also to focus on the dosage form. They need to bring to pharmaceutics the strengths and skills of their disciplines in the handling and evaluation of products containing the newer polypeptides, monoclonal antibodies, and hormones, enzymes, and other cell process regulators and catalysts. My suggestions of studies appropriate for the present and the future hark back to the beginnings of physical and biophysical pharmacy. They underscore the importance of the educational programs in pharmacy that produce pharmaceutical scientists qualified to work in these areas.

Sid Riegelman, who we remember in this Symposium, was close to the physical and biophysical pharmacy developments during his entire professional lifetime. He spoke frequently on these topics, published many original articles in the field, strongly influenced its direction, and was one of its leading academic authorities. It is a pleasure to recall my close associations with him, Louis Busse, and Tak Higuchi during our early years together at Wisconsin.

REFERENCES

1. U.S. Patent 2,952,792. Sustained Release Pharmaceutical Tablets, J.V. Swintosky, Perkiomenville, Pa., assignor to Smith Kline & French Laboratories, Continuation of application Ser. No. 449,880, Aug. 16, 1954.
2. R. Dominguez and E. Pomerene, Calculation of the rates of absorption of exogenous creatinine, Proc. Soc. Exp. Biol. Med. 60:173-181 (1945).
3. G.E. Boxer, V.C. Jelinek, R. Tompsett, R. Dubois and A.O. Edison, Streptomycin in the blood: chemical determination after single and repeated intra-muscular injections, J. Pharmacol. Exp. Ther. 92:226-235 (1948).

4. J. Axelrod and J. Reichenthal, The fate of caffeine in men and a method for its estimation in biological materials, J. Pharmacol. Exp. Ther. 107:519–523 (1953).

5. T. Teorell, The kinetics of distribution of substances administered to the body, Part 1. The extra vascular modes of administration, Arch. Intern. Pharmacodynamie 57:205–240 (1937).

6. J.V. Swintosky, Illustrations and pharmaceutical interpretations of first-order drug elimination rate from the blood-stream, J. Amer. Pharm. Assoc., Sci. Ed. 45:395–400 (1956).

7. E.L. Foltz, J.V. Swintosky and M.J. Robinson, Absorption, distribution and fate of sulfaethylthiadiazole administered orally and intravenously, Fed. Proc. 15:422 (1956).

8. J.V. Swintosky, Excretion equations and interpretation for digitoxin, Nature 179:98–99 (1957).

9. J.V. Swintosky, M.J. Robinson, E.L. Foltz and S.M. Free, Sulfaethylthiadiazole I. Interpretations of human blood level concentrations following oral doses, J. Amer. Pharm. Assoc., Sci. Ed. 46:399–403 (1957).

10. J.V. Swintosky, M.J. Robinson and E.L. Foltz, Sulfaethylthiadiazole II. Distribution and disappearance from the tissues following intravenous injection, J. Amer. Pharm. Assoc., Sci. Ed. 46:403–411 (1957).

11. J.V. Swintosky, E.L. Foltz, A. Bondi Jr. and M.J. Robinson, Sulfaethylthiadiazole III. Kinetics of absorption, distribution and excretion, J. Amer. Pharm. Assoc., Sci. Ed. 47:136–141 (1958).

12. J.V. Swintosky, A. Bondi, Jr. and M.J. Robinson, Sulfaethyltiadiazole IV. Steady state blood concentration and urinary excretion data following repeated oral doses, J. Amer. Pharm. Assoc., Sci. Ed. 47:753–756 (1958).

13. J.V. Swintosky, Design of oral sustained release dosage forms, Indian J. Pharm. 25:360–367 (1963).

14. J.V. Swintosky, Biologic half-life and tissue concentrations, Proceedings of Pharmacy Teachers Seminar, AACP, Madison, Wisconsin 13:140–156 (1961).

15. J.B. Portnoff, J.V. Swintosky and H.B. Kostenbauder, Control of urine pH and its effect on drug excretion in humans, J. Pharm. Sci. 50:890 (1961).

16. H.B. Kostenbauder, J.B. Portnoff and J.V. Swintosky, Control of urine pH and its effects on sulfaethidole excretion in humans, J. Pharm. Sci. 51:1084–1089 (1962).

17. J.V. Swintosky and F.M. Sturtevant, Exponential disappearance of pharmacologic activity, J. A. Ph. A. Sci. Ed. 49:685–686 (1960).

18. D.R. Reese, C.W. Chong and J.V. Swintosky, Physical properties of lipids used in pharmacy. I. Screening raw materials via photomicrography, J. Amer. Pharm. Assoc., Sci. Ed. 49:85–89 (1960).

19. D.R. Reese, P.N. Nordberg, S.P. Eriksen and J.V. Swintosky, Technique for studying thermally induced phase transitions, J. Pharm. Sci. 50:177-178 (1961).

20. S.P. Eriksen, D.R. Reese and J.V. Swintosky, Physical properties of lipids used in pharmacy II. Use of heating-cooling curves to study lipid materials, J. Pharm. Sci. 51:843-850 (1962).

21. U.S. Patent 3,412,131. Alkyl carbonates of salicylic acid. J.V. Swintosky, Perkiomenville, Pa., assignor to Smith Kline & French Laboratories, filed August 2, 1966.

22. L.W. Dittert, H.C. Caldwell, T. Ellison, G.M. Irwin, D.E. Rivard and J.V. Swintosky, Carbonate ester prodrugs of salicylic acid. Synthesis, solubility characteristics, in vitro enzymatic hydrolysis rates, and blood levels of salicylate following oral administration to dogs, J. Pharm. Sci. 57:828-831 (1968).

23. A. Misher, H.J. Adams, J.J. Fishler and R.G. Jones, Pharmacology of the hexylcarbonate of salicylic acid, J. Pharm. Sci. 57:1128-1131 (1968).

Chapter 8

MODERN PHARMACEUTICAL DOSAGE FORMS

Arnold H. Beckett

Chelsea College
Manresa Road
London, England

The topic allocated to me for my contribution to this Symposium indicates that change is occurring, or has occurred, in our design of dosage forms, because otherwise the word "modern" in the title would be superfluous. Why is change necessary in the use of classical forms of drug presentation such as tablets, capsules, solutions or simple formulations in which the physico-chemical characteristics of the drug molecule control the absorption, distribution and elimination of the drug? Obviously, because some drugs have short biological half-lives; some, long half-lives. The administration schedules necessary to produce appropriate therapeutic concentrations of drug may vary greatly; problems follow therefrom.

One of the main problems in drug administration today, in most countries, is the lack of patient compliance in taking the classical drug products prescribed. Thus, the impact of all the advances in the production of new, potent and selective agents by industry, and the knowledge gained by physicians about how these agents should be used is substantially reduced upon application to treatment of patients. This lack of patient compliance is hardly surprising due to two factors: the need for different dosage regimens, especially if more than one product must be taken (1,2), and the side effects which may make the patient feel worse than the medical problem that is affecting him. The confusion of one elderly woman who had to take eight different products each day probably exemplifies the difficulties. Each day, she dutifully took the eight dosage forms from the separate containers, mixed them in a bowl and at random selected four which she took in the morning and left the remaining four to be taken at night.

Something must be done to change the crazy schedules of drug administration often necessitated by the different half-lives of drugs. The solution to the problem is to produce dosage forms in which the rate of drug delivery is properly controlled. The aim for most products should be to dose once every 24 hours (or once every 12 hours in certain circumstances) when the oral route is used. Preferably, the dosage form should be such that drug release is not affected by food or liquid intakes.

The problem of intersubject variation caused by extensive first-pass metabolism is another factor which necessitates the change to modern dosage forms. Oral dosage forms, however, cannot overcome this problem; the introduction of transdermal, rectal and intranasal dosage forms, which can also be designed to control the rate of drug input, represent the modern approaches which are proving to be successful.

The ever rising cost of medical care programs, in all countries, is increasing the demand that the primary health care responsibility be placed more on the individual and on nonmedical staff. In fact, this is the advice given by the World Health Organization. Thus, the use of medical staff time must be reserved for important aspects of health care and must not be wasted on trivia as is often the case today. In other words, self-medication will increase in all countries. This will increase the emphasis on patient involvement, but suitable, safer forms of the most effective drugs currently available only by medical prescription must be produced. Controlled drug delivery will thus be employed for the oral route of self-medication because, in this way, side effects are reduced and drug administration made convenient.

Today there are fewer new drug molecules being approved each year for marketing as pharmaceutical products. There will probably be even fewer in the future. Thus, the emphasis will be on more efficient design of pharmacological testing and use of structure-activity relationships to lead to a suitable drug. At present, much of the testing and relationships are of doubtful value when the metabolites of the molecule being tested are active or cause side effects and when their plasma concentration-time profiles are different from that of the administered molecule. Since the ratios of the various species will vary with time after drug administration, the pharmacological response at different times cannot be correlated with plasma concentrations of the drug. The rate of drug input must be controlled for suitable periods of time so that there are direct concentration relationships between drug and metabolite and all aspects are at steady state. When a molecule has been selected for clinical trial, the drug needs to be incorporated into modern dosage forms exhibiting controlled delivery so that the intersubject variation in response might be reduced and side effects lessened. Fewer patients would then be required for assessment of the potential of the new molecule.

I hope I have presented sufficient reasons to justify my interpretation of modern dosage forms as "those forms in which the rate of release of the drug is controlled in a predictable manner, irrespective of whether the oral, rectal, transdermal or another route of administration is used." In summary, the purposes of controlling the rate and location of drug input into man are:

1. To reduce side effects of drugs whether they be local, systemic or both.

2. To provide more effective utilization of a dose of the drug.

3. To minimize the influence of first-pass metabolism and thus intersubject variation in response to a drug.

4. To minimize the influence of food, drink and physical activity on drug absorption.

5. To deal with circadian rhythm, in the manifestation of a disease, by having suitable drug plasma concentrations at appropriate times.

6. To make product administration convenient for the patient, irrespective of the biological half-life of the drug and the numbers of products to be taken.

7. To facilitate drug administration in hospitals and to reduce the costs of such administration.

All this means that life becomes easier for the patient and the prescriber.

I now propose to present some examples of the approach to the design of modern pharmaceutical dosage forms using the oral route of administration. There are many different approaches to the design of oral controlled release products: matrix tablets, ionic bonded drugs in tablets, osmotic pumps, pellets which erode slowly, pellets with membranes which slowly rupture or with membranes through which the drug diffuses, and others. However, the design must take into account the changing characteristics and conditions of the gastrointestinal tract, and the rate at which the different products pass through the gastrointestinal tract.

If the dose is in a single delivery system, such as a tablet, this unit may reside for very different times in the stomach and small intestine. In general, the transit time to the feces is too

short to give good bioavailability if the unit maintains its
integrity throughout the transit. It is preferable in the design
of a 24-hour product to incorporate the drug into a system of many
subunits, such as pellets, which, when administered in a capsule,
become many small drug depots as the capsule shell readily
dissolves. These drug depots become widely scattered in the
gastrointestinal tract so that, within an hour or two after
administration, systemic drug input involves absorption of drug
throughout the whole of the small intestine. The distribution of
pellets with a density above 1.5 at one, four and eight hours after
administration is shown in Figure 1; some 40-50% of the pellets are
in the colon even 24 hours after the dose (3,4). It is preferable
to use diffusion through a membrane (a process which can be made
predictable) as the rate-controlling step for drug release, rather
than to depend upon erosion or the older method of membrane rupture
to release the drug (processes which are less predictable in the
gastrointestinal tract).

If diffusion is used as the rate-controlling step and dosage
once every 24 hours is planned, it is important that the pellets
release the drug faster in the colon where there are less fluid
conditions than in the upper gastrointestinal tract. It is also
important that none of the pellets carry their drug into the feces;
otherwise, bioavailability will be reduced relative to a solution
or tablet dose. The slow release of drug from each pellet and the
wide scattering of the pellets ensure that a high concentration of

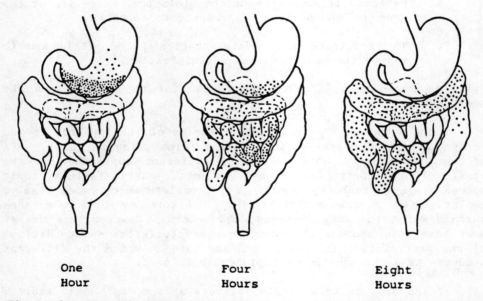

One   Four   Eight
Hour   Hours   Hours

Figure 1. Distribution of pellets in the gastrointestinal tract in
            man at various times after oral administration.

drug locally in the gastrointestinal tract does not occur. Also, the sum of the separate release rates controls the rate of systemic drug delivery. An in vitro test using a pH gradient profile to simulate the changing pH conditions of the gastrointestinal tract can be used to produce in vitro/in vivo correlations and thus may be used to set in vitro specifications for production. It is impossible for a capsule of pellets designed to meet such specifications to "dump" the whole drug content in the gastrointestinal tract. Thus, it is much safer to use such pellet formulations of drug rather than conventional dosage forms or controlled release tablets in which the drug is presented in a single unit.

The reduction of local irritation using controlled release pellets rather than a controlled release tablet formulation has been demonstrated (in rabbits and monkeys) for potassium chloride, a substance which is corrosive to mucous membranes (4). Controlled release pellets of theophylline, designed for administration once every 12 hours, produce much less gastrointestinal tract disturbance than does theophylline in a conventional dosage form (Hadzija et al., to be published). More recently, it has been demonstrated that pellets of theophylline designed for administration once every 24 hours result in very little difference between the plasma concentrations during the broad plateau and the troughs, upon repeated doses. In addition, a dose of more than one gram can be given all at once without causing significant side effects. L-Hyoscyamine has been used successfully in 2 mg doses in controlled release pellet form to prevent vomiting in cancer patients receiving anticancer drugs; side effects from this dose in this form are negligible (Beckett et al., unpublished observation). Nicotinic acid may be given in large doses (1 to 2 g) in controlled release pellet formulation without producing flushing (Beckett et al., unpublished observation). The above examples indicate that controlling drug release in a predictable way using many small subunits may reduce both local and systemic side effects and establishes the feasibility of a once every 24 hours (or once every 12 hours) dosing regimen.

I will now describe, in some detail, the design of a controlled release product of the anti-inflammatory acid, ketoprofen. This compound, along with certain other nonsteroidal anti-inflammatory drugs (NSAIDs) such as ibuprofen, indomethacin and diclofenac, is eliminated rapidly from the body (Fig. 2) in humans and is, therefore, short acting (5-8). Because urine is more alkaline in the first few hours after going to bed, some 60-80% of a dose is excreted within four hours of going to bed (9). Therefore, there will be little drug left in the body when it is most needed; for example, before getting up in the morning, when joint stiffness is greatest in arthritic patients (10). In addition, with conventional dosage forms, the drug is released all at once and is quickly absorbed in the stomach and duodenum. As a

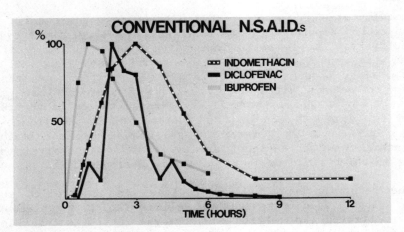

Figure 2. Plasma concentration-time curves for three nonsteroidal anti-inflammatory drugs following oral administration of conventional dosage forms. (Plasma concentration relative to maximum concentration observed.)

result, sensitive tissues are exposed to high concentrations of irritant drug and local irritation and even damage may occur. For a drug such as ketoprofen, the use of a conventional dosage form leads to peaks above and troughs below the therapeutic range even when a dose is given every 6 hours (Fig. 3).

A once every 24-hour dosing schedule would, therefore, require a suitable controlled release form of a known drug (use of a physical method), or the synthesis of a completely new drug molecule having a long biological half-life in humans (use of chemical

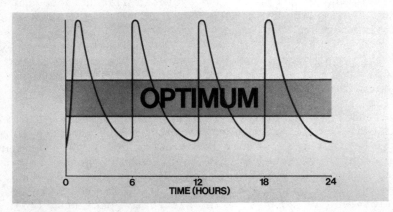

Figure 3. Plasma concentration-time profile following administration of ketoprofen every 6 hours.

method). In the latter case, using a conventional dosage form, the physico-chemical characteristics of the drug molecule itself are important, but the peak plasma concentration is likely to occur 1-3 hours after administration and there may be substantial inter-subject variations in the time of the peak and the rate of elimination. By using controlled delivery of a known and estab-lished drug of shorter biological half-life, a suitable plasma profile can result from correct product design (Fig. 4), and there will be less intersubject variation in response; also, steady state will be achieved more quickly upon multiple dosing of this product than when using a drug of long biological half-life. The use of an enteric coating to physically alter drug delivery does not give a controlled delivery and is likely to produce substantial differ-ences in response (8) (Fig. 5).

Medical opinion stresses that an anti-inflammatory acid that is given each night before going to bed should be designed so as to produce a broad drug plasma concentration plateau from about 5-12 hours after the dose, and lower concentrations throughout the day until the next dose is taken. This drug release pattern would correspond to the circadian rhythm in the symptoms (10) (Fig. 6) and provide for maximum utilization of drug with the minimum dose for each 24-hour period. The anti-inflammatory acid should not be released in the stomach, so it need not be taken with food. Con-trolled release pellets of ketoprofen are designed to conform to this drug release pattern: dosing is required once every 24 hours, at night, and the bioavailability is comparable to that of the

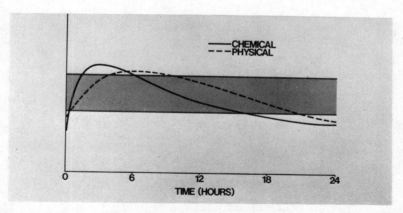

Figure 4. Plasma concentration-time profiles of drug after hypo-thetical adjustment of drug release profile for a drug with a short half-life (physical) and chemical modifica-tion of drug to increase half-life (chemical) (see text).

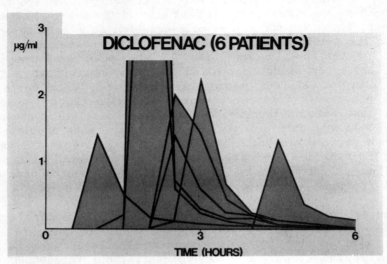

Figure 5. Variation in plasma concentration-time profiles for diclofenac after administration of an enteric coated oral dosage form to six patients (8).

conventional dosage form (Fig. 6). The use of controlled release pellets in the product Oruvail® leads to less loss of drug from the body in the first four hours after administration (Fig. 7), less intersubject variation in plasma levels (Fig. 8) and less fecal blood loss (Fig. 9) than the conventional dosage form of ketoprofen (Nielsenaud and Raulov, 1981, May & Baker Ltd. files).

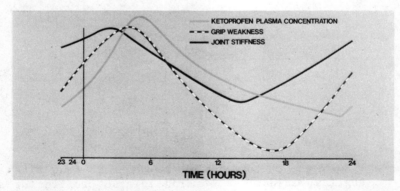

Figure 6. Circadian variations of arthritic symptoms compared to concentration-time profile of ketoprofen from commercial once a day dosage form (Oruvail®).

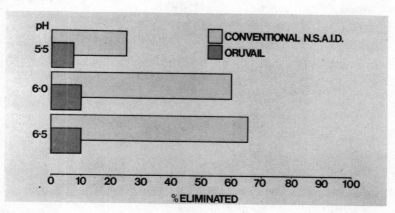

Figure 7. Four-hour urinary elimination of ketoprofen after administration of Oruvail® versus a conventional dosage form.

Space limitations preclude the presentation of other examples,
but there is no doubt, in my opinion, that the need for development
of modern pharmaceutical dosage forms is now recognized and the
technology is available to meet this need in the interests of
patients and prescribers.

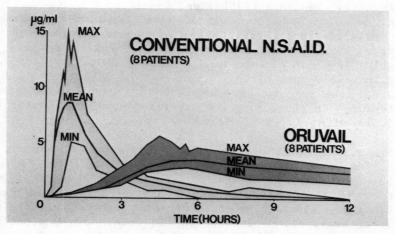

Figure 8. Intersubject variation of ketoprofen plasma concentrations after administration of two different types of
dosage forms.

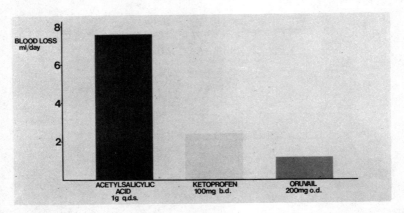

Figure 9. Fecal blood loss following administration of aspirin (1 g) four times a day, ketoprofen (100 mg) in conventional dosage form twice a day and ketoprofen (200 mg) as Oruvail® once a day.

REFERENCES

1.   R.B. Stewart and L.E. Cluff, A review of medication errors and compliance in ambulent patients, Clin. Pharmacol. Ther. 13:463–468 (1973).

2.   B. Blackwell, Patient compliance, N. Engl. J. Med. 289:249–252 (1973).

3.   A.H. Beckett, Important formulation factors influencing drug absorption, in: "Drug Absorption, Procedings of the Edinburgh International Conference," L.F. Prescott and W.S. Nimmo, eds., ADIS Press, New York (1981), pp. 133–143.

4.   A.H. Beckett, Newer methods of administration of nitrates to man to give a more predictable therapeutic response, in: "Nitrates III, Cardiovascular Effects," P.R. Lichtlen, H.-J. Engel, A. Schrey and H.J.C. Swan, eds., Springer-Verlag, Berlin (1981), pp. 61–65.

5.   O.R.W. Lewellen and R. Templeton, The pharmacokinetics of ketoprofen in man during and after repeated oral dosing (50 mg q.i.d.) with "Orudis", Scand. J. Rheumatol. Suppl. 14:53–62 (1976).

6.   P.S. Collier, P.F. D'Arcy, D.W.G. Harron and N. Morrow, Pharmacokinetic modelling of ibuprofen, Br. J. Clin. Pharmacol. 5:528–530 (1978).

7.   K.C. Kwan, G.D. Breault, E.R. Umberhauer, F.G. McMahon and D.E. Duggan, Kinetics of indomethacin absorption, elimination and enterohepatic circulation in man, J. Pharmacokinet. Biopharm. 4:255–280 (1976).

8.   J.V. Willis, M.J. Kendall, R.M. Flinn, D.P. Thornhill and P.G. Welling, The pharmacokinetics of diclofenac sodium following

intravenous and oral administration, Eur. J. Clin. Pharmacol. 16:405-410 (1979).

9. A. Khayat, Pharmacokinetic study of ketoprofen, Ph.D. Thesis, University of London (1981).

10. J.A.L. Harkness, M.B. Richter, G.S. Panayi, K. Van de Pette, A. Unger and R. Pownall, Circadian variation in disease activity in rheumatoid arthritis, Br. Med. J. 284:551-554 (1982).

Chapter 9

SPECIFICITY OF ESTERASES AND EFFECT OF STRUCTURE OF PRODRUG ESTERS OF ACYLATED ACETAMINOPHEN ON HYDROLYTIC REACTIVITY

Takeru Higuchi, Pradeep Niphadkar and Takeo Kawaguchi

Department of Pharmaceutical Chemistry
University of Kansas
Lawrence, Kansas

INTRODUCTION

The transient modification of active drug structures to enhance their efficient delivery is now a widely practiced method (1). Although initial efforts were generally applied to drug substances that had already been introduced, it has become increasingly common for drug developers to incorporate this concept at the earliest stages of development. The art and science of providing a temporary chemical cloak for the active drug species to aid in their delivery is now such a common practice that many, if not most, future drugs will be prodrugs and the term itself may eventually disappear since prodrugs are drugs.

The application of the concept will probably be pursued even more vigorously as we become more adept at its use. In particular, more contrived utilization of endogenous enzymic systems to regenerate the active species at any chosen point in the delivery pathway offers interesting opportunities for future development. Various oxidative, reductive, phosphorylative and hydrolytic enzymes can, and have, been used for this purpose. The enzymes in the last category, however, continue to receive the most attention.

In this report, the specificities of a limited variety of esterases towards acylated acetaminophen (APAP) were examined. The purpose of the study was to determine whether ester prodrugs can be designed to cleave at certain selected sites within the body or preferentially along the pathway, for example, from the gut to the brain. Various prodrug modifications of APAP and the interactions of these prodrugs with various crude esterase preparations have

already been studied by Dittert et al. (2) and Swintosky et al.
(3). Although these reports dealt primarily with the possible use
of the derivatives as a means of delivering APAP, the results provided a hint of structural specificity in the rate of enzymatic
cleavage of these esters.

An attempt was made in the present study to determine specifically the comparative selectivity of crude gut, gut wall, liver,
blood and brain preparations obtained from the rat, and other partially purified esterases as hydrolytic catalysts toward model neutral, cationic and anionic esters of acetaminophen. The data
obtained may help in the selection of acyl functions which would
release other model drugs at a selected point in a sequence such as
that shown in Figure 1. The methods employed were admittedly crude
in that no serious efforts were made to separate soluble and cell-
bound enzymes when tissue homogenates were used. Nevertheless, the
results are presented since they offer interesting insights into
the extent of structural specificity existent in these reactions.

METHODS

Materials

All the esters were synthesized directly from acetaminophen,
following published methods (2,3), and characterized by elemental
analysis, NMR, and so forth. The individual substrates were subjected to HPLC analysis to establish their essential purity.

Rat plasma was obtained from EDTA-treated fresh blood of male
Sprague-Dawley rats. The blood was centrifuged at 1000 x g for 15-
20 minutes and the resulting plasma stored at 0-5°C for no more
than 30 hours before use.

Rat liver, brain and intestinal homogenates were prepared in
0.05 M .phosphate buffer, pH 7.00. One gram of fresh tissue was
homogenized with 10 ml of the phosphate buffer for 10-30 minutes, with a glass homogenizer and a Teflon pestle having radial

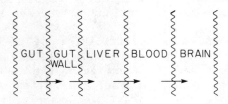

Figure 1. Schematic of esterase gauntlet barrier for a prodrug
ester acting eventually in the brain.

serrations. During the preparation and storage of the tissue homogenates, the temperature was maintained at 0–5°C to prevent inactivation. Again, these preparations were kept no longer than 30 hours.

Rate Studies

The hydrolytic rates of the enzyme substrates were determined in the presence of the various enzymic preparations, diluted appropriately with 0.05 M phosphate buffer, pH 7.00 (in some cases 6.00). The increase in concentration of released APAP was followed by periodic sampling of the reaction mixture and HPLC analysis. Samples were injected directly onto a C–18 µBondapak column fitted with a guard precolumn. The half-lives were estimated from the resulting first-order relationship.

Systems Studied

The substrates studied are shown in Table I. The acetaminophen esters' structures are shown along with their nonenzymatic hydrolytic rates. The slow chemical hydrolytic rates shown for the neutral esters (E–1 to E–4) reflect considerable uncertainty in that they were determined by following the initial rates of formation of free APAP. The overall kinetics of formation over a longer period of time exhibited strong autocatalytic effects resulting from what appears to be a free radical mechanism. Since elucidation of the mechanism of the chemical reaction was not the major purpose of the study, this aspect of the chemistry of the system is not treated here. It is sufficient to note that the neutral esters are relatively stable with half-lives of well over 100 hours at pH 7.0. The branched species showed even greater stability, as expected. The cationic ester (E–5) showed a predictable greater sensitivity. The dicarboxylic acid monoesters (last structure shown in Table I) were quite labile toward chemical hydrolysis because of significant intramolecular participation; the glutarate (n = 1) half-life was less than 10 hours (the succinate half-life was less than 3 minutes, data not shown). Dittert et al. (2) have reported a longer half-life (approximately 660 minutes) for the nonenzymatic cleavage of the glutarate in 0.10 M phosphate buffer, pH 7.4 at 37°C. The 3 minute half-life observed in the present study was obtained at 25°C and in 0.05 M phosphate buffer, pH 7.0. The latter value appears to be more consistent with results reported by Bruice and Pandit (4) for related systems.

The various esterase preparations used in these studies are listed in Table II. The homogenates were prepared fresh for each series of runs, and measurements were carried out more or less simultaneously with various ester substrates, using APAP propionate as the control. The reaction rates were adjusted to convenient ranges by varying the homogenate concentration in the reaction

Table I. Structures and chemical hydrolytic half-lives of APAP esters studied.

Compound	Structure	Half-life (hr) (pH=7.0, T=25°C)
E-1	$-O-C-CH_2-CH_3$ $\parallel$ O	> 248
E-2	$-O-C-(CH_2)_4-CH_3$ $\parallel$ O	> 462
E-3	CH_3 $\vert$ $-O-C-C-CH_3$ $\parallel$ $\vert$ O CH_3	> 1386
E-4	CH_3 $\vert$ $-O-CH_2-O-C-C-CH_3$ $\parallel$ $\vert$ O CH_3	> 3465
E-5	$CH_2-CH_2-CH_3$ $\vert$ $-O-C-CH_2-CH_2-N \cdot HCl$ $\parallel$ $\vert$ O $CH_2-CH_2-CH_3$	0.65
	$-O-C-CH_2-(CH_2)_n-CH_2-C-O^-\ H^+$ $\parallel$ $\parallel$ O O	> 8.33[a]

[a] $n = 1,2,3$.

Table II. Esterase systems studied.

Rat liver homogenate
Rat intestinal homogenate
Rat brain homogenate
Rat plasma
Partly purified porcine liver esterase[a]
Partly purified horse serum butyryl cholinesterase[b]

---

[a]Sigma E-9627.
[b]Sigma C-7512.

mixture, since the catalytic activities varied enormously with the chemical nature of the esters. Measurements were made at several catalyst concentrations, and plots, such as shown in Figure 2 and Figure 3, were obtained for each system. The values reported later, in Tables III-V, are the ratios of the slopes of these relative to the propionate slope (E-1). For these studies the substrate concentrations were kept below 4 x 10^{-5} moles/liter.

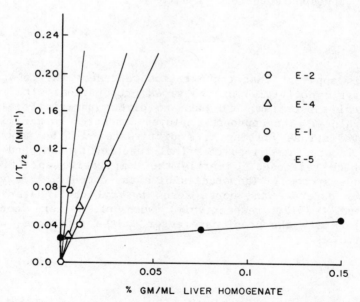

Figure 2. Plot of reciprocal of observed half-lives of several APAP esters and concentration of rat liver homogenate in 0.05 M phosphate buffer, pH 7.00 at 25°C (APAP esters defined in Table I).

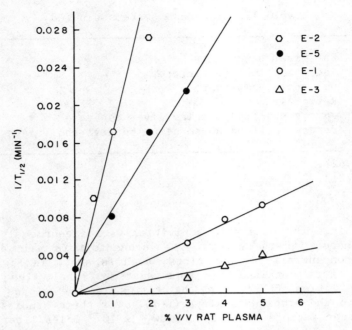

Figure 3. Plot of reciprocal of observed half-lives of several APAP esters and concentration of rat plasma in 0.05 M phosphate buffer, pH 7.00 at 25°C.

It is apparent that these ratios represent the relative over-all catalytic activities of the gross preparations with respect to the several substrates, and have no direct numerical relationship to K_{cat} values. The approach employed attempted to minimize experimental variations arising from differences in the amount of the esterase incorporated into the final reaction system, and to obtain values which reflected primarily the comparative specificities of these crude systems. The studies with the commercial enzymes (porcine liver esterase and horse serum butyryl cholinesterase, Sigma E-9627 and C-7512, respectively) were of a more conventional nature, but with the propionate ester as the reference, were still comparative.

RESULTS

Response to Commercial Enzymes

The relative catalytic behavior of the partly purified liver and serum esterases towards the cationic and neutral esters is shown in Table III. Both enzyme preparations were quite active toward the esters, with the exception of the two pivalates (E-3 and E-4) in the presence of the serum esterase. It may be that for both enzyme preparations the deacylation of the receptor enzyme in the presence of the pivalates may be the rate-determining process, in that the catalytic rates for both E-3 and E-4 are essentially the same in both enzyme systems. If this is the case, it would appear that the rate of deacylation of the cholinesterase is substantially slower than that of the liver esterase. On the other hand, the apparently similar response of both systems to the pivalate esters may be fortuitous. The increased sensitivity of the caproate ester (E-2) over that of the propionate is probably attributable to its greater hydrophobicity.

The aminoester (E-5) showed a significantly lower rate with these enzyme preparations than the propionate ester. The catalytic activities of both esterase preparations toward this substrate were so low compared to the rapid chemical loss experienced by the ester that the relative catalytic constants could not be accurately determined.

Response to Rat Tissue Homogenates and Plasma

The observed relative catalytic activities of the tissue homogenates and plasma with the amino and the neutral esters of APAP are shown in Tables IV and V. The liver and intestinal preparations exhibited some significant differences, the latter being more active toward the hydrophobic caproate ester (E-2) and less active toward the two pivalates (E-3 and E-4). The liver homogenate also seemed to be significantly more active than the intestinal preparation toward the cationic ester, but both were less effective with these substrates than with the neutral esters.

As can be seen in Table IV, the esterase specificity of rat plasma was markedly different from that seen with the two homogenates. The specificity of rat plasma toward the dipropyl aminoester is approximately 1000 times that of the intestinal, and 100 times that of the liver preparation relative to the propionate ester. Whether this situation exists for human plasma as well has not been tested, but the observation certainly merits further exploration. With the plasma, as with the two homogenates, the response with the two pivalate esters was remarkably similar.

The catalytic activity of the brain homogenate toward the several esters is shown in Table V. The observed esterase activity of the preparation was relatively low with measurable activity seen only for the two fatty acid derivatives.

Table III. Relative hydrolytic catalytic rates with partially purified commercial enzymes.

Compound	Structure	Catalytic Rate Ratio[a]	
		Porcine Liver Esterase	Horse Serum Butyryl Cholinesterase
E-1	$-O-C-CH_2-CH_3$ with $\parallel$ O	1.00, 1.00[b]	1.00, 1.00[c]
E-2	$-O-C-(CH_2)_4-CH_3$ with $\parallel$ O	5.60, 3.70	2.50, 3.40
E-3	$-O-C-\overset{CH_3}{\underset{CH_3}{C}}-CH_3$ with $\parallel$ O	1.70, 1.30	0.02, 0.016
E-4	$-O-CH_2-O-C-\overset{CH_3}{\underset{CH_3}{C}}-CH_3$ with $\parallel$ O	1.10, 1.80	0.014, 0.017
E-5	$-O-C-CH_2-CH_2-\overset{CH_2-CH_2-CH_3}{\underset{CH_2-CH_2-CH_3}{N}}$ · HCl with $\parallel$ O	0.04, 0.07	0.19, 0.14

[a]Duplicate determinations; rate relative to propionate (E-1).

[b]$t_{1/2}$ range: 36-19 minutes.

[c]$t_{1/2}$ range: 18-8 minutes.

Table IV. Relative rates of hydrolysis of several APAP esters catalyzed by rat tissue preparations.

Compound[b]	Relative Rates[a] (pH 7.00, 25°C)		
	Intestinal Homogenate	Liver Homogenate	Plasma
E-1	1.00[c]	1.00[d]	1.00[e]
E-2	6.0 ± 0.9	2.7 ± 0.7	8.9 ± 0.8
E-3	0.49 ± 0.07	1.3 ± 0.5	0.37 ± 0.04
E-4	0.48 ± 0.08	1.1 ± 0.25	0.42 ± 0.03
E-5	0.0038 ± 0.0005	0.023 ± 0.006	3.3 ± 0.6

[a]Data are expressed as the average ± SEM relative to propionate (E-1); n = 4 for liver and intestinal preparations; n = 5 for plasma. The propionate rate is arbitrarily taken as 1.00.
[b]See Table III for structures.
[c]$t_{1/2}$ range: 20-7.5 minutes.
[d]$t_{1/2}$ range: 40-25 minutes.
[e]$t_{1/2}$ range: 24-9 minutes.

Table V. Relative rates of hydrolysis of several APAP esters catalyzed by rat brain homogenate.

Compound[a]	Catalytic Rate Ratio[b]
E–1	1.00^c
E–2	10.1, 12.3, 7.2
E–3	<0.05, <0.05, <0.05
E–4	<0.05, <0.05, <0.05
E–5	0.002, 0, 0

[a]See Table III for structures.
[b]Triplicate determinations; rate relative to propionate (E-1).
[c]$t_{1/2}$ range: 120–92.5 minutes.

Dicarboxylate Monoesters and Porcine Liver Esterase

The apparent K_m and K_{cat}/K_m values for the acid esters studied, and for the propionate ester with the porcine liver esterase preparation are shown in Table VI. These were calculated from Lineweaver-Burk plots in the usual manner. Comparable measurements with the homogenates were not attempted because it was not possible to obtain meaningful plots with these systems. The reversal in the pH dependence of the catalytic activity (K_{cat}/K_m) for the carboxylic esters compared to that of the neutral propionate strongly suggests that it is the unionized form of the dicarboxylic acid monoester which is acted on by the enzyme. Thus, the anionic esters seem to be substantially more resistant toward esterase activity than the neutral species. Although explicit data are not available at this time, preliminary examinations with other esterase preparations lead to a similar conclusion.

Although the K_m values could only be estimated for the longer members of the series, the results suggest that these are more poorly bound than the glutarate, which in turn binds better than the propionate. The degree of binding for the charged esters may not be greatly different from that of their neutral counterparts. The apparent binding tendency of these esters seems to run contrary to their catalytic activities.

Table VI. Binding and catalytic constants for dicarboxylic monoesters of APAP with porcine liver esterase.

APAP Ester	pH 6.00		pH 7.00	
	K_m (mM)	$[K_{cat}/K_m] \times 10^{-2}$ (min^{-1}U^{-1})	K_m (mM)	$[K_{cat}/K_m] \times 10^{-2}$ (min^{-1}U^{-1})
$-O-\overset{O}{\overset{\|}{C}}-CH_2CH_3$ propionate	0.97	35	2.27	105
$-O-\overset{O}{\overset{\|}{C}}-(CH_2)_3COOH$ glutarate	0.18	1.6	0.24	0.82
$-O-\overset{O}{\overset{\|}{C}}-(CH_2)_4COOH$ adipate	1.1	5.3	10	3.6, 4.0
$-O-\overset{O}{\overset{\|}{C}}-(CH_2)_5COOH$ pimelate	7[a]	15	10; 40[a]	6.1

[a]K_m for the pimelate system could not be determined with any great
precision due to the limited solubility of the ester acid and its
weak binding tendency.

Comparative Catalytic Response

In Figures 4-8, the catalytic rates of the various esters are compared graphically. From these charts and earlier observations, the following generalizations appear to be valid:

1.   The neutral esters were substantially more easily cleaved enzymatically.

2.   The more hydrophobic neutral esters were more suscepti- ble. The sterically hindered (pivalate) esters were, surprisingly, quite rapidly hydrolyzed in the two liver preparations, but not in the others.

3.   Both cationic and anionic esters were very much more slowly attacked in most instances. The shift from the diethyl to the dipropyl amino group produced a very

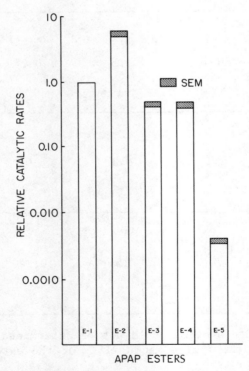

Figure 4. Semilogarithmic plot of mean relative catalyzed hydro- lytic rates (± SEM) of APAP esters in the presence of intestinal homogenate, pH 7.00 at 25°C. The rate of APAP propionate is arbitrarily taken as 1.0.

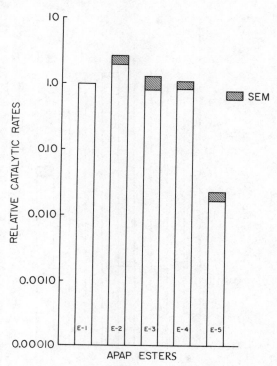

Figure 5. Semilogarithmic plot of mean relative catalyzed hydrolytic rates (± SEM) of APAP esters in the presence of
rat liver homogenate, pH 7.00 at 25°C. The rate for
APAP propionate is arbitrarily taken as 1.0.

significant increase in the cleavage rate in most of the
systems studied.

4.   Rat plasma esterase was relatively highly effective in
cleaving the aminoester, in contrast to other esterase
sources, but the same effect was not seen with the commercial cholinesterase preparation.

5.   Esterase activity in the rat brain homogenate was low
compared to other tissues.

6.   With partly purified porcine liver esterase (which displayed behavior very similar to the crude rat liver
homogenate), the free carboxyl containing glutarate,
adipate and pimelate monoester forms, rather than their
anionic species, seem to undergo hydrolytic reactions.

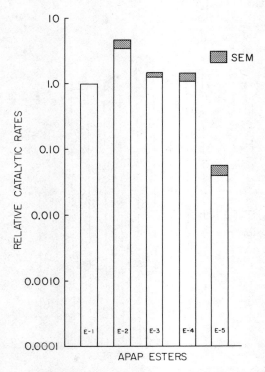

Figure 6. Semilogarithmic plot of mean relative catalyzed hydrolytic rates (± SEM) of APAP esters in the presence of
partly purified porcine liver esterase, pH 7.00 at
25°C. The rate of APAP propionate is arbitrarily taken
as 1.0.

DISCUSSION

The observations listed above can only be considered valid for
APAP esters at this point. They do, however, strongly suggest that
considerable specificity can be built into such prodrugs. Minor
changes in the chemical structure appear to lead to significant alterations in the observed enzyme catalyzed rates. It is of some
interest to note the similarity in behavior of the two liver preparations. Further detailed studies with other systems are indicated, however, to determine the generality of these observations.

The present investigation has, in a preliminary way, attempted
to determine the extent of specificity and nonspecificity existent
in the gauntlet of esterases present, from the gut to the brain, in
one animal species. No serious attempts were made to separate and
purify the enzymes since it was assumed that the mixed systems were
at least partially representative of the tissue domain from which

they were obtained. Furthermore, it must be recognized that under in vivo conditions the relative specificities are probably significantly affected by differences in the transport properties of the substrate esters. Studies of this nature are needed, however, if we are ever to gain the ability to design prodrugs based on endogenous biochemical systems to overcome barriers to effective drug delivery.

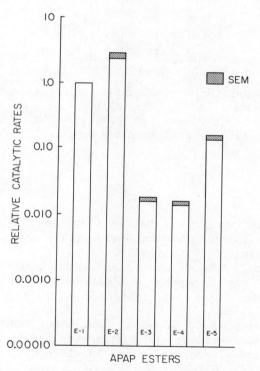

Figure 7. Semilogarithmic plot of mean relative catalyzed hydrolytic rates (± SEM) of APAP esters in the presence of partly purified horse serum butyryl cholinesterase, pH 7.00 at 25°C. The rate for APAP propionate is arbitrarily taken as 1.0.

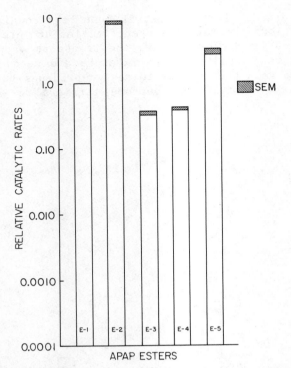

Figure 8. Semilogarithmic plot of mean relative catalyzed hydrolytic rates (± SEM) of APAP esters in the presence of
diluted rat plasma, pH 7.00 at 25°C. The rate for APAP
propionate is arbitrarily taken as 1.0.

REFERENCES

1. "Prodrugs as Novel Drug Delivery Systems," T. Higuchi and V.
    Stella, eds., ACS Symposium Series (14), American Chemical So-
    ciety, Washington, D.C. (1975).
2. L.W. Dittert, H.C. Caldwell, H.J. Adams, G.M. Irwin and J.V.
    Swintosky, Acetaminophen prodrugs I: Synthesis, physico-
    chemical properties and analgesic activity, J. Pharm. Sci.
    57:774-780 (1968).
3. J.V. Swintosky, H.C. Caldwell, C.W. Chong, G.M. Irwin and L.W.
    Dittert, 4-Acetamidophenyl 2,2,2-trichloroethyl carbonate syn-
    thesis, physical properties and in vitro hydrolysis, J. Pharm.
    Sci. 57:752-756 (1968).
4. T.C. Bruice and U.K. Pandit, The effect of geminal substitu-
    tion ring size and rotamer distribution on the intramolecular
    nucleophilic catalysis of the hydrolysis of monophenyl esters
    of dibasic acids and the solvolysis of the intermediate anhy-
    drides, J. Am. Chem. Soc. 82:5858-5865 (1960).

Chapter 10

TRANSDERMAL ABSORPTION: A UNIQUE OPPORTUNITY FOR DRUG DELIVERY

D.L. Azarnoff, A. Karim, H. Lambert, J. Boylan and
G. Schoenhardt

Research and Development Division
G.D. Searle and Co.
Chicago, Illinois

The amount of drug absorbed from the gastrointestinal (GI) tract into the systemic circulation with conventional tablet and capsule dosage forms is dependent on the quantity and type of food in the stomach, GI motility and GI microbial flora. Furthermore, for drugs with a high hepatic extraction ratio, the drug may be largely deactivated by first-pass metabolism before reaching the systemic circulation. Drug absorption from the GI tract can, therefore, result in variable and/or unpredictable plasma concentrations. Some of this variability can be minimized by administering controlled release tablet and capsule formulations. However, these dosage forms cannot eliminate the inherent variability associated with first-pass metabolism.

An important recent advance in biopharmaceutics has been the utilization of controlled delivery of drugs through the intact skin to the systemic circulation. During transdermal absorption the drug traverses the layers of the skin, then enters capillaries which lead to the general circulation (Fig. 1). Since drug transport through human skin is primarily passive diffusion, and since the GI variables mentioned previously are absent, one can expect more constant drug concentrations in the plasma. Transdermal drug delivery approaches zero-order drug input, which is equivalent to administering a constant intravenous infusion. Controlled transdermal drug administration:

1.   Avoids the risk and inconvenience of intravenous therapy.

2. Avoids the variable absorption and metabolism sometimes associated with oral therapy.

3. Permits use of pharmacologically active agents with short biological half-lives.

4. Permits lower daily dosage of drug because of reduced liver metabolism and continuous drug input.

5. Diminishes chance of over or underdosing because of the prolonged, preprogrammed delivery of drug as required by therapeutic need.

6. Provides for a simplified medication regimen.

7. Allows rapid termination of drug input by removal of the system from the surface of the skin.

The transdermal route, however, is not suitable for drugs that irritate or sensitize the skin, and is restricted by the surface area of the delivery system to potent drugs that need to be administered on a chronic basis.

KINETICS OF TRANSDERMAL ABSORPTION BY PASSIVE DIFFUSION

The amount of drug absorbed by passive diffusion per cm^2 per hour (flux) can be described by Fick's law (1), which is given in Equation (1):

$$J = k_p \cdot \Delta C = \frac{D \cdot k}{e} \Delta C \qquad (1)$$

where:

J   represents the flux or quantity of drug absorbed per unit of area and unit of time.

k_p is the permeability constant $\left(= \frac{D \cdot k}{e} \right)$.

ΔC is the difference between the concentration above (C_1) and below (C_2) the membrane. (C_2 is generally negligible compared to C_1.) Since J is directly proportional to ΔC, the amount of drug absorbed transdermally will depend on the concentration of the dissolved drug in the vehicle, as well as on the surface area of the application site, provided that the skin has no capacity to sequester drug.

D   is the diffusion constant of the drug in the rate-limiting barrier. D is inversely proportional to both the size of the molecules and the viscosity of the barrier medium (6).

k   is the stratum corneum/vehicle partition coefficient of the drug. Because of the lipid material present, the stratum corneum has lipophilic characteristics and, therefore, k will be high for lipophilic drugs.

e   represents the thickness of the stratum corneum.

FACTORS AFFECTING TRANSDERMAL ABSORPTION

A major problem with the use of the skin as a portal of entry for drugs is that this organ ordinarily serves as a relatively impermeable barrier that protects the body. For a large number of drugs, the stratum corneum (outermost 10-15 mµ layer of the skin) is the main barrier to drug transport by passive diffusion (Fig. 1). Stripping away the stratum corneum usually results in a considerable increase in the permeability of the skin (2-5).

When the surface of the skin is occluded, transdermal water loss is inhibited and the stratum corneum becomes hydrated. When fully hydrated, the permeability of the stratum corneum increases severalfold (6). Solutes and solvents other than water can also interact with skin and substantially modify its permeability. One well-known agent having this effect is dimethylsulfoxide which can enhance drug transport through the skin by at least one order of magnitude (7,8).

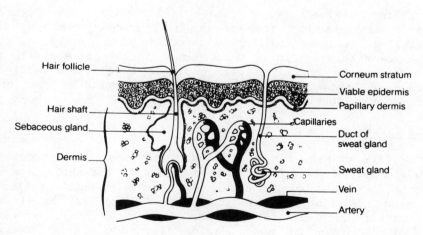

Figure 1. The structure of skin.

Penetration of drugs through the skin may increase with the number of hair follicles present in the skin and the extent of blood flow under the skin (Fig. 1). Permeability of skin may therefore differ widely for different sites on the body in the same subjects and for the same site in different subjects (9-11).

Drug permeability through the skin is also known to be influenced by temperature, age, sex and racial factors (6). The irritant action of anionic and cationic surfactants, as well as pathological conditions such as eczema and psoriasis, can also result in altered skin permeability (6).

Superficial and Deep Retention of Drugs Applied to the Skin

The existence of a depot in the skin for some topically applied agents such as corticosteroids, griseofulvin and estradiol has been demonstrated (12). This phenomenon, called the "reservoir effect," is a property of the cornified cells. Some of the molecules stored are slowly absorbed over a period of several days; some are removed by repeated washing and skin desquamation. The reservoir effect can result in very prolonged pharmacological effects of some potent topically applied drugs.

CONTROLLED RELEASE TRANSDERMAL SYSTEMS

The controlled release transdermal systems currently available fall into two main categories; those in which the drug is stored in a membrane sealed reservoir, and those in which the drug is stored in a matrix.

Reservoir System

In the reservoir system, the drug is stored in a single compartment or reservoir from which it migrates through a rate-controlling membrane to the absorption site. The principal advantage of this system is the constant release rate of the drug. The disadvantage is that a tear or break in the rate-controlling membrane can result in "dose dumping" or a rapid release of the entire drug content.

Matrix System

In this system, the drug is uniformly dispersed throughout a polymeric matrix through which it diffuses to the absorption site. Depending on the physico-chemical parameters which define the system and the drug, release from such matrices may be via zero-order or more complex kinetics. The advantage of matrix systems is the lack of danger of dose dumping since the polymer cannot be ruptured.

Microsealed Drug Delivery System

The "Microsealed Drug Delivery" (MDD) system (Fig. 2), developed by Searle, combines the principles of the reservoir and matrix systems. In the MDD system, the drug is dispersed throughout a polymer in microcompartments which serve as tiny reservoirs. The system allows for zero-order release of drug without the danger of dose dumping. The amount of drug released can be controlled by altering the solubility of the drug in the liquid compartment, the physico-chemical properties of the system, or the size and/or structure of the silicone polymer.

TRANSDERMAL DELIVERY OF NITROGLYCERIN

Nitroglycerin (NG) is an ideal candidate for transdermal drug delivery. It is a potent, lipophilic, neutral compound with a low molecular weight. It undergoes extensive first-pass metabolism following oral administration (13). NG has a short elimination half-life of 2.8 minutes, a high apparent distribution volume of 3.3 liters/kg, and a high plasma clearance of 0.72 liters/min/kg (14). A topical dosage form of NG is already available as a 2% ointment (15,16). The ointment is messy to use and the applied dose, based on the concentration and the surface area, is subject to significant variability (17).

During the course of evaluating the transdermal absorption of NG, we have encountered several practical problems and unusual pharmacokinetics of the topically applied NG. For example:

1. The reference standard of NG is not available as a pure crystalline chemical but only as a 10% NG lactose adsorbate. The standard curve was prepared with pure NG that was collected by sublimation and weighed.

2. NG is rapidly adsorbed to (18) and hydrolyzed by (19) red blood cells. Therefore, immediate inhibition of the hydrolases, centrifugation and extraction of plasma samples following blood collection is necessary.

3. The therapeutic plasma concentrations of NG are very low (< 1 ng/ml), so a highly accurate and sensitive assay method capable of detecting 0.05 ng/ml is required.

4. NG has numerous side effects including headache, postural hypotension, flushing, tachycardia and dizziness. The dose of NG used in a human bioavailability study therefore cannot be too high or the subject dropout rate may be excessive.

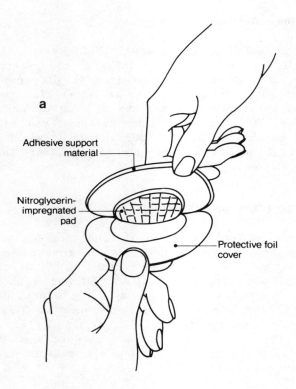

a

Adhesive support material

Nitroglycerin-impregnated pad

Protective foil cover

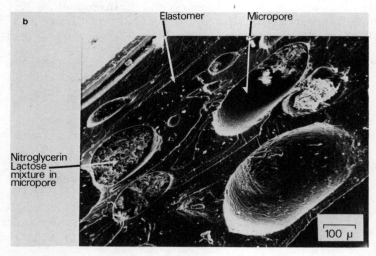

b

Elastomer   Micropore

Nitroglycerin Lactose mixture in micropore

100 μ

Figure 2. Microsealed drug delivery system for nitroglycerin (MDD-NG); a = MDD-NG system, b = electron micrograph of MDD-NG system illustrating the presence of microcompartments which serve as tiny reservoirs for nitroglycerin.

In the studies described below, plasma concentrations of NG were determined by a quantitative gas-liquid chromatographic method using isosorbide dinitrate as the internal standard and electron capture detection.

Surface Area and Concentration

The relationship between the transdermal absorption of NG and the surface area of the application site was evaluated in healthy subjects with the study design outlined in Figure 3. Four to 16 cm^2 (2 mg NG/cm^2) experimental microsealed drug delivery-nitroglycerin (MDD-NG) pads or 0.5 to 1.0 inch Nitro-Bid® ointment (8-16 mg NG) spread over 53 cm^2 were applied on the volar surface of the left wrist and plasma concentrations of NG were determined in the ipsilateral and contralateral antecubital veins for 24 hours. The ipsilateral plasma concentrations were expected to be higher, and thus easier to measure, than the contralateral concentrations as a result of being closer to the site of absorption. The contralateral plasma concentrations, representing the systemic concentrations, were expected to be lower due to the extensive distribution and metabolism of NG. Application of neither the MDD-NG (16 cm^2) nor a therapeutic dose (20) of Nitro-Bid® ointment (one inch) produced systemic plasma concentrations of NG that were above the limit of detection, even though the ipsilateral concentrations were as high as 12 ng/ml (Fig. 4).

The ipsilateral plasma concentrations of NG increased as the surface area of the applied MDD-NG was increased from 4 to 16 cm^2. An approximately linear relationship was found between the

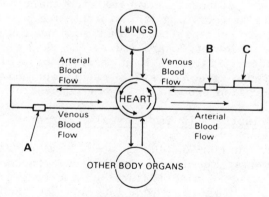

Figure 3. Procedure for evaluating transdermal absorption of nitroglycerin in man. MDD-NG is applied on the volar surface of the wrist (C) and NG plasma concentrations are determined in the ipsilateral (B) and the contralateral (A) forearm antecubital veins.

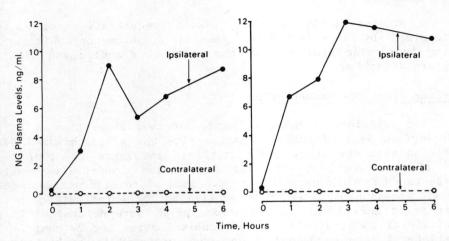

Time, Hours

Figure 4. Relationship between plasma concentrations of NG in the antecubital veins of the ipsilateral and contralateral forearms. Each value is a mean of five healthy male subjects. MDD-NG (32 mg NG over 16 cm^2; left panel) or 2% ointment (one inch, 16 mg NG over 53 cm^2; right panel) were applied on the volar surface of the left wrist in a cross-over study. The sensitivity of the assay for NG was 0.1 ng/ml.

area under the plasma concentration-time curve (AUC) and the surface area of the applied MDD-NG (Fig. 5).

The ipsilateral plasma concentrations of NG following application of the ointment increased with the concentration of NG applied. While maintaining the surface area of 53 cm^2, the ipsilateral plasma concentrations increased approximately 1.5-fold when the concentration of NG applied to the skin was increased from 0.15 to 0.30 mg/cm^2 (Fig. 6). This observation applies only to the concentration range studied since saturation may occur in the transdermal absorption process at higher concentrations.

Intersubject Variability in Transdermal Absorption

Application of MDD-NG (16 mg over 8 cm^2) pads to the volar surface of the wrist resulted in continuous transdermal absorption of NG and a constant mean ipsilateral plasma concentration of about 4 ng/ml for up to 32 hours. High intersubject, but less intrasubject, variability in the rate of transdermal absorption was found (Fig. 7). This variability may be due to individual differences in skin characteristics or NG clearance.

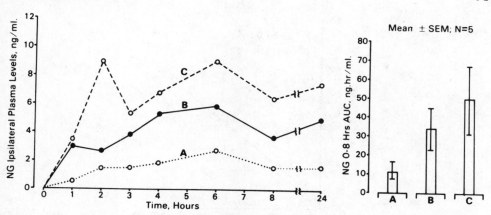

Figure 5. Relationship between the surface area of the application site and the ipsilateral plasma concentrations of nitroglycerin. Each value is a mean of five healthy male subjects and vertical bars represent the standard error of the mean. MDD-NG systems were applied on the volar surface of the left wrist in a cross-over study. A = 8 mg NG over 4 cm^2 (2 mg/cm^2), B = 16 mg NG over 8 cm^2 (2 mg/cm^2), C = 32 mg NG over 16 cm^2 (2 mg/cm^2).

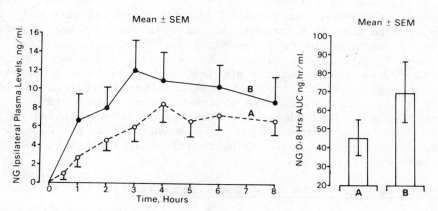

Figure 6. Relationship between the applied NG concentration and the ipsilateral plasma concentrations of nitroglycerin. Nitro-bid® ointment (2%) was applied on the volar surface of the left wrist. A = 1/2 inch, 8 mg NG over 53 cm^2 (0.15 mg/cm^2), n = 23; B = 1 inch, 16 mg NG over 53 cm^2 (0.30 mg/cm^2), n = 6.

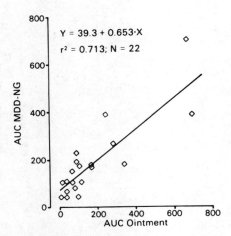

Y = 39.3 + 0.653·X
r² = 0.713; N = 22

Figure 7. Relationship between 0–48 hours ipsilateral areas under the plasma concentration-time curves (AUC, ng·hr/ml) following application of MDD–NG (16 mg over 8 cm²) or 2% ointment (8 mg over 53 cm²) on the volar surface of the left wrist of 22 healthy male subjects in a randomized, cross-over study.

Systemic Plasma Concentrations

The systemic plasma concentrations of NG (contralateral antecubital veins) were below the detection limit of the assay following application of either MDD–NG or ointment to the left wrist. Therefore, the study was repeated in additional subjects with the NG applied to the chest (precordial region). Each subject received MDD–NG (32 mg over 16 cm²) and Nitro-Bid® ointment (one inch (16 mg) over 53 cm²) in a randomized, balanced, cross-over manner. Mean NG plasma concentrations of about 0.3 ng/ml were attained in the left and the right antecubital veins after application of MDD–NG (32 mg over 16 cm²) and the ointment (16 mg over 53 cm²) to the chest (Fig. 8). These doses were the same as those applied to the wrist. The mean systemic plasma concentrations of 0.3 ng/ml remained constant for up to 32 hours following application of MDD–NG to the chest (Fig. 9).

Site-Related Differences in Systemic Availability

The above findings suggest a site-related difference in the systemic availability of the transdermally applied NG. In addition, a first-pass blood vessel uptake of NG has been demonstrated recently (21,22) in rats when the drug is injected directly into the blood perfusing the vessels. Furthermore, the uptake of NG in the aorta was less extensive than the uptake in the inferior vena

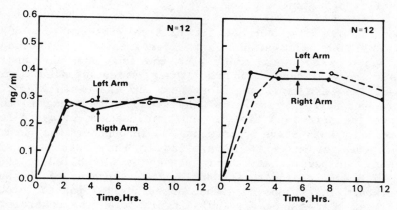

Figure 8. Plasma concentrations of nitroglycerin in the left and right forearm antecubital veins following application of MDD-NG (32 mg over 16 cm^2; left panel) or 2% ointment (one inch, 16 mg over 53 cm^2; right panel). Each point is the mean of 12 subjects; the two preparations were applied on the precordial region of the chest in a randomized, balanced, cross-over study.

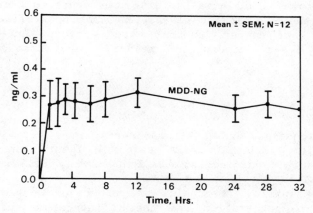

Figure 9. Mean systemic plasma concentration-time curve of nitroglycerin in 12 healthy male subjects following application of MDD-NG (32 mg over 16 cm^2) on the precordial region of the chest.

cava.   Differences in blood vessel uptake and/or metabolism of
topically applied NG may account for the site-related systemic
availability differences we observed for NG.

Our results also support the clinical observations of Hansen
et al. (23) who noted significant differences in the responses of
normal subjects to NG ointment when the same dose was applied to
different body sites.   Of the three sites studied (the mid-
forehead, the left lower anterior chest and the medial left ankle),
the forehead uniformly produced the greatest response in terms of
incidence, severity and time to onset of changes in systolic blood
pressure and subjective complaints.   Throughout the dose range
studied, the responses to NG applied to the chest were slightly
less than, but paralleled, the responses to NG applied to the forehead. With application to the ankle, the responses of the subjects
were markedly less pronounced than after application to forehead or
chest sites, and were nearly indistinguishable from controls.

FUTURE APPLICATION OF TRANSDERMAL DRUG DELIVERY

The transdermal delivery of other drugs could provide useful
therapy in many disease states. A major constraint in the application of the transdermal system is the need for drugs that are
therapeutically potent in doses on the order of a few milligrams a
day. Fortunately, a wide range of important potent drugs, suitable
for transdermal delivery, already exists in several significant
areas of therapeutics. In the cardiovascular area, the transdermal
system may prove valuable in administering drugs to treat hypertension or peripheral vascular disease.   Other possibilities include
the treatment of cancer, central nervous system and respiratory
malfunctions,   and   conditions   related   to   steroidal   hormone
deficiency.

REFERENCES

1.   A.S. Michaels, S.K. Chandrasekaran and J.E. Shaw,   Drug
      permeation through human skin.   Theory and in vitro
      experimental measurement, Am. Inst. Chem. Eng. J.   21:985-996
      (1975).
2.   R.J. Scheuplein, Mechanism of percutaneous absorption.   I.
      Routes of penetration and the influence of solubility, J.
      Invest. Dermatol. 45:334-346 (1965).
3.   R.J. Scheuplein, Mechanism of percutaneous absorption.   II.
      Transient diffusion and the relative importance of various
      routes of skin penetration, J. Invest. Dermatol. 48:79-88
      (1967).
4.   R.J. Scheuplein and I.H. Blank, Permeability of the skin,
      Physiol. Rev. 51:702-747 (1971).

5. R.J. Scheuplein and I.H. Blank, Mechanism of percutaneous absorption. IV. Penetration of nonelectrolytes (alcohols) from aqueous solutions and from pure liquids, J. Invest. Dermatol. 60:286–296 (1973).

6. J.E. Wahlberg, Percutaneous absorption, Curr. Probl. Dermatol. 5:1–36 (1973).

7. H. Baker, The effects of dimethylsulfoxide, dimethylformamide and dimethylacetamide on the cutaneous barrier to water in human skin, J. Invest Dermatol. 50:283–288 (1968).

8. S.K. Chandrasekaran, P.S. Campbell and A.S. Michaels, Effect of dimethylsulfoxide on drug permeation through human skin, Am. Inst. Chem. Eng. J. 23:810–816 (1977).

9. R.J. Feldmann and H.I. Maibach, Regional variation in percutaneous penetration of cortisol-^{14}C in man, J. Invest. Dermatol. 48:181–183 (1967).

10. H.I. Maibach, R.J. Feldmann, T.H. Milby and W.F. Serat, Regional variation in percutaneous penetration in man. Pesticides, Arch. Environ. Health 23:208–211 (1971).

11. J.E. Shaw and S.K. Chandrasekaran, Controlled topical delivery of drugs for systemic action, in: "Drug Metabolism Reviews" (Vol. 8), F. DiCarlo, ed., Marcel Dekker, New York (1978), pp. 223–233.

12. C.F.H. Vickers, Stratum corneum reservoir for drugs, in: "Pharmacology and the Skin," W. Montagna, R.B. Stoughton and E.J. Van Scott, eds., Appleton Century Crofts, New York (1972), pp. 177–189.

13. P.W. Armstrong, J.A. Armstrong and G.S. Marks, Blood levels after sublingual nitroglycerin, Circulation 59:585–588 (1979).

14. E.F. McNiff, A. Yacobi, F.M. Young-Chang, L.H. Golden, A. Goldfarb and H.-L. Fung, Nitroglycerin pharmacokinetics after intravenous infusion in normal subjects, J. Pharm. Sci. 70:1054–1058 (1981).

15. J.A. Franciosa, R.C. Blank, J.N. Cohn and E. Mikulic, Hemodynamic effects of topical, oral and sublingual nitroglycerin in left ventricular failure, Curr. Ther. Res. 22:231–245 (1977).

16. P.W. Armstrong, J.A. Armstrong, G.S. Marks, J. McKinven and S. Slaughter, Pharmacokinetic-hemodynamic studies of nitroglycerin ointment in congestive heart-failure, Am. J. Cardiol. 46:670–676 (1980).

17. S. Sved, W.M. McLean and I.J. McGilveray, Influence of the method of application on pharmacokinetics of nitroglycerin from ointment in humans, J. Pharm. Sci. 70:1368–1369 (1981).

18. C. Wu, T. Sokoloski, M.F. Blanford and A.M. Burkman, Absence of metabolite in the disappearance of nitroglycerin following incubation with red blood cells, Int. J. Pharm. 8:323–329 (1981).

19. J.A. Armstrong, S.E. Slaughter, G.S. Marks and P.W. Armstrong, Rapid disappearance of nitroglycerin following incubation with human blood, Can. J. Physiol. Pharm. 58:459–462 (1980).

20. Nitro-Bid® Ointment (2% nitroglycerin), "Physicians' Desk
     Reference," Med. Economics Co. (1980), p. 1093.
21. A. Kamiya and H.-L. Fung, First-pass uptake of nitroglycerin
     by rat blood vessels after intra-vessel injections, Abstract,
     American Pharmaceutical Association Meeting, April (1981).
22. H.-L. Fung and A. Kamiya, Disposition of nitroglycerin in rat
     plasma and selected blood vessels, Abstract #1087, Eighth
     International Congress of Pharmacology, Tokyo, July (1981), p.
     552.
23. M.S. Hansen, S.L. Wood and R.E. Wills, Relative effectiveness
     of nitroglycerin ointment according to site of application,
     Heart Lung 8:716-720 (1979).

Chapter 11

PHARMACOKINETICS AND PHARMACEUTICAL TECHNOLOGY

H. Sucker

Pharmacy Research and Development
Sandoz Limited
Basel, Switzerland

When a new dosage form is to be developed from either a new or a familiar active ingredient, the following aims are pursued in the formulation:

1. Maximum therapeutic effectiveness
2. Freedom from unacceptable side effects
3. Patient acceptance
4. Compliance with physical and chemical specifications
5. Stability
6. Avoidance of batch to batch variation

The first two points are concerned with therapeutic effect and are therefore problems of pharmacology and pharmacokinetics. Their connection with points 4 to 6, which are typical problems of pharmaceutical technology, is illustrated in Scheme I. Point 3, the question of patient acceptance, presents a psychological problem which may have different solutions in different geographical areas. For example, suppositories are widely used and accepted in central and southern Europe but are not very popular in English speaking countries.

Biopharmaceutics and pharmacokinetics have become the major challenges in pharmaceutical technology. They have greatly increased the demands made on the quality of the drug and also on the knowledge and competence of the formulator. On the other hand, application of these disciplines has helped improve the efficacy of our dosage forms.

Scheme II shows the route taken by a drug molecule with respect to its biological availability. Formerly, measurement of

97

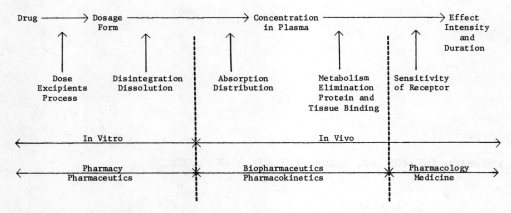

Scheme I. Disciplines involved in development of drug formulations.

the disintegration time of a tablet was the only test applied which had a bearing on the ability of the drug to be absorbed by the body.   Today, not only is an adequate dissolution rate required, but the formulator is also expected to employ some technique to enhance absorption of the drug in the gastrointestinal tract (GIT).

Having thus seen the general fate of a drug molecule in the body, we now proceed to Scheme III, which shows the many ways pharmacokinetic data may be applied to the technological development of dosage forms.   In addition to determinations of bioavailability and bioequivalence, great use is made of simulation.   Simulation is employed, even before practical formulation work begins, to obtain

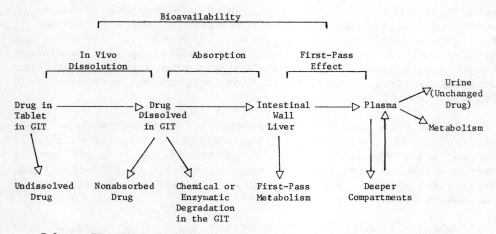

Scheme II. Flow diagram for an orally ingested dosage form.

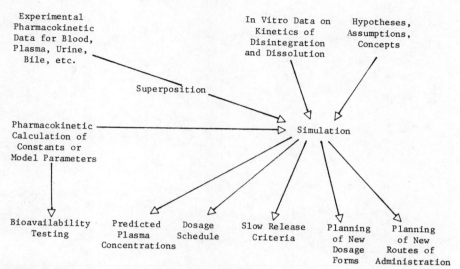

Scheme III. Ways in which pharmacokinetic data may be applied to the technological development of dosage forms.

an idea of the possibilities and the limitations of the drug, to provide a guide to the required or desirable dissolution profile, to determine the ratio of the initial dose to the retard dose and to answer other questions.

In our experiments, a very simple model (Scheme IV) has proved satisfactory in almost every case for preformulation work. We use a function defining the dissolution rate followed by the Bateman function which defines the first-order kinetics of absorption and elimination. More complicated models incorporating deeper compartments do not result in more accurate prediction. For simple programming of the dissolution rate function for retard tablets, even an approximation based on first-order kinetics has proved satisfactory in many cases (Fig. 1). For example, using the pH change after two hours, or linearization by means of the RRSB (Rosin, Rammler, Sperling and Bennet) distribution (which in English-speaking countries is also known as the Weibull distribution), a drug combination containing phenylpropanolamine was one product for which simulation was successfully used (Fig. 2).

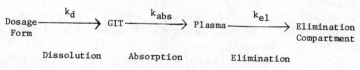

Scheme IV. Simulation model for preformulation.

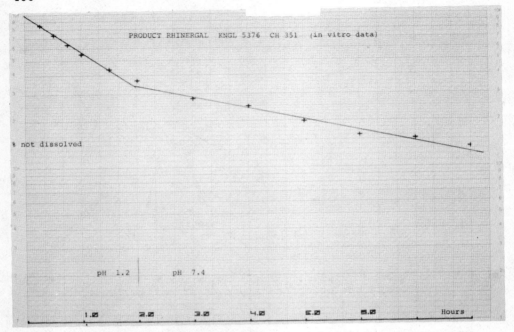

Figure 1. Dissolution rate linearized with first-order kinetics.

Another example of such a simulation is the case of a new dosage form that was proposed and subsequently tested, namely Visken® Retard (pindolol) press-coated tablets. On the basis of this simulation study (Fig. 3), a dosage form was designed to provide a specified dissolution profile by supplying an initial dose and a gastric juice-resistant retard core. The very first batch with the desired dissolution profile which was submitted for biological evaluation produced a blood concentration curve departing by no more than ± 20% from the simulated value at any point.

It should, of course, be pointed out that there are a number of physiological constraints and that such "textbook" simulations cannot be achieved in every case. The results just described must not blind us to the fact that, in general, the correlation of in vitro and in vivo behavior constitutes one of the most difficult problems and one which must be tackled afresh for every drug. The most important limitations are listed in Table I. The gastro-intestinal tract does not absorb active compounds uniformly throughout its whole length, in part because the intestinal contents increase in viscosity as they pass through the tract, but mainly because the lower intestine has a much smaller specific surface area. Special significance therefore attaches to the

Table I. Problems for retard formulations.

---

1. Physiologically available residence time

   $\tau \leqslant 6 - 10$ hr

2. Active absorption stage — the absorption window

   $\tau \leqslant 2$ hr

3. Declining absorption rate in the large intestine

   $k_{abs} \neq$ constant

4. Dissolution rate varying as a function of pH

   $k_d(pH) \neq$ constant

5. High elimination rate — very high retard dose required

6. First-pass effect

   Dose response $\neq$ f (Dose)

7. Response $\neq$ f (C_{plasma})

---

computation of the absorption kinetics by means of deconvolution, using impulse analysis; a program for this was devised in our laboratories by Tobler and Regez (unpublished), which has since been described by Shipley et al. (1). If the blood concentration curve after an intravenous (i.v.) injection (impulse) is known, any other blood curve may be represented as a chronological sequence of such increments of various magnitudes, the sum of which is equal to the _in vivo_ dissolution rate of that proportion of the product which is absorbed. Where the kinetics are linear, this method provides a valuable insight into the _in vivo_ process.

What is the optimal drug concentration profile? If the minimum effective concentration is known, as it is for antibiotics and sulfonamides, for example, this question is easily answered. The concentration should remain above the minimum effective concentration for as long as possible. Blood concentrations shooting far above this level do not provide increased efficacy, but are often the cause of unpleasant side effects. Attempts to achieve the highest possible dissolution rate and thus rapid absorption and high peak concentrations (but short durations of

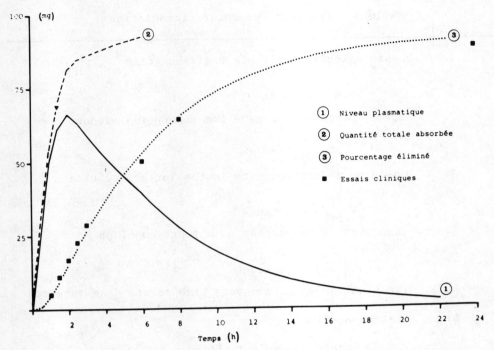

Figure 2. Simulation of the blood concentration curve of phenyl-propanolamine.

action), are justified only when the usable proportion of the physiological residence time is limited; for example, because there is an "absorption window." If elimination is extremely slow, with a half-life of 12 hours or more, for example, then the blood concentration profile at steady state is not significantly influenced by the absorption rate profile. On the other hand, for many drugs having a half-life of absorption of about 20 minutes and a half-life of elimination of a few hours, the dissolution profile assumes considerable importance. In our laboratories, therefore, we have devised a nomenclature covering the various oral dosage forms, which has been approved by the Association of Swiss Industrial Pharmacists (Table II). We have developed the following numerical criteria for the quantitative evaluation of retard forms:

1.   Comparison of half-life bands

$$R\Delta = \frac{\Delta_{1/2} \text{ retard form}}{\Delta_{1/2} \text{ normal form}} \geq 1.5 \ldots 3$$

where $\Delta_{1/2}$ is the length of time plasma concentrations remain above half the maximum plasma concentration.

2.   Comparison of peak blood concentrations

$$R_c = \frac{C_{max} \text{ retard form}}{C_{max} \text{ normal form}} \leq 1$$

3.   Comparison of specific bioavailability

$$R_{BA} = \frac{AUC_R / D_R}{AUC_N / D_N} \geq 1$$

where AUC is the area under the plasma concentration-time curve; D is dose.

Figure 4 depicts the differences in these parameters for a dibenzepin retard formulation as compared to a quick release dosage form of the drug.   A great variety of methods may be used in

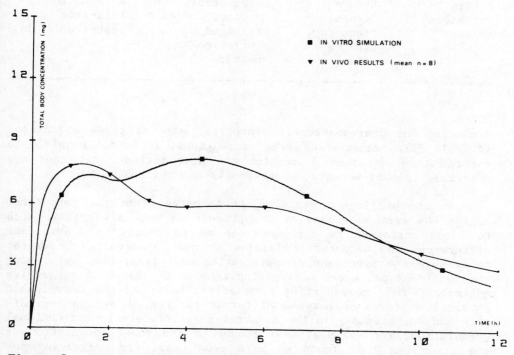

Figure 3. Simulation of the blood concentration curve of pindolol (Visken®) retard formulation.

Table II. Nomenclature for controlled release dosage forms.

Type	Objective	Principle	Remarks
Quick release	Rapid onset of effect	Rapid disintegration, rapid dissolution	Solid solutions or effervescent tablets
Forte	Stronger and longer effect	Higher dose and, in some cases, a smaller first-pass effect	Longer duration of effects especially with slow elimination kinetics
Slow release	Avoid side effects at start	Avoid initial peak by slowing absorption	
Retard sustained release	Reduce dosage frequency, prolong effect	Lower absorption constant and/or prolonged absorption in the GIT	Elimination half-life less than 12 hr

producing the pharmacokinetic prototype; some of these are listed in Table III. Because of space limitations, it is not possible to enter into a detailed discussion of these methods, but they are described in many monographs, textbooks and reviews.

At the scaling-up stage it is important that the formulator design the various stages of the process in such a way that batch to batch variation is not so great as to result in significant differences in therapeutic effect. In our laboratories we prefer to measure the important process variables, rather than specifying the machine type, speed and running time on the basis of subjective estimates, thus compensating more effectively for the unavoidable physical differences between different batches of active ingredients and excipients. In the manufacture of tablets by conventional granulation, for example, measurement of the power consumption of the mixer has been found to be a good basis for estimating the noncritical volume of granulation liquid, the minimum quantity of

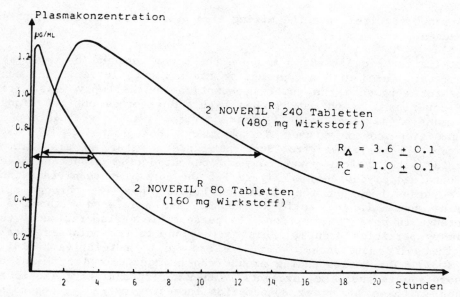

Figure 4. Example of retard criteria of dibenzepin retard formulation.

Table III. Interactions of drug and excipients with respect to the absorption kinetics.

Wetting
Hydrophilization
Hydrophobization
Surface
Pore structure
Viscosity

Hydrophilic
Amphiphilic } Solid solution
Hydrophobic

pH value
Complexation

Coating

---

lubricant required, and the mixing time over which the second phase is added.

The technique used to measure the power consumption employs a voltmeter linked with a compensator and a chart plotter. The compensator subtracts the power consumption of the empty mixer from the power used by the mixer when full and smoothes out the signal by means of an electronic filtering device. With a granulate of a composition commonly used in pharmacy (86% lactose, 10% corn starch, 4% polyvinylpyrrolidone as binder, water as granulation liquid), the typical power consumption curve of a planetary mixer is obtained as depicted in Figure 5. The curve can be divided into five phases based on the amount of liquid added (S_2 through S_5). During phase I, the solid components are moistened without any increase in power consumption. No perceptible agglomeration of the primary particles occurs. This corresponds to the moisture uptake of the solid substances, which are exposed to a relative humidity of 100%. The corresponding amount can be ascertained by means of adsorption isotherm measurements. When more granulating liquid is added in phase II, power consumption increases markedly, depending on the composition, as the solid particles begin to agglomerate. During phase III, power consumption tends to level off. Our findings indicate that usable granulates can be produced only within

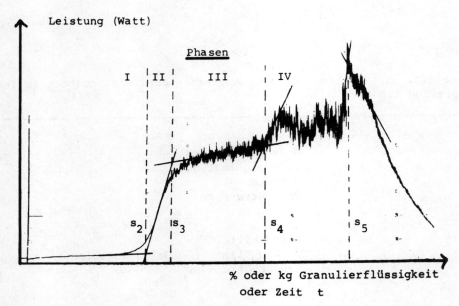

Figure 5. Power consumption curve of a granulation process in a planetary mixer. Plot of power consumption in watts versus time in hours as granulating liquid is added during the different phases.

the range of this plateau. Below S_3, the agglomerates are too soft
after drying, while at S_4 the mass is too moist for further processing.

Today, we use power consumption measurement for in-process
control in the Production Department in order to compensate automatically for differences in the quantity of the granulating liquid
required. The uncritical quantity $(S_3 + S_4)/2$ is replaced by $S_3 +$
S_{add} where:

$$S_{add} = \frac{S_4 - S_3}{2}$$

The normal power signal (curve a, Fig. 6) is converted to a filtered signal (curve b) in which the rapid oscillations are damped.
The signal is then used to produce a differentiated signal (curve
c). At the first power increase, the differentiated signal gives a
clearly recognizable peak. From this time on, the calibrated pump
runs for an adjustable time (t_{add}) which corresponds to the
granulating liquid S_{add}, and then it shuts off. After a further
preselected kneading time, the mixer automatically switches off.
We have been able to show that S_{add} can be taken as $4.5 \pm 1.2\%$ of

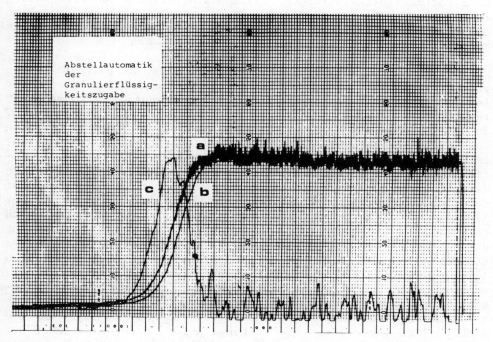

Figure 6. Power consumption curve of an automated granulation
process.

S_3, even if it is not possible to overwet a batch to determine the values of S_3 and S_4. To rapidly determine the quantity of granulation liquid required, we therefore determine S_3 electronically, as described, and allow the calibrated pump to continue to run for the adjustable time (t_{add}) corresponding to the quantity 4.5%.

With the same device, we can measure the decrease in the electrical power consumption of a mixer after the addition of lubricants. This allows the determination of both the minimum amount of lubricant required and the mixing time. Magnesium stearate reduces the power consumption significantly even at very low concentrations. Very often the minimal power consumption is reached using 0.1% magnesium stearate (Figs. 7 and 8). With this concentration it is possible to make tablets which do not stick and which require a minimum force for ejection. For stearic acid, however, higher concentrations (Fig. 9) and longer mixing times are required. In all cases, with increasing quantities of lubricant, the expected prolonged disintegration time and reduced dissolution rate, and a sharp fall in radial tensile strength were observed. Measurements of power uptake allow the correct conditions to be found for obtaining both reproducible granulates with defined porosity, strength and good tableting properties, and tablets with good radial tensile strength, rapid disintegration and high dissolution rate. The power measurement technique, therefore, seems to be a better guide to processing conditions than other variables measured in powder technology.

In order to obtain good reproducibility of pharmacokinetic properties, it is important that granulates be dried to a constant level of residual moisture. In our experience, more consistent results are obtained by fluidized bed drying than by oven drying. In the fluidized bed method, process control is based on measurement of the temperature of the fluidization air, since the material being dried is in equilibrium with the air (Fig. 10). In calibration experiments, temperature measurements are made in order to establish the difference between the temperature $v_{2,e}$ measured at the time when a sample having the desired residual moisture content is taken, and the moist solid temperature that is identical with the wet bulb temperature v_k measured during the period of constant drying rate. For a given material, the drying process is always stopped when the fluidized bed temperature, v_2, has risen to a level exceeding the moist solid temperature measured during the constant rate period by the quantity Δv. The cutout may be controlled either manually or electronically. This technique automatically compensates for variations in the humidity of the inlet air to the dryer. The criteria which in our experience are important determinants of the pharmacokinetic properties of the end product are summarized in Table IV.

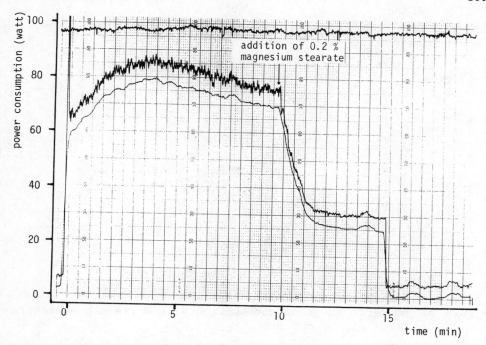

Figure 7. Decrease in power consumption of a dry mix after addition of magnesium stearate, 0.2%.

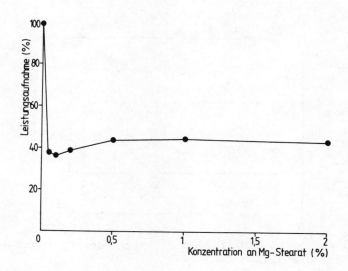

Figure 8. Decrease in power consumption with different concentrations of magnesium stearate.

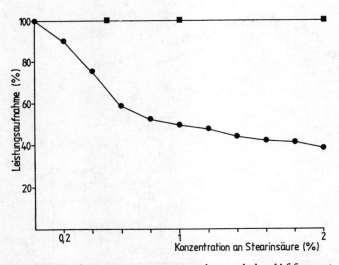

Figure 9. Decrease in power consumption with different concentrations of stearic acid.

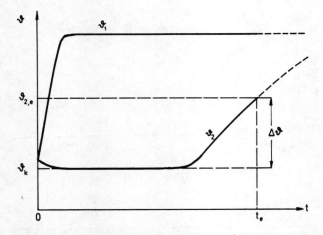

Figure 10. Automated fluidized bed drying (see text for explanation
of symbols).

Table IV. Criteria important for process control at different stages of tablet manufacture.

Drug and auxiliaries	Particle size distribution
Wet granulation	Power consumption
Fluidized bed drying	Fluidized bed temperature
Addition of external phase	Power consumption
Tableting	Pressure control and speed

In the 29 years since the term pharmacokinetics was first introduced by Dost, the application of pharmacokinetic thinking has become most important in the development of drug dosage forms. As a tribute to my friend Sid Riegelman, I have attempted to demonstrate how this thinking can be applied in the daily routine work of a formulator.

REFERENCE

1.   R.A. Shipley and R.E. Clark, "Tracer Methods for In Vivo Kinetics; Theory and Applications," Academic Press, New York (1972).

Chapter 12

BIOAVAILABILITY AND PHARMACOKINETICS IN DRUG DEVELOPMENT

Bernard E. Cabana

International Drought Registration, Inc.
Gaithersburg, Maryland

Bioavailability and pharmacokinetic studies should be considered an integral part of drug disposition studies and should play an important role in every phase of drug development, starting with preclinical studies and proceeding through the various IND clinical phases (phases I-III).

Although a great deal of attention has been given to the subject of drug bioavailability in recent years (1), the issue of bioequivalence or generic equivalence, and not clinical pharmacokinetics, was of primary focus. In 1972, the APhA Academy of Pharmaceutical Sciences published its first guideline (2) entitled, "Guidelines for Biopharmaceutic Studies in Man." This guide dealt mainly with the issue of bioequivalence and the methods of conducting such studies. Since that time, the APhA has published several "Bioavailability Monographs" on important drugs. In recent years, the FDA has prepared comprehensive guidelines for bioequivalence studies.

The purpose of this presentation is to briefly describe important considerations pertaining to bioavailability/pharmacokinetic studies involving new chemical entities, new drug delivery systems, or new indications. It is not intended that this presentation serve as a checklist of what must be done for every new drug. Nor is it intended that it be complete in every detail or attempt to answer all questions about all drugs. Rather, my purpose is to provide a brief summary of important questions that need to be raised and facts that perhaps need to be obtained during the various phases of the IND drug development. Also, I am commenting on the types of studies that should be carried out from the viewpoint of a scientist rather than a regulator. In other words, firms can and do obtain FDA approval by doing less than I describe in this chapter. At the same time, I want to stress that good biopharma-ceutic product research is more than just good science, it is good economics, especially when the drug reaches the marketplace and becomes available to a wide variety of patients. When properly conducted, in a timely fashion, bioavailability/pharmacokinetic studies can contribute a great deal toward the prevention of serious toxicity or drug ineffectiveness during clinical trials which may ultimately foster better patient compliance and product acceptance.

Although there are numerous considerations that need to be given to IND drug development, space does not permit me to discuss them all. Table I summarizes the elements of greatest importance to be considered in IND/NDA drug development.

BIOPHARMACEUTIC CONSIDERATIONS AND ASSESSMENT FOR POTENTIAL BIO-AVAILABILITY PROBLEMS

Biopharmaceutics is a relatively new scientific discipline concerning the relationship between the physical and chemical pro-perties of an active drug ingredient (and its dosage form) and the biologic (therapeutic or toxic) effects observed following the administration of a drug. Biopharmaceutic considerations bear directly on the safety and efficacy of a drug product. It is well documented in the scientific literature that, if not given the proper consideration, these factors can and do render drugs both unsafe and/or ineffective for their intended uses. The effects of

Table I. Elements to be considered in IND/NDA drug development.

---

1. Biopharmaceutic consideration and assessment for potential bioavailability problem.

2. Bioavailability/pharmacokinetics and their relationship to therapeutics.

3. Dose-independent kinetics versus Michaelis-Menten kinetics.

4. Effect of diseased state.

5. Special patient populations.

6. Concomitant drug administration/environmental factors.

---

an alteration of the physical composition of a drug are often not appreciated. The importance of these factors to therapeutics was vividly demonstrated with griseofulvin (3) and chloramphenicol (4). With both of these drugs, the extent of bioavailability was altered significantly by changing the particle size. In the case of griseofulvin, the FDA and USP required micronization of the drug. The FDA resolved the differences in bioavailability associated with chloramphenicol by specifying the polymorphic crystalline form and by imposing a bioavailability requirement on all manufacturers.

The above examples are not isolated instances. Similar problems have been reported for phenytoin (5), an anticonvulsant, and digoxin (6), a potent cardiotonic drug. In the latter case, a change in drug particle size was associated with a 2 to 3-fold difference in plasma concentration of digoxin in human subjects.

In my opinion, it is imperative that a manufacturer assess a drug's potential for bioavailability problems early in the drug development scheme, preferably during preclinical or phase I tolerance trials. It should be stressed that it is necessary to determine the inherent bioavailability properties of both the drug and the dosage form to be employed during clinical trials. The investigator may gather a great deal of information about the inherent absorption properties of a drug initially from comparative oral and i.v. studies in animal models (beagle dogs, for example) and later from radiotracer studies in phase I clinical trials. Radiotracer studies permit the assessment of total absorption and an estimate of first-pass metabolism. Administration of a drug in a readily soluble form permits a proper estimate of the absorption characteristics of the drug itself and appropriate pharmacokinetic parameters in the absence of interfering inert excipients. Many drugs have an inherently poor bioavailability profile because of pKa considerations, localized absorption, GI instability or first-pass metabolism.

From the physico-chemical and pharmacokinetic properties of a drug one can often predict potential bioavailability problems and thus design a dosage form which will optimize drug delivery. Ignoring physico-chemical parameters (such as pH-solubility profile, particle size, dissolution rates), and pharmacokinetic parameters (such as first-pass metabolism or rapid metabolic or renal clearance), may lead to poor dosage form design or inappropriate drug delivery which ultimately can result in poor clinical trials associated with a high incidence of ineffectiveness or manifestations of toxicity.

Such biopharmaceutic considerations should not be limited to the pure drug substance, but should also include the drug delivery system. The most frequent cause of bioavailability problems and therapeutic failures is associated with changes in the composition of drugs involving inert ingredients contained in the dosage form. Phenytoin (DPH) best exemplifies two types of problems associated with bioinequivalent drugs. A report before a congressional investigating committee (7) in 1967 revealed that six Veterans Administration hospitals experienced an increase in reported convulsive seizures when the brand of DPH was changed, indicating an underdosage with the new formulation. At about the same time, reports from Australia indicated an increase in the incidence of anticonvulsant intoxication, or overdosage as a direct result of a simple change in inert ingredients (8). The change, which resulted in intoxication of 51 epileptic patients in Brisbane, Australia, produced a significant increase in DPH plasma concentrations in the patients. This occurred as a result of simply replacing calcium sulfate dihydrate with lactose in the formulation.

Recently, the FDA has stressed the importance of drug dissolution testing to assure drug bioavailability (9) and has advised manufacturers on the importance of assessing pH-dissolution rate profiles. This advice is based on findings with chlorpropamide and furosemide (10). In the latter case, the Agency identified as a potential hazard an unapproved furosemide product due to the large amount of dicalcium phosphate present in the formulation. This product, when compared to Lasix®, demonstrated significant differences in dissolution rate at low pH and was associated with several clinical failures in the U.S. A bioavailability study revealed the product to be grossly inferior to Lasix®; the plasma concentrations obtained were only 60-65% of those achieved with Lasix®.

In recent years the FDA has determined that it can no longer rely solely on the comparison of mean plasma concentrations in rendering a bioequivalence determination. It has promulgated in the Federal Register the use of a "75/75 Percent Rule" for bioequivalency of several drug classes. This rule utilizes each individual subject as his own control in comparing a test drug to a reference drug for in vivo bioavailability assessment (12). Such new considerations stem directly from FDA sponsored studies on tetracycline, digitoxin (9) and phenytoin (11) which clearly demonstrated to the Agency the unreliability of mean dissolution rate data and average plasma concentrations as a basis for new drug approval.

This unreliability can best be illustrated by comparing mean plasma concentrations of generic brands of tetracycline hydrochloride tablets (Fig. 1) with plasma concentrations obtained in individual subjects (Table II). Such a comparison clearly shows that unsatisfactory plasma concentrations were obtained in certain subjects with one product: 6 out of 12 subjects had a bioavailability of less than 50% (in some instances less than 25%). These

Table II. Tetracycline relative bioavailability.

Subject	M/L[a]	R/L	U/L
1	0.91	0.10	0.97
2	0.80	0.10	1.01
3	0.56	1.17	0.83
4	0.86	0.71	0.69
5	1.45	0.91	1.68
6	0.79	0.10	0.61
7	0.87	0.84	0.92
8	0.74	0.44	1.03
9	0.94	0.71	0.73
10	0.83	0.03	1.56
11	0.85	0.86	0.46
12	1.29	0.25	1.22
Mean	0.90	0.52	0.98
CV%	28.2	76.1	37.4

[a]Key: L–Lederle, M–Mylan, R–Rachelle, U–UpJohn, (see Fig. 1).

plasma concentrations, if maintained, would undoubtedly have resulted in therapeutic failures. Further dissolution studies showed that there was a direct correlation between the incidence of in vitro dissolution rate failure and the in vivo failure rate. In each instance, the failure rate was approximately 50%.

The results of this in vitro/in vivo study are consistent with comparative bioavailability data for individual patients using other tetracycline products. Shah and co-workers reported in 1975 that there was a direct relationship between the dissolution rate performance of tetracycline hydrochloride capsules and the percentage of subjects achieving satisfactory bioavailability (Fig. 2). Brands of tetracycline that dissolved less than 60% in 30 minutes, using the FDA paddle method with water as the medium, would have excessive bioavailability failure rates (30–50% of individual subjects).

The predictive capability of the latter approach (13) was also reported for digitoxin (9). FDA collaborative studies with Wood (9,14) have shown that slowly dissolving brands of digitoxin (Fig. 3) are associated with excessive failure rates ranging from 30 to 90%. For instance, brands that dissolved less than 60% in 60 minutes (employing USP method I) were associated with a failure

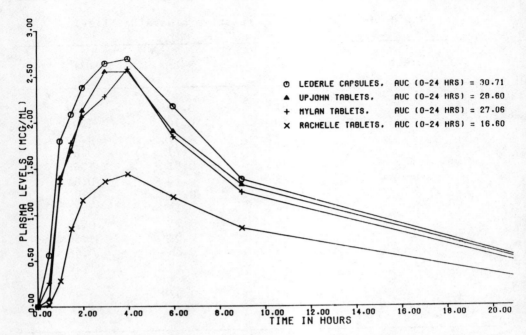

Figure 1. Mean plasma concentration of tetracycline in 12 healthy human volunteers following oral administration of different products.

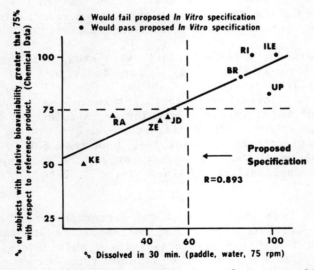

Figure 2. In vitro/in vivo correlation of tetracycline employing the 75/75 Rule. Reprinted from (9), with permission.

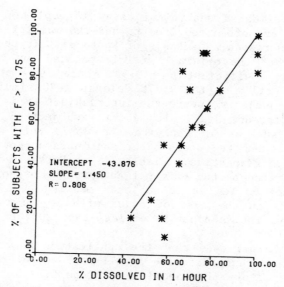

Figure 3. In vitro dissolution rate versus in vivo bioavailability of digitoxin tablets. Reprinted from (9), with
permission.

rate of greater than 80% in individual subjects; that is, greater
than 80% of the subjects tested would have a bioavailability of
less than 75% relative to an oral digitoxin solution. In contrast,
drug products that dissolved more than 80% in one hour were
associated with a failure rate of less than 20%. The underlying
principle assumed in the use of the 75/75 Rule is that the
bioavailability of a rapidly dissolving drug product or oral
solution will tend to replicate itself in the individual subjects.
In contrast, slowly dissolving drug products will tend to be more
erratically absorbed and thus will result in higher failure rates.

    In the recent past the new 75/75 Rule proposed by the FDA for
"Bioequivalency Studies" came under criticism as being scientifically invalid and unpredictable in bioavailability studies involving subjects with large inter- and intrasubject coefficients of
variation; that is, intersubject coefficient of variation (CV) of
60% (15). Although the FDA does not disagree with the calculated
results for hypothetical problems in the published article or the
application of the Pittman-Morgan Test, the authors of the proposed
FDA 75/75 Rule do disagree with the author's underlying assumption
that such large variations are the norm in bioequivalency studies.
It has been the experience of the Agency that, for the large
majority of drugs for which bioavailability data is submitted as
part of a New Drug Application, the CV is generally less than 40%

if a properly validated analytical assay is employed. Drugs that have a large CV are often required to undergo multiple dose steady-state study comparisons as a basis of approval. It should be noted that the author of the original article pointed out that, given a true correlation coefficient $\rho = 0.90$, there is a probability of 90% success in utilizing the 75/75 Rule in 1000 simulated studies on groups of 24 subjects, where the intersubject CV is 40% for both the test and reference drug, with an intrasubject CV of 30%. The probability of success in applying the 75/75 Rule will signifi-cantly increase when the intersubject and intrasubject variation is below 40% and 30% respectively (Table III). Furthermore, utilizing the method described by the original author, the proportion of 1000 studies involving as few as 12 subjects meeting the 75/75 Rule is greater than 88% in the case of drugs with an intersubject CV of less than 40% and intrasubject CV of less than 20%.

It should be stressed that the application of the 75/75 Rule is only valid for drugs that have a well-defined reference standard which has reproducible pharmacokinetic properties in terms of ab-sorption and clearance. To achieve these results, the FDA often utilizes an oral solution as the basis for comparison when the re-ference drug has poor bioavailability. It should also be stressed that the 75/75 Rule is only applied in conjunction with a proper analysis of variance.

BIOAVAILABILITY AND PHARMACOKINETICS AND THEIR RELATIONSHIP TO THERAPEUTICS

An important consideration, which is often overlooked from a regulatory perspective, is the fact that manufacturers may often alter the drug dosage form and employ a large variety of formula-tions during the course of clinical trials. This is particularly prevalent among multi-national companies that conduct studies abroad and in the U.S. It is often discovered, after completion of such clinical studies, that the dosage forms employed in the pivotal clinical trials were either inadequate in terms of their bioavailability profile, or unstable or not defined relative to the dosage forms proposed for marketing. Therefore, in addition to requiring that the final dosage form proposed for marketing be com-pared to an absolute standard (for example, either i.v. or oral solution), it is necessary to do an additional bioequivalence comparison of the dosage forms employed in pivotal clinical trials to the formulation proposed for marketing. When significant differences in bioavailability profiles of these dosage forms are found, relabeling considerations will be required (which always causes a delay in FDA approval) and at times additional clinical trials in the U.S. may even be required, either prior to approval or as phase IV studies.

Table III. Proportion of 1000 simulated studies with nine hypothetical drugs meeting 75/75 Rule.

Drug	N	Inter-subject CV[a] CV TP	CV RP	Intra-subject CV	Proportion of 1000 Studies Meeting 75/75 Criterion ρ = 0	ρ = 0.5	ρ = 0.7	ρ = 0.8	ρ = 0.9
D1	24	60	60	30	0.15	0.26	0.35	0.43	0.52
D2	24	40	40	30	0.72	0.81	0.86	0.88	0.90
D3	24	60	40	30	0.29	0.36	0.39	0.41	0.43
D1	12	60	60	20	0.24	0.35	0.47	0.54	0.66
D2	12	40	40	20	0.55	0.69	0.79	0.82	0.88
D3	12	60	40	20	0.38	0.47	0.53	0.56	0.59
D4	12	30	30	15	0.74	0.87	0.91	--	0.98
D5	12	15	15	13	1.00	1.00	1.00	--	1.00
D6	12	30	15	13	0.84	0.86	0.88	--	0.89
D7	12	30	30	10	0.68	0.86	0.94	--	0.99
D8	12	15	15	10	1.00	1.00	1.00	--	1.00
D9	12	30	15	10	0.80	0.86	0.89	--	0.91

[a]N = Number of subjects, TP = test product, RP = reference product.

Obviously, the relationship of bioavailability to therapeutics is of immense significance. The more critical a drug, the greater the need to obtain a definable, reproducible dosage form. Figure 4 shows plasma concentrations of triamterene obtained in human subjects following administration of two solid dosage forms and a fine suspension of triamterene-hydrochlorothiazide. Whereas formulation A is equivalent to the fine suspension, formulation B yielded a 2.5-fold lower plasma concentration-time area for triamterene. Close examination of the literature indicates that the administration of triamterene-hydrochlorothiazide to patients in daily doses of 100 mg triamterene/50 mg hydrochlorothiazide is associated with approximately a 12% incidence of hyperkalemia in the geriatric population (16,17) and an even higher incidence in diabetics.

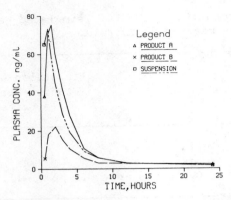

Figure 4. Bioavailability comparison of different triamterene-hydrochlorothiazide formulations.

Let us now suppose that clinical trials had been initiated with formulation B and thereafter the patients were switched to formulation A. What could one predict about the likelihood of hyperkalemia? It is my belief that the incidence of hyperkalemia in geriatrics could be expected to be much greater. Let us now consider a clinical trial involving a fully bioavailable furosemide product. What therapeutic consequences might result from simply switching brands to a less bioavailable form during clinical trials? The sudden administration of a deficient furosemide product to certain patients might well result in clinical failures as evidenced by a lack of diuresis, and therefore edema and congestive heart failure. Several such clinical failures have been documented by the FDA in the past two years. In certain instances, the physician was unable to assess the clinical situation and even death ensued.

Concern about the therapeutic consequences of the substitution of a poorly defined dosage form during the course of clinical trails should not be limited to "poor formulations" but also to dosage forms which result in greater bioavailability. The latter can best be illustrated with chlorthalidone. In this instance, a new formulation of a 100 mg dosage form of chlorthalidone was associated with 1.6 to 1.7 times higher plasma concentrations than those of the reference standard and a 1.5-fold increase in urinary drug recovery. Unfortunately, this dosage form could not be approved by the FDA since the Agency had served notice in the Federal Register (18) to remove this dosage strength from the market based on a higher incidence of decreased serum potassium and increased serum uric acid, with no greater benefit in terms of hypotensive effects (19,20). Given the steeper dose-response curve for decrease in serum potassium compared to a flat dose-response for chlorthalidone's effect on sodium excretion and blood pressure, a more bioavailable dosage form at this dosage strength is, in my opinion, clearly contraindicated.

Concern should not be limited only to the bioavailability of a dosage form, but also to the pharmacokinetics of a drug in any given patient population. Without appropriate knowledge of the pharmacokinetics of the ADME processes of a new drug, the clinical pharmacologist is flying blind as to the potential toxicity or lack of efficacy that might result. This author is aware of clinical trials where serious toxicity was encountered during multiple dose studies because the plasma clearance of the parent drug and/or active metabolite(s) was totally ignored in designing the dosing regimen, and toxic concentrations of drug occurred. Knowledge of the drug's pharmacokinetic profile and careful patient monitoring is particularly important for drugs such as phenytoin that exhibit Michaelis-Menten kinetics.

Recently, the Food and Drug Administration, in cooperation with the United States Pharmacopeia (USP), established two separate monographs for prompt release and extended release phenytoin sodium USP capsules. The Agency further established separate new drug requirements with separate labeling requirements for such dosage forms. The basis for the dual requirements stems from in vitro/in vivo correlative studies in normal human volunteers (9,21) and clinical pharmacokinetic studies performed in epileptic patients (11,22). Dissolution studies conducted by the FDA revealed a significant difference in dissolution profile among several marketed brands ranging from less than 60% dissolution in 1 hour for Dilantin® to 100% in 15 minutes for some generic brands. Single dose bioavailability studies using these same brands revealed that there was a direct relationship between rates of absorption, as measured by T_{max} and C_{max}, and the dissolution rate at 30 minutes employing the USP rotating basket method at 100 rpm with water as the dissolution medium (9). An excellent correlation was obtained relating the time to peak (T_{max}), r = 0.944, p < 0.001, and peak concentration (C_{max}), r = 0.902, p < 0.001, to the dissolution rate. No significant difference in the extent of bioavailability was noted among these products. Slowly dissolving products, such as Dilantin®, achieved peak concentrations in 5-6 hours and were associated with a significantly reduced C_{max} in comparison to the quickly dissolving products which generally peaked within 2-3 hours.

The consequences of different rates of absorption were not initially appreciated by all within the Agency due to the assumption that the long biologic half-life of phenytoin (18-24 hours) would soon mask any differences associated with differences in rates of absorption. However, reconsideration of the scientific issues involved was stimulated by the approval of new labeling instructions for Dilantin® allowing for once-a-day administration.

These new labeling claims were based on multiple dose steady-state studies performed by Parke-Davis that demonstrated equivalent steady-state plasma concentrations after once-a-day and more frequent therapy. Examination of the scientific literature indicated that, due to the Michaelis-Menten kinetics which prevail with phenytoin, patients might be placed at risk by switching to a rapidly absorbed drug product, particularly if it is administered only once a day.

A study was undertaken in epileptic patients to determine the role that differences in absorption rate might play in therapeutic effect (22). Three oral preparations, differing significantly in their rate of absorption but having a total bioavailability of 95-97% based on single dose bioavailability studies in healthy volunteers, were employed in this study. The three oral preparations, an oral solution, a rapidly dissolving capsule (Zenith) and an extended release capsule (Dilantin®), were each administered for 2 weeks to 24 epileptic patients over a 6-week period according to a completely randomized study design. Eighteen patients were administered 100 mg every 8 hours, and 6 subjects received 200 mg every 12 hours. In addition to continuous plasma concentration monitoring, neurologic examinations for signs of nystagmus, ataxia, and mental symptoms were performed at each visit to the clinic. Phenytoin and its major metabolite, unconjugated p-HPPH, were analyzed in plasma using a high pressure liquid chromatographic assay (22).

The administration of the more rapidly absorbed phenytoin drug products resulted in significantly higher steady-state plasma concentrations (Fig. 5). On the average, the differences in plasma concentrations observed were in the range of 2-3 µg/ml which should be expected to have no clinical significance. However, utilization of the new FDA promulgated 75/75 Rule for both trough values (C_{min}) and areas under the steady-state plasma concentration-time curves for each patient revealed that 7 of 18 (39%) patients who received the 300 mg per day dose and 2 of 6 who received the 400 mg per day dose of phenytoin differed by more than 25%. In certain epileptic patients, the "apparent bioavailability" of the extended release capsule was about 50-60% that of the oral solution and resulted in C_{min} values that were 55-65% that of the oral solution. Close examination of each patient's plasma profile revealed that 3 separate patient categories could be distinguished among the initial 18 subjects who received the 300 mg per day dose. One category did not appear to manifest any dosage form-related difference in DPH steady-state plasma concentrations. The second category exhibited significant differences in trough plasma concentrations of DPH. The C_{min} values fell from 10-12 µg/ml for the oral solution to potentially subtherapeutic concentrations, during the last dosing period, of 4-6 µg/ml for the more slowly absorbed extended release capsule. The third category of patients

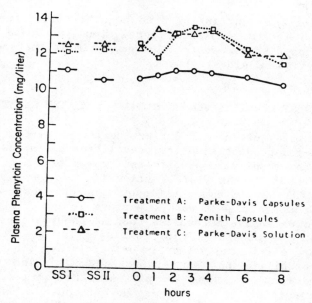

Figure 5. Mean steady-state plasma phenytoin concentrations in eighteen epileptic patients administered 300 mg per day doses of three different phenytoin preparations.

(2 subjects) showed the opposite effect; plasma concentration <u>increased</u> from therapeutic levels (C_{min} = 12-15 µg/ml) to potentially toxic levels (C_{min} = 18-27 µg/ml).

It should be noted that use of the more rapidly absorbed oral solution by the latter two patients was associated with increased nystagmus and mental symptoms. However, one cannot rule out that these side effects could be associated with the presence of ethyl alcohol and propylene glycol in the oral solution vehicle. Similar findings were also noted with the rapidly absorbed Zenith drug product. Although experts familiar with these data do not agree about their interpretation, given that the bioavailability of these phenytoin drug products (after single dose administration) was 95-97% relative to an i.v. solution, they generally believe that single dose studies are inappropriate to define the bioavailability of drugs exhibiting Michaelis-Menten kinetic properties. Further more, it is obvious that the use of mean plasma data is totally inappropriate for assessing the bioavailability of such drugs.

It is imperative to assess the pharmacokinetic properties of the drug delivery system if one wishes to optimize a new drug. For example, use of a pseudo-zero-order transdermal drug delivery system for scopolamine (23) can prevent serious toxicity and side effects. Similarly, by taking into account differences in clearance values in various patient populations, such as pediatrics, geriatrics, and diseased state, one can optimize therapeutic trials and design optimal dosing regimens.

DOSE—INDEPENDENT KINETICS VERSUS MICHAELIS—MENTEN KINETICS

An assumption often made during the course of drug development is that dose-independent kinetics prevail for all drugs. That this is not true can readily be ascertained from a review of the literature (24-33). In recent years, during the course of IND/NDA drug review, the FDA has noted significant departure from dose proportionality for many drugs. Such departure is not limited to drugs which undergo extensive metabolism such as phenytoin (26), propranolol (29,30) and lorcainide (31), but has also been observed with drugs that are eliminated primarily or partly by urinary excretion, such as piperacillin (27) and naproxen (32). The total plasma clearance and renal clearance of piperacillin decrease as the dose increases (resulting in a greater AUC) because of saturation of active renal tubular secretion. In the case of naproxen the plasma clearance is increased at high doses because of saturation of plasma protein binding.

Assessment of dose proportionality is of prime importance in drug development, particularly in dealing with critical drugs that have a narrow therapeutic index or drugs which require close patient monitoring such as anticonvulsants, antiarrythmics, anticoagulants, and so forth. When a departure from dose linearity is observed, an attempt should be made to delineate the underlying causes, such as saturation of drug metabolism, change in hepatic extraction, protein binding saturation, saturation of tubular secretion, and so forth, and to include this information in the drug product literature. Such studies should permit the design of the appropriate dosing regimen for subsequent clinical trials, thereby avoiding unanticipated manifestations of toxicity resulting from unanticipated drug and/or metabolite(s) accumulation.

EFFECT OF DISEASED STATE

During clinical trials, the diseased state may result in a significant alteration in total plasma clearance due to concomitant renal or hepatic disease. The possibility of alteration of drug binding by pathologic states and its effect on plasma clearance needs to be considered. Such findings are often associated with manifestations of toxicity due to greater drug accumulation (34). An alteration in renal clearance can generally be detected by an elevation in serum creatinine or a decrease in creatinine and inulin clearance. Differences in metabolic clearance are not always indicated by clinicopathology findings and are more difficult to deal with since such occurrences can often be related to drug interactions or interactions with dietary factors.

The clinical significance of renal disease should not be underestimated in designing trials on new drug entities. Recent studies have shown that the biologic half-life of atenolol can vary 15-fold ranging from 6 hours to over 100 hours with progressive renal failure (35). The plasma clearance of atenolol in uremic patients was directly correlated to creatinine clearance and serum creatinine and blood concentrations increased over a 21-day dosing period. The volume of distribution of atenolol was also correlated to creatinine clearance. The volume of distribution of atenolol decreased significantly (2 to 3-fold) in uremic and anephric patients. The effects of renal disease are not limited solely to the excretion of drugs, but may also influence drug metabolism. Thus, certain metabolic pathways are significantly reduced in uremia, for example, acetylation of sulfisoxazole (36), reduction of cortisol (37) and hydrolysis of procaine (38). The role of protein binding also needs to be considered in uremic patients. Riedenberg (39) has shown that the half-life of phenytoin is decreased in uremic patients because of a significant reduction in binding to plasma protein.

Renal function can also affect the elimination and the volume of distribution of a drug which is extensively metabolized. This was readily demonstrated with pindolol (40,41); both the volume of distribution and the renal clearance were significantly reduced with decreased creatinine clearance. Similar findings were recently reported for fenbufen, a new nonsteroidal anti-inflammatory analgesic which is extensively metabolized (42). Uremic patients with creatinine clearances of 3-20 ml/min exhibited a more rapid rate of metabolism of fenbufen, but a decreased renal clearance of polar metabolites resulting in greater accumulation of certain metabolites.

The effects of liver disease on the disposition kinetics of new drugs have not been as extensively studied as the effects of renal disease. This is perhaps due to the complexity of the physiological kinetic model systems, which indicate a potential for alteration of drug metabolism kinetics, hepatic blood flow and volume of drug distribution, and saturation of the drug extraction ratio. However, in my judgment, lack of drug monitoring in such patients could result in serious toxicity due to drug accumulation.

Liver cirrhosis has been shown to result in a 5-fold increase in the biologic half-life of verapamil (from 170 to 815 min) (43), a 3-fold increase in the half-life of chlordiazepoxide (from a mean of 10 hr to 34.9 hr) (44) and more than a 2-fold difference in propoxyphene plasma concentrations (45). In the case of verapamil, the cirrhotic patients showed a 2-fold increase in the steady-state volume of distribution. Perhaps the most significant finding in these three studies is that the variance of the estimated kinetic parameters in the cirrhotic patients was 5 to 10-fold greater than in normal healthy volunteers, indicating a need for close patient monitoring in cirrhotics to avoid drug accumulation and toxicity.

Investigators of a new drug should be mindful of the fact that other diseases may alter the ADME pharmacokinetic parameters of a drug either by altering its absorption, protein binding or metabolism. Thus, for instance, achlorhydric patients or patients suffering from GI disease could be expected to have an altered bioavailability profile for a drug either due to poor dissolution of certain drug formulations, such as formulations requiring acidic milieu (dicalcium phosphate or calcium sulfate, for example), or due to an alteration in GI transit time for a drug that exhibits a window effect (site specific absorption). Thyroid dysfunction could be expected to result in significant alteration in the elimination of a drug which is eliminated by metabolism (46). From these many examples it should be obvious to all investigators that clinical pharmacokinetics may play an immense role in the clinical evaluation of a drug in the diseased state.

SPECIAL PATIENT POPULATIONS

Additional bioavilability and pharmacokinetic studies may be required to define a new drug in pediatric and/or geriatric patient populations. Changes in drug disposition kinetics associated with the aging process are of potential clinical importance in that the more rapid metabolic clearance often seen in pediatric patients may result in a lack of efficacy, whereas a decrease in plasma clearance in the elderly could lead to excessive drug accumulation and the possibility of exaggerated clinical response or toxicity (47).

COMCOMITANT DRUG ADMINISTRATION AND ENVIRONMENTAL FACTORS

In his evaluation of a new drug the clinical investigator must often contend with the use of concomitant drugs and environmental or dietary factors such as smoking, alcohol, pollutants, pesticides, and so forth, which may influence drug disposition kinetics and at times require dosage adjustment. Alteration in drug disposition kinetics can result from a decrease in renal tubular secretion, (the probenecid-ampicillin interaction); enzyme induction, (phenobarbital); displacement from protein binding sites, (the phenytoin-dicumerol interaction); and alterations in gastrointestinal absorption, (the antacid-tetracycline interaction). Other environmental or dietary factors may also influence the bioavailability or pharmacokinetics of a drug. Consumption of ethanol, for instance, has been shown to enhance the oral absorption of diazepam (48) and to increase plasma concentrations of intravenously administered diazepam (49). The latter effect was associated with a decrease in N-demethylation of the drug. The effect of smoking on drug disposition and its potential clinical implications in therapeutics has been the subject of a major review by the Department of Health (50). In recent years, the FDA has become aware of the potential effects of smoking on the pharmacokinetics and pharmacodynamics of therapeutically important drugs such as theophylline, phenacetin, imipramine and propoxyphene, and has required special labeling for theophylline.

In summary, there are a number of important questions that an investigator needs to ask concerning any drug during the course of IND drug development. The bioavailability/pharmacokinetic studies to be undertaken should be dictated by the physico-chemical and pharmacological properties of the drug itself. There is no one single guide for drug development. They can only be developed by appropriate application of the research method.

REFERENCES

1. Drug Bioequivalence Study Panel Report ("Drug Bioequivalence") to the Office of Technology Assessment, Congress of the United States, July (1974).

2. "Guidelines For Biopharmaceutic Studies in Man," APhA Academy of Pharmaceutical Sciences, Washington, D.C., February (1972).

3. R.M. Atkinson, C. Bedford, K.J. Child and E.G. Tomich, The effect of griseofulvin particle size on blood levels in man, Antibiotic Chemother. 12:232-238 (1962).

4. A.J. Glazko, A.W. Kinkel, W.C. Alegnani and E.L. Holmes, An evaluation of the absorption characteristics of different chloramphenicol preparations in normal human subjects, Clin. Pharmacol. Ther. 9:472-483 (1967).

5. A.J. Glazko, in: "Proceedings of the Conference on Bioavailability of Drugs," National Academy of Sciences of the United States, Washington D.C. (1971), pp. 163-177.

6. A.J. Jounela, P.J. Pentikäinen and A. Sothmann, Effect of particle size on the bioavailability of digoxin, Europ. J. Clin. Pharmacol. 8:365-370 (1975).

7. D.G. Hall, in: "Hearing Before the Subcommittee on Monopolies Select Committee on Small Business," U.S. Senate, Government Printing Office, Washington D.C. (1967), pp. 258-281.

8. J.H. Tyrer, M.J. Eadie, J.M. Sutherland and W.D. Hooper, Outbreak of anticonvulsant intoxication in an Australian city, Brit. Med. J. 2:271-273 (1970).

9. B.E. Cabana, Bioequivalence and in vitro testing of drug formulations in: "Towards Better Safety of Drugs and Pharmaceutical Products," D.D. Breimer, ed., Elsevier/North Holland, Amsterdam (1980), pp. 301-322.

10. V.K. Prasad, R.S. Rapaka, P. Knight and B.E. Cabana, Dissolution test medium — a critical parameter to identify bioavailability problems of furosemide tablets, Int. J. Pharm. 11:81-90 (1982).

11. B.E. Cabana, E.D. Purich and J. Hunt, Therapeutic plasma levels of phenytoin in epileptic patients as a function of absorption rate, Proceedings of the First European Congress of Biopharmaceutics and Pharmacokinetics, Clermont-Ferrand, France (1981).

12. B.E. Cabana, E.D. Purich, R.S. Rapaka, W.B. Schary and V.K. Prasad, Biopharmaceutic considerations and new drug approval, World Conference on Clinical Pharmacology and Therapeutics, London, August (1980).

13. W.R. Fairweather, Investigating relationship between in vivo and in vitro pharmacological variables for purpose of prediction, J. Pharmacokin. Biopharm. 5:405-418 (1977).

14. J.H. Wood, Bioequivalency establishment of marketed digitoxin products, APhA Academy of Pharmaceutical Sciences 23rd Meeting, Phoenix, Arizona, November (1977).

15. J.D. Haynes, Statistical simulation study of new proposed uniformity requirement for bioequivalency studies, J. Pharm. Sci. 70:673-675 (1981).

16. K.B. Hansen and A.D. Bender, Changes in serum potassium levels occurring in patients treated with triamterene and a triamterene-hydrochlorthiazide combination, Clin. Pharmacol. Ther. 8:392-399 (1967).

17. A.D. Bender, C.L. Carter and K.B. Hansen, Use of diuretic combination of triamterene and hydrochlorthiazide in elderly patients, J. Am. Geriatrics Soc. 15:166-173 (1967).

18. Chlorthalidone, in: "Federal Register," 44:54124-54127, September 18 (1979).

19. M.G. Tweeddale, R.I. Ogilvie and J. Ruedy, Antihypertensive and biochemical effects of chlorthalidone, Clin. Pharmacol. Ther. 22:519-527 (1977).

20. B.J. Materson, J.R. Oster, U.F. Michael, S.M. Bolton, Z.C. Burton, J.E. Stambaugh and J. Morledge, Dose response to chlorthalidone in patients with mild hypertension, Clin. Pharmacol. Ther. 24:192-198 (1978).

21. A.P. Melikian, A.B. Straughn, G.W.A. Slywka, P.L. Whyatt and M.C. Meyer, Bioavailability of eleven phenytoin products, J. Pharmacokin. Biopharm. 5:133-146 (1977).

22. R.J. Sawchuk and R.J. Gumnit, Pharmacokinetic and overt toxicity of phenytoin sodium products in clinical patients, FDA Contract 223-76-3019, Final Report.

23. J. Shaw and J. Urquhart, Programmed systemic drug delivery by the transdermal route, in: "Trends in Pharmacological Sciences," April (1980), pp. 208-211.

24. J.G. Wagner, A modern view of pharmacokinetics, J. Pharmacokin. Biopharm. 1:363-401 (1973).

25. W.J. Jusko and M. Gretch, Plasma and tissue protein bindings of drugs in pharmacokinetics, Drug Metab. Rev. 5:43-140 (1976).

26. T.M. Ludden, J.P. Allen, L.W. Schneider and S.A. Stavchansky, Rate of phenytoin accumulation in man: A simulation study, J. Pharmacokin. Biopharm. 6:399-415 (1978).

27. T.B. Tjandramaga, A. Mullie, R. Verbesselt, P.J. De Schepper and L. Verbist, Piperacillin: Human pharmacokinetics after intravenous and intramuscular administration, Antimicrob. Agents Chemother. 14:829-837 (1978).

28. G.H. Evans and D.G. Shand, Disposition of propranolol V. Drug accumulation and steady-state concentrations during chronic oral administration to man, Clin. Pharmacol. Ther. 14:487-493 (1973).

29. D.G. Shand and R.E. Rangno, The disposition of propanolol I. Elimination during oral administration in man, Pharmacology 7:159-168 (1972).

30. T. Walle, E.C. Conradi, U.K. Walle, T.C. Fagan and T.E. Gaffney, The predictable relationship between plasma levels and dose during chronic propranolol therapy, Clin. Pharmacol. Ther. 24:668-677 (1978).

31. E. Jahncen, H. Bechtold, W. Kasper, F. Kersting, H. Just, J. Heykants and T. Meinertz, Lorcainide, I. Saturable presystemic elimination, Clin. Pharmacol. Ther. 26:187-195 (1979).

32. R. Runkel, E. Forchielli, H. Sevelius, M. Chaplin and E. Segre, Nonlinear plasma level response to high doses of naproxen, Clin. Pharmacol. Ther. 15:261-266 (1973).

33. P.J. Meffin, E.W. Robert, R.A. Winkle, S. Harapat, F.A. Peters and D.C. Harrison, Role of concentration dependent plasma protein binding in disopyramide disposition, J. Pharmacokin. Biopharm. 7:29-46 (1979).

34. B.E. Cabana and L.W. Dittert, Drug absorption and disposition as monitors of safety and efficacy, J. Pharmacokin. Biopharm. 3:143-158 (1975).

35. J. McAinsh, B.F. Holmes, S. Smith, D. Hood and D. Warren, Atenolol kinetics in renal failure, Clin. Pharmacol. Ther. 28:302-309 (1980).

36. M.M. Reidenberg, H. Kostenbauder and W.P. Adams, Rate of drug metabolism in obese volunteers before and during starvation and in azotemic patients, Metabolism 18:209-213 (1969).

37. E. Englert Jr., H. Brown, D.G. Willardson, S. Wallach and E.L. Simons, Metabolism of free and conjugated 17-hydroxycorticoids in subjects with uremia, J. Clin. Endocrinol. Metab. 18:36-48 (1958).

38.   M.M. Reidenberg, M. James and L.G. Dring, The rate of procaine
      hydrolysis in serum of normal subjects and diseased patients,
      Clin. Pharmacol. Ther. 13:279–284 (1972).

39.   M.M. Reidenberg, I. Odar-Cederlöf, C. von Bahr, O. Borga and
      F. Sjöqvist, Protein binding of diphenylhydantoin and
      desmethylimipramine in plasma for patients with poor renal
      function, N. Engl. J. Med. 285:264–267 (1971).

40.   E.E. Ohnhaus, E. Nüesch, J. Meier and F. Kalberer, Pharmaco-
      kinetics of unlabeled and ^{14}C-labeled pindolol in uremia,
      Europ. J. Clin. Pharmacol. 7:25–29 (1974).

41.   S. Øie and G. Levy, Relationship between renal function and
      elimination kinetics of pindolol in man, Europ. J. Clin.
      Pharmacol. 9:115–116 (1975).

42.   H.J. Rogers, J.P. Savitsky, B. Glenn and R.G. Spector,
      Kinetics of single dose of fenbufen in patients with renal
      insufficiency, Clin. Pharmacol. Ther. 29:74–80 (1981).

43.   B.G. Woodcock, I. Rietbrock, H.F. Vöhringer and N. Rietbrock,
      Verapamil disposition in liver disease and intensive care
      patients: kinetics, clearance and apparent blood flow rela-
      tionship, Clin. Pharmacol. Ther. 29:27–34 (1981).

44.   E.M. Sellers, D.J. Greenblatt, H.G. Giles, C.A. Naranjo, H.
      Kaplan and S.M. MacLeod, Chlordiazepoxide and oxazepam dispo-
      sition in cirrhosis, Clin. Pharmacol. Ther. 26:240–246 (1979).

45.   K.M. Giacomini, J.C. Giacomini, T.P. Gibson and G. Levy,
      Propoxyphene and norpropoxyphene concentrations after oral
      propoxyphene in cirrhotic patients with and without surgically
      constructed portacaval shunt, Clin. Pharmacol. Ther. 28:417–
      424 (1980).

46.   M. Eichelbaum, Drug metabolism in thyroid disease, Clin.
      Pharmacokin. 1:339–350 (1976).

47.   D.P. Richey and A.D. Bender, Pharmacokinetic consequences of
      aging, Ann. Rev. Pharmacol. Toxicol. 17:49–65 (1977).

48.   D.J. Greenblatt, R.I. Shader, D.R. Weinberger, M.D. Allen and
      D.S. MacLaughlin, Effect of a cocktail on diazepam absorption,
      Psychopharmacology 57:199–203 (1978).

49.   E.M. Sellers, C.A. Naranjo, H.G. Giles, R.C. Frecker and M.
      Beeching, Intravenous diazepam and oral ethanol interactions,
      Clin. Pharmacol. Ther. 28:638–645 (1980).

50.   J.A. Califano, "Smoking and Health – A Report of the Surgeon.
      General", U.S. Department of Health, Education and Welfare,
      January 11, 1979, pp. 27–50.

Chapter 13

CLEARANCE — MODELS, VALIDATION AND IMPLICATIONS

Malcolm Rowland

Department of Pharmacy
University of Manchester
Manchester, England

The utility of clearance (CL) as the parameter to relate rate
of elimination to measured drug concentration is now well established in pharmacokinetics. The concept of clearance was first
proposed by Möller et al. (1) to characterize the handling of urea
by the kidney, and subsequently applied to quantitate the removal
of substances by the liver, gastrointestinal tract and other eliminating organs. Today, clearance measurements are used to assess
organ function, to predict steady-state concentrations following
constant rate regimens, to predict the degree of hepatic first-pass
loss of orally administered drug, and to assess the extent of drug
absorption (2,3). The application of clearance concepts in pharmacokinetics has come with the measurement of concentrations of drug
and metabolites in plasma and blood.

A DEFINITION

As originally developed, clearance is a steady-state concept.
In its simplest form it is defined by the relationship:

$$\text{Clearance} = \frac{\text{Rate of drug elimination}}{\text{Drug concentration}} \tag{1}$$

and has units of volume per unit time. For a given rate of elimination, the value of clearance depends on the medium assayed:
plasma, whole blood or plasma water. Thus:

$$\text{Rate of elimination} = CL \cdot C = CL_b \cdot C_b = CLu \cdot Cu \tag{2}$$

where CL, CL_b and CLu refer to clearance based on measurement of
drug in plasma (C), whole blood (C_b) and plasma water (Cu), respectively. Pharmacologically, unbound drug is the most important
species, whilst total plasma concentrations are the most commonly
measured. Clearance may thus be viewed as the effective volume of
measured fluid that is cleared of drug per unit time.

In Equation (1), drug concentration refers to that entering
the eliminating organ; this is usually in an artery (an inconve-
nient sampling site). Measurement of drug in a peripheral, and
more convenient, venous site usually suffices because at steady
state, following constant rate administration, the concentration of
drug in vein and artery are equal in the usual case in which venous
drainage is from a noneliminating tissue (2). For linear systems,
that is, those in which the pharmacokinetics do not change with
either drug concentration or time, organ clearance can also be
assessed from the area under the concentration-time curve following
a bolus dose of drug (3).

A PHYSIOLOGIC VIEW

An alternative and more physiological view of organ clearance
has been gained by expressing clearance in terms of organ blood
flow (Q) and extraction ratio (E):

$$CL_b = Q \cdot E \tag{3}$$

This relationship requires that clearance be defined with respect
to measurement of drug in blood because the organ receives blood,
not just plasma. An exception is when all drug is restricted to
the plasma, in which case the extraction ratio is given by the
ratio of plasma clearance to organ plasma flow.

The liver and kidneys are the major eliminating organs for
most drugs. These organs are arranged in parallel and, therefore,
total clearance (CL) is the sum of the individual clearances,
hepatic (CL_H) and renal (CL_R):

$$CL = CL_H + CL_R \tag{4}$$

The gut wall and the lungs are occasionally organs of elimination
and these are in series with the liver and the rest of the body
respectively. The overall availability of drug across organs in
series (F) is the product of the availability across the (n) individual organs, F_i:

$$F = \prod_{i=1}^{n} F_i \tag{5}$$

and since $F_i = 1-E_i$, the overall extraction ratio, $E = (1-F)$, is given by (4):

$$E = 1 - \prod_{i=1}^{n} (1 - E_i) \tag{6}$$

By administering drug at a site directly before each organ in series (into the gastrointestinal tract and portal vein for the gut wall-liver system, for example) and assessing the resultant systemic availability, the extraction ratio across each organ can be determined. Using this approach, Cassidy and Houston (5) demonstrated that, in the rat, phenol is extracted by the gut wall and lungs, as well as by the liver.

Classifying drugs in terms of their extraction ratios has proven useful. For those of high extraction, clearance approaches and is sensitive to changes in organ blood flow, a perfusion limitation. Any binding of drug within blood clearly could not be limiting the extraction of such drugs. Furthermore, predictably, if the eliminating organ is the liver, these high extraction drugs exhibit a low oral bioavailability due to a substantial first-pass presystemic hepatic loss (3). In contrast, the clearance of drugs of low extraction is not usually limited by perfusion. The limitation in this case is normally cellular (enzymatic) activity, but occasionally may be membrane permeability, diffusion out of red blood cells or conceivably dissociation of a drug-protein complex, if the drug has an extremely high affinity for plasma proteins (6). Glomerular filtration is sensitive to renal blood flow. The renal clearance of drugs that are filtered, but neither secreted nor reabsorbed, will therefore vary with renal perfusion even though the organ extraction ratio is low, since glomerular filtration rate is such a small percentage (8%) of total renal blood flow. Nonetheless, in all instances in which the extraction ratio is low, a linear dependence is predicted between clearance, assessed with respect to total plasma drug concentration, and the degree of plasma binding (7):

$$CL = fu \cdot CLu \tag{7}$$

where fu is the fraction of unbound drug in plasma and CLu is the unbound clearance of the drug. Figure 1 illustrates this linear relationship with tolbutamide, a drug of low extraction. Under such conditions CLu is a direct measure of the rate-limiting step, usually cellular activity.

While helpful in appreciating the general influences of perfusion, binding within blood and cellular activity on clearance, the analysis in the preceding paragraph deals only with the limiting conditions of high and low extraction. It allows no quantitative

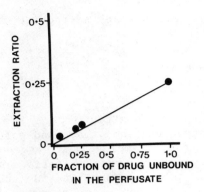

Figure 1. Linear dependence of the extraction ratio of tolbutamide on the binding of the drug in the perfusate of an
isolated perfused rat liver in situ preparation (28).

prediction of changes in clearance due to changes in a physiologic
parameter over the entire range of extraction ratio values. This
has been demonstrated with indocyanine green in the rat. The
extraction ratio, high at a low rate of hepatic perfusion,
decreases in a curvilinear manner with increasing hepatic blood
flow (8). For this and other reasons, classification of drugs
simply in terms of extraction ratio has been questioned (9).

MODELS OF HEPATIC CLEARANCE

To overcome the stated limitations, several simple models of
clearance that relate elimination to intracellular events have been
proposed for the liver, the major eliminating organ for most drugs
(Fig. 2). One model, commonly referred to as the well-stirred or
venous equilibrating model, represents the liver in terms of one or
more compartments, with drug in the emergent venous blood in
equilibrium with that in the hepatic compartment closest to it.
This model, originally used by Bischoff and Dedrick (10), has been
extensively explored (11,12) and is the most widely used in physiological pharmacokinetic modeling (13). The second model, commonly
referred to as the sinusoidal perfusion or parallel tube model, has
its origins in hepatic physiology (14) and assumes that elimination
occurs in hepatocytes lining directionally perfused sinusoidal
tubes. As such, the concentration of drug within the sinusoids and
hepatocytes decreases continuously in the direction of the hepatic
vein. In both models, an "intrinsic clearance" (CL_{int}) is defined
as the rate of drug elimination divided by the unbound drug concentration at the enzymatic site. In terms of simple enzyme kinetics,
intrinsic clearance is given by:

$$CL_{int} = \Sigma \frac{Vm_i}{Km_i + Cu_H} \tag{8}$$

where Vm_i and Km_i are the maximum velocity and Michaelis–Menten constant, respectively, of the ith enzyme, and Cu_H is the unbound drug concentration at the enzymatic site. The two models differ as to how this concentration is related to the measured incoming and venous drug concentrations. In the well-stirred model this concentration is considered equal to the unbound emergent concentration, whereas in the second model it is defined as the logarithmic mean of the unbound input and output concentrations.

Pang and Rowland (11) have examined theoretically, by graphical means, ways of discriminating between the two models. Both models predict the same behavior in clearance and other parameters when the extraction ratio of the drug is low. Differences in predictions emerge only with drugs of high extraction, particularly with regard to systemic availability, area under the curve following a single oral dose or average concentration at steady state during chronic oral dosing. One can also examine this problem

Model I

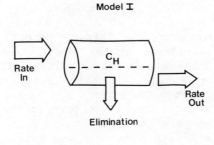

Model II

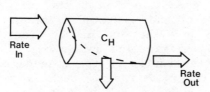

Figure 2. Diagrammatic representation of two simple models of hepatic elimination, the well-stirred model (model I) and the parallel tube model (model II). The dashed lines represent unbound hepatic drug concentration.

numerically, defining a discrimation function as the difference in the predictions of the two models. Differences between the two models' predictions will be greatest when the discrimination function is maximum. This maximum value is found by differentiating the function with respect to the parameter of interest (blood flow, for example), and solving for the value of the parameter numerically (15).

The experimental data dealing with this problem of discrimination are sparse and conflicting at present. Most of the studies involve altered hemodynamics. Using a single-pass isolated perfused rat liver preparation with portal vein infusion, changes in emergent venous concentrations of lidocaine (a very highly extracted drug, E~0.995, in this animal) with changes in hepatic blood flow were better described by the venous equilibrating model than by the parallel tube model (16).

According to the venous equilibrating model, the rate of elimination is given by:

$$\text{Rate of elimination} = CL_{int} \cdot Cu_{out} \tag{9}$$

where Cu_{out} is the unbound concentration of drug in the effluent venous blood. Since intrinsic clearance is independent of perfusion, according to this model, the value of Cu_{out} and the resultant systemic concentration in vivo at steady state should be independent of perfusion when drug is infused directly into the liver. This hypothesis was supported by the observations of Shand et al. (17), and recently confirmed by Ahmad (18), using lidocaine as a highly extracted model substrate in the recirculating perfused rat liver preparation. As shown in Figure 3, the concentration of drug in the reservoir is relatively insensitive to changes in perfusion. In contrast, changes in the emergent venous drug concentration, but consistency of the logarithmic average concentration, were observed for galactose at steady state in the same animal model, a finding more consistent with the sinusoidal perfusion model (19).

The influence of altered plasma protein binding on clearance has been mentioned. An examination of the influence of a change in binding on the ratios of the predicted extraction ratios, and hence clearance (Fig. 4), shows that one cannot discriminate between the two models of hepatic elimination unless one is dealing with drugs of very high extraction ratio, in the absence of binding, and can vary binding over a very wide range. Such large changes in binding may not occur or even be possible to achieve experimentally in vivo. Guentert and Øie, for example, found that under normal conditions, despite a high degree of plasma binding, the hepatic extraction ratio of quinidine in rabbits was extremely high; clearance was perfusion rate-limited (20). Up to a threefold change in binding was achieved through depletion of plasma proteins

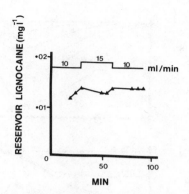

Figure 3. Lack of change in the reservoir concentration of lidocaine with changes in blood flow in a recirculating
isolated perfused rat liver preparation in which
lidocaine is infused via the portal vein (18).

by bleeding, but no change in clearance was observed. The
observation is important therapeutically for drugs given by
constant rate infusion. The unbound (and pharmacologically active)
concentration in plasma at steady state is determined by the
unbound clearance. If blood clearance (CL_b) is unchanged but the
unbound fraction of drug in blood (fu_b) varies, it follows from the
relationship (see Eq. (2)):

$$CLu = CL_b/fu_b \qquad\qquad\qquad (10)$$

that the unbound steady-state concentration will change reciprocal-
ly with any change in binding. Total steady-state blood clearance
will not be changed. At the other extreme are drugs of low extraction. Since the unbound clearance of these drugs does not change
with plasma protein binding, there should be no change in the
unbound concentration at steady state. However, the corresponding
total plasma drug concentration will vary with alterations in
binding.

Further examination of Figure 4 indicates that the systemic
availability, rather than the extraction ratio, is more sensitive
to relatively modest changes in binding. This is especially true
for drugs of high extraction ratio in the absence of binding, although there is an optimal range of binding to discriminate between
the two models. At higher degrees of binding the extraction ratio
becomes so low that availability approaches unity for both models.
The need to monitor unbound drug is evident.

Much larger changes in plasma binding can be achieved in the
isolated organ system. The liver appears to maintain its integrity

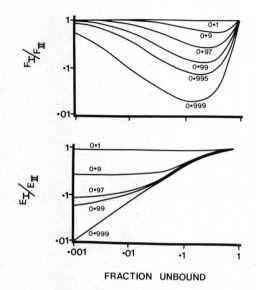

Figure 4. Ratio of extraction ratios (bottom) and availabilities
(top), as predicted by models I and II (see Fig. 2) with
changes in unbound drug in the perfusate while operating
under linear conditions and assuming that hepatic blood
flow = 1.0 ml/min/g liver.   The number next to each
curve is the extraction ratio when there is no binding
in the perfusate (fu = 1).

with respect to drug metabolism in the absence of protein in the
perfusing medium.   Drug binding can thus be varied and controlled
by varying the protein concentration in the perfusate.   Figure 5
shows how, in the single-pass isolated perfused rat liver system,
the extraction ratio of diazepam varies from almost one, in the
absence of albumin (the binding protein), to a very low value when
binding is high.   Distinction between the two models of hepatic
clearance is now possible, especially when one considers the
differences in the predicted availability (F = 1−E) rather than
extraction ratio.   In the absence of protein, the availability of
diazepam is only 1% (E = 0.99).   Examination of Figure 4 indicates
that major differences in the predictions of the models exist when
the unbound fraction decreases towards 0.1.   As illustrated in
Figure 6, the data are better fitted by the parallel tube model
than the well-stirred model; the latter is unable to predict the
very large change observed in availability over the twentyfold
range of binding values (fu = 0.05−1).   It may be argued that
such systems with altered binding are superior to those involving
altered perfusion for discrimination between the models, since
altered perfusion may cause concomitant alterations in intrahepatic
microcirculation as well as in oxygen tension.   Such secondary perturbations may also affect drug elimination.

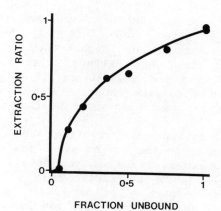

Figure 5. Changes in the extraction ratio of diazepam in the single-pass isolated perfused rat liver <u>in situ</u> preparation with changes in binding. Binding was changed by altering the albumin concentration in the perfusate.

ADDITIONAL COMPLEXITIES

The events in the liver are clearly more complex than those portrayed in the simple models in Figure 2. The liver receives two blood supplies, one from the hepatic portal vein and the other from the hepatic artery. Both models assume that complete mixing of

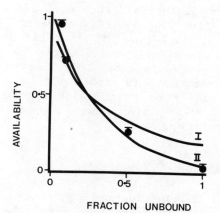

Figure 6. The observed data (circles ± SD) and predictions based on model I and model II (see Fig. 2) of changes in availability of diazepam in a single-pass perfused liver preparation with changes in binding within the perfusate.

these blood supplies occurs before they reach the sinusoidal bed and hence the hepatocytes, but this may not be so. The availability of lidocaine is much higher when perfused through the hepatic artery (9%) than when perfused through the portal vein (0.5%) of isolated perfused rat livers (21). Furthermore, by varying the ratio of lidocaine entering the liver via the portal vein and hepatic artery one can vary the availability of this drug.

These observations suggest that either not all of the arterial supply enters at the beginning of the sinusoids (as sometimes seen in scanning electron micrographs of the hepatic microcirculation (22)), or that some of the arterial supply perfuses liver cells that have a different density of enzymes. Operationally, the observed changes in lidocaine concentration leaving the liver that occurred with changes in both total perfusion flow and varying ratios of portal to hepatic arterial input were better predicted by a model in which the liver was divided into two well-stirred compartments, with portal flow entering one compartment and arterial flow entering the other, than by a corresponding parallel tube model (Fig. 7).

The question of uneven distribution of enzymes has also been raised. Using retrograde perfusion experiments, Pang and Terrel (23) showed that sulfate conjugation of acetaminophen occurs predominantly in the periportal region, while O-deethylation of phenacetin (to acetaminophen) occurs preferentially in the centrilobular region of the liver. Heterogeneous distribution of other hepatic enzymes has also been demonstrated. These types of observations raise serious doubts as to our ability to accurately model the events in the liver. Indeed, the well-stirred model has been questioned on physiological grounds, and a more elaborate and perhaps more realistic distributed perfusion sinusoidal model, which considers the distribution of sinusoids of differing length and enzyme density, has been proposed (24). However, the complex three-dimensional organization of the hepatic microcirculation (22), and the heterogeneous distribution of the hepatic enzymes, both of which are likely to change with altered physiologic and pathologic states, makes any proposed model a gross over-simplification of reality.

MODELS OF RENAL EXCRETION

The other major eliminating organ, besides the liver, is the kidney. Any model of renal clearance must take into account the glomerular filtration of all drug molecules and the possibility of secretion, reabsorption or both also occurring. For compounds like inulin and mannitol that are neither secreted nor reabsorbed, renal clearance, corrected for any binding, must equal the glomerular filtration rate (GFR). Active secretion, a saturable process, has

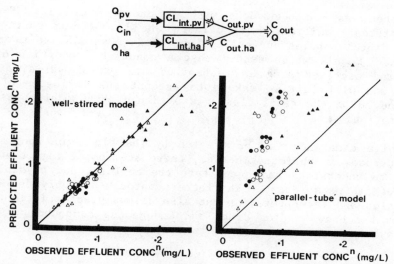

Figure 7. Observed versus predicted effluent lidocaine concentrations calculated assuming functionally separate portal venous and hepatic arterial streams (see inset) for the well-stirred model (model I, left) and the parallel tube model (model II, right), using the single-pass isolated perfused rat liver <u>in situ</u> preparation. The total blood flow was fixed at 10 ml/min and the portal vein: hepatic arterial perfusate flow ratio was fixed at 9:1 (filled circles), 7:3 (open circles), 5:5 (filled triangles), throughout an experiment, or was varied (open triangles). Kindly supplied by Anis Ahmad and Peter Bennett.

been modeled in an analogous manner to the well-stirred model (25) and the tubular model (26) used to describe hepatic clearance. Definitive experiments that distinguish between these two models for active transport have not been reported, although it is likely that, as with the liver, any model will be a gross over-simplification of reality. It is frequently stated that secretion is independent of binding but, as with hepatic elimination, this is likely to be true only when the secretion process is so efficient that it becomes limited by perfusion.

Many lipophilic drugs are reabsorbed from the lumen of the nephron. The kinetics of reabsorption are governed by the permeability characteristics of the luminal membrane with respect to the drug, and the concentration gradient of the diffusing species. Reabsorption of water and changes in membrane permeability, which take place along the entire length of the nephron, would need to be considered, as has been done with regard to urea (27). For weak electrolytes, modification of urinary pH, which occurs particularly in the distal tubules and collecting ducts, must also be taken into account. Models which assume that a constant proportion of filtered and secreted drug is reabsorbed are gross over-simplifications, and will fail to take into account the influence of urine flow and pH on the renal clearance of drugs that undergo extensive reabsorption.

While clearance may be treated by the black-box approach for many purposes in pharmacokinetics, there are compelling reasons for trying to understand and quantitate the cellular and physiological basis of its measurement. The latter approach not only facilitates prediction and interpretation but also allows greater insights into the way the body handles drugs and endogenous compounds. Only in this way can true advances in this subject be made.

REFERENCES

1. E. Möller, J.J. McIntosh and D. Van Slyke, Studies of urea excretion, J. Clin. Invest. 6:427-446 (1929).

2. M. Rowland, L.Z. Benet and G.G. Graham, Clearance concepts in pharmacokinetics, J. Pharmacokin. Biopharm. 1:123-126 (1973).

3. M. Rowland, Effect of some physiological factors on bioavailability of oral dosage forms, in: "Current Concepts in the Pharmaceutical Sciences: Dosage Form Design and Evaluation," J. Swarbrick, ed., Lea and Febiger, Philadelphia (1973), pp. 182-230.

4. D. Cutler, A linear recirculatory model for drug disposition, J. Pharmacokin. Biopharm. 7:101-116 (1979).

5. K. Cassidy and B. Houston, In vivo assessment of extrahepatic conjugative metabolism in first-pass effects using the model compound phenol, J. Pharm. Pharmacol. 32:57-59 (1980).

6. J.A. Jansen, Influence of plasma protein binding kinetics on hepatic clearance assessed from a "tube" model and a "well-stirred" model, J. Pharmacokin. Biopharm. 9:15-25 (1981).

7. T.N. Tozer, Concepts basic to pharmacokinetics, Pharmac. Therap. 12:109-132 (1981).

8. R.W. Brauer, G.F. Leung, R.F. McElroy Jr. and R.H. Holloway, Circulatory pathways in the rat liver as revealed by P^{32} chromic phosphate colloid uptake in the isolated perfused liver preparation, Am. J. Physiol. 184:593-598 (1956).

9. S. Keiding and P.B. Andreasen, Hepatic clearance measurements and pharmacokinetics, Pharmacology 19:105-110 (1979).

10. K.B. Bischoff and R.L. Dedrick, Thiopental pharmacokinetics, J. Pharm. Sci. 57:1346-1351 (1968).

11. K.S. Pang and M. Rowland, Hepatic clearance of drugs. I. Theoretical considerations of a "well-stirred" and a "parallel tube" model. Influence of hepatic blood flow, plasma and

blood binding and hepatocellular enzyme activity on hepatic drug clearance, J. Pharmacokin. Biopharm. 5:625-653 (1977).

12. G.R. Wilkinson and D.G. Shand, Commentary: A physiological approach to hepatic drug clearance, Clin. Pharmacol. Ther. 18:377-390 (1975).

13. K.J. Himmelstein and R.J. Lutz, A review of the applications of physiologically based pharmacokinetic modeling, J. Pharmacokin. Biopharm. 7:127-145 (1979).

14. K. Winkler, L. Bass, S. Keiding and N. Tygstrup, The effect of hepatic perfusion on assessment of kinetic constants, in: "Regulation of Hepatic Metabolism," L. Lundquist and N. Tygstrup, eds., 6th Alfred Benzon Symposium, Munksgaard, Copenhagen (1974), pp. 797-807.

15. B. Mannervik, Design and analysis of kinetic experiments for discrimination between rival models, in: "Kinetic Data Analysis," L. Endrenyi, ed., Plenum Press, New York (1981), pp. 235-270.

16. K.S. Pang and M. Rowland, Hepatic clearance of drugs. II. Experimental evidence for acceptance of the "well-stirred" model over the "parellel tube" model using lidocaine in the perfused rat liver in situ preparation, J. Pharmacokin. Biopharm. 5:655-679 (1977).

17. D.G. Shand, D.M. Kornhauser and G.R. Wilkinson, Effects of route of administration and blood flow on hepatic elimination, J. Pharmacol. Exp. Ther. 195:424-432 (1975).

18. A.B. Ahmad, Ph.D. thesis, University of Bath, England (1982).

19. S. Keiding and E. Chiarantini, Effect of sinusoidal perfusion on galactose elimination kinetics in perfused rat liver, J. Pharmacol. Exp. Ther. 205:465-470 (1978).

20. T.W. Guentert and S. Øie, Effect of plasma protein binding on quinidine kinetics in the rabbit, J. Pharmacol. Exp. Ther. 215:165-171 (1980).

21. A.B. Ahmad, P.N. Bennett and M. Rowland, The influence of varying arterial flow contributing to the perfused rat liver on systemic availability of lignocaine, Brit. J. Pharmacol. 74:244P-245P (1981).

22. R.H. Kardon and R.G. Kessel, Three-dimensional organization of the hepatic microcirculation in the rodent as observed by scanning electron microscopy of corrosion casts, Gastroenterology 79:72-81 (1980).

23. K.S. Pang and J.A. Terrell, Retrograde perfusion to probe the heterogeneous distribution of hepatic drug metabolizing enzymes in rats, J. Pharmacol. Exp. Ther. 216:339-346 (1981).

24. L. Bass, P. Robinson and A.J. Bracken, Hepatic elimination of flowing substances: the distributed model, J. Theoret. Biol. 72:161-184 (1978).

25. F. Kiel, Dynamics of renal proximal tubular secretion, Nature 189:927-928 (1961).

26. S. Øie and L.Z. Benet, Altered drug disposition in disease
     states, Ann. Rep. Med. Chem. 15:277–287 (1980).

27. L.G. Wesson, A theoretical analysis of urea excretion by the
     mammalian kidney, Amer. J. Physiol. 179:364–371 (1954).

28. W.L. Shary, Ph.D. thesis, University of Manchester, England
     (1979).

Chapter 14

ESTIMATION OF AN EFFECTIVE HALF-LIFE

K.C. Kwan, N.R. Bohidar and S.S. Hwang

Merck Institute for Therapeutic Research
Merck Sharp & Dohme Research Laboratories
West Point, Pennsylvania

In pharmacokinetics, the apparent or effective half-life of a drug may be a manifestation of the kinetics of elimination, the kinetics of absorption, the kinetics of disappearance from the site of application, some complex function of elimination and distribution, or a combination of the above. Regardless of the physical or biological realities (or one's conception of them), the half-life is an important, if not the sole, determinant of drug accumulation. On repeated administration according to a given regimen, drugs with longer half-lives will accumulate more slowly but to a greater extent.

The half-life of a drug is usually determined experimentally by monitoring changes in plasma concentration or the rate of urinary excretion as a function of time. For linear systems, a semilogarithmic plot of the time course of change may be polyphasic but will be terminally linear and concentration-independent. Difficulties may be encountered with drugs that undergo extensive enterohepatic circulation in that the reentry process contributes to drug accumulation and is usually sporadic, giving rise to discontinuities in log-linear decay. Thus, the conventional method of estimating half-lives is fraught with uncertainties in the presence of enterohepatic circulation. On the other hand, attempts to circumvent these perturbations, either surgically by exteriorizing the bile duct or analytically by selecting the steepest common slope (1), lead to estimates of half-life that obtain in the absence of enterohepatic circulation. Such estimates are not useful in predicting the rate and extent of drug accumulation under normal circumstances. The concept of an effective half-life for drug accumulation has been applied to indomethacin (2) and sulindac (3), drugs that are known to undergo extensive enteroheptic

147

circulation. The experimental strategy in each case is to estimate the mean plasma concentration (or AUC) of the drug over two dosing intervals during chronic drug administration. Since the regimen is known, the ratio of the AUC's is a measure of the rate of drug accumulation. By definition, therefore, an effective half-life ($t_{1/2,n}$), is that which is consistent with the observed accumulation by a known regimen. The purpose of this chapter is to examine the assumptions and limitations attendant on the concept of an effective half-life and its experimental determination.

THEORETICAL

Given that the kinetics of drug absorption and disposition are constant with time, the rate and extent of drug accumulation upon chronic administration should be predictable solely as a function of the dosage regimen. If, in addition, the dosing sequence recurs in a cyclical manner, a steady state is achieved wherein the time course of change in plasma concentration or urinary excretion becomes invariant from one cycle to the next. Under these circumstances, the approach to and attainment of steady state are both deterministic and perfectly predictable.

Enterohepatic circulation, on the other hand, is sporadic and unpredictable. As such, it may be viewed as a second regimen in which the amount to be reabsorbed ("dose") is variable and the timing of reabsorption is irregular. Both regimens contribute to drug accumulation. However, the stochastic nature of enterohepatic circulation precludes any expectation of an experimentally observable steady state. Instead, the observed accumulation at any time represents a statistical sample of the mean accumulation for the population at that time. The average rate of drug accumulation, and therefore the drug's effective half-life, can be deduced and characterized by repeated sampling. The effective half-life of the drug can then be used to predict the average steady state and the average time course of accumulation by some other regimen.

Pharmacokinetic Considerations

Suppose a fixed dose, D, of drug is administered chronically at intervals of time, τ. Assuming linear kinetics, the ratio of areas under the plasma concentration curve (AUC) during any dosing intervals, i and j, can be approximated (3) by Equation (1):

$$\frac{AUC_\tau^j}{AUC_\tau^i} = \frac{1-e^{-jn\tau}}{1-e^{-in\tau}} \tag{1}$$

where n is the effective rate of drug accumulation such that $t_{1/2,n} = \ln 2/n$. Furthermore, AUC_τ following any dose is related to that at steady state, AUC_τ^{ss} (4-6) in accordance with Equation (2):

$$AUC_\tau^{ss} = \frac{AUC_\tau^i}{1-e^{-i\eta\tau}} = \frac{AUC_\tau^j}{1-e^{-j\eta\tau}} \qquad (2)$$

Finally, since AUC_τ^{ss} is equivalent to the total area under the curve after a single dose, AUC_∞^1, we can write:

$$AUC_\infty^1 = \frac{AUC_\tau^1}{1-e^{-\eta\tau}} \qquad (3)$$

or

$$\eta = -\frac{1}{\tau} \ln\left(1 - \frac{AUC_\tau^1}{AUC_\infty^1}\right) \qquad (4)$$

In principle, therefore, the experimental determination of $t_{1/2,\eta}$ can be achieved by the ratio of AUC_τ at two dosing intervals in the course of chronic drug administration or by the ratio of AUC over a convenient interval τ to AUC_∞ after a single dose. However, because of random perturbations associated with enterohepatic circulation, individual AUC_τ^i and AUC_τ^j must be considered as samples of their true values at intervals i and j. Estimates of AUC_τ^i and AUC_τ^j may be obtained by sampling plasma concentrations following the ith and jth dose in the same subject or by sampling the ith interval in one panel and the jth interval in another comparable panel of subjects. In either event, the mean and variance of the resulting $t_{1/2,\eta}$ are functions of the mean and variance associated with the individual observations of AUC_τ^i and AUC_τ^j.

The estimation of $t_{1/2,\eta}$ following a single dose of drug is dependent on a proper estimate of AUC_∞^1. The presence of enterohepatic circulation precludes the use of extrapolations based on observed plasma concentration profiles in that the effective half-life is in fact the unknown. However, providing that drug is excreted in the urine, AUC_∞^1 can be estimated by Equation (5) because:

$$AUC_\infty^1 = \frac{U_\infty}{CL_R} \qquad (5)$$

where U_∞ is the total amount of drug recovered unchanged in the urine and CL_R is the renal clearance, which can be estimated from the ratio of urinary excretion for a finite interval to the corresponding area under the plasma concentration curve over the same interval. As in the multiple-dose situation, each estimate of $t_{1/2,\eta}$ after a single dose represents a sample of the true value.

Statistical Considerations

The overall objective is to find unbiased estimates of the true effective half-life and its variance. We will examine situations whereby sample estimates of AUC required for the solution of Equations (1) or (3) are derived from different subjects (the independent case), from the same subjects (the correlated case), and from single-dose experiments. We will also consider the joint estimation of $t_{1/2,\eta}$ from AUC_τ^i or AUC_τ^j derived from more than one panel of subjects. The common strategy is to place confidence limits on the accumulation ratio from which the mean and the limits of η can be deduced.

Let AUC_τ^i be sample estimates with variance $V(AUC_\tau^i)$ associated with N_i independent observations; AUC_τ^j, $V(AUC_\tau^j)$ and N_j are similarly defined. Suppose AUC_τ^i values are normally and independently distributed with mean μ_i and variance σ_i^2, the minimum variance unbiased estimators of the location parameter μ_i and of the scaler parameter σ_i^2 (adjusting for the appropriate degrees of freedom) are given by the solutions to the following simultaneous equations:

$$\frac{\partial L}{\partial \mu_i} = 0 \tag{6}$$

and

$$\frac{\partial L}{\partial \sigma_i} = 0 \tag{7}$$

where

$$L = -\frac{N_i}{2} \ln (2\pi\sigma_i^2) - \sum_k (AUC_{\tau,k}^i - \mu_i)^2 / 2\sigma_i^2$$

In accordance with the maximum likelihood estimation principle, the minimum variance unbiased estimators of the location parameter and of the scaler parameter associated with AUC_τ^j are derived in the same manner. We denote the respective solutions of the location parameter by θ_i and θ_j and the scaler parameter by $V(\theta_i)$ and $V(\theta_j)$.

The accumulation ratio (ρ) is a fixed point in a two-dimensional parameter space such that:

$$\rho = \frac{\theta_j}{\theta_i} \tag{8}$$

Equation (8) can be expressed as a homogeneous equation in the form:

$$\theta_j - \rho\theta_i = 0 \tag{9}$$

Given that a linear function of normally distributed variables is also normally distributed, let the mean and the variance be implicitly defined as $E(\theta_j - \rho\theta_i)$ and $V(\theta_j - \rho\theta_i)$, respectively. Furthermore, the ratio of a squared normal variate over the variance of the same normal variate is distributed as the Snedecor F central distribution with $\nu_1 = 1$ and ν_2 degrees of freedom. Hence:

$$[V(\theta_j - \rho\theta_i)]F_{1,\nu_2(\alpha)} = [\theta_j - \rho\theta_i]^2 \tag{10}$$

where $100(1-\alpha)$ is the desired probability associated with the confidence statement on the parameter ρ. Whereas the mean can be explicitly stated as:

$$E(\theta_j - \rho\theta_i) = \mu_j - \rho\mu_i \tag{11}$$

in each case, the expression for variance depends on the design of the experiment.

  The Independent Case. Since AUC_τ^i and AUC_τ^j are sample estimates from different panels of subjects, the estimation of θ_i is totally unrelated to the estimation of θ_j and vice versa. The variance in this case is:

$$V(\theta_j - \rho\theta_i) = [\frac{\partial(\theta_j - \rho\theta_i)}{\partial\theta_j}]^2 V(\theta_j) + [\frac{\partial(\theta_j - \rho\theta_i)}{\partial\theta_i}]^2 V(\theta_i)$$

$$= V(\theta_j) + \rho^2 V(\theta_i) \tag{12}$$

Substituting Equation (12) into Equation (10), we have, after rearrangement:

$$[\theta_i^2 - F_{1,\nu_2(\alpha)}V(\theta_i)]\rho^2 - 2\theta_i\theta_j\rho + [\theta_j^2 - F_{1,\nu_2(\alpha)}V(\theta_j)] = 0 \tag{13}$$

The two solutions to Equation (13) represent the upper and lower $100(1-\alpha)\%$ confidence limits of ρ; they are:

$$\rho = \frac{\theta_i\theta_j \pm \{\theta_i^2\theta_j^2 - [\theta_i^2 - F_{1,\nu2(\alpha)}V(\theta_i)][\theta_j^2 - F_{1,\nu2(\alpha)}V(\theta_j)]\}^{\frac{1}{2}}}{\theta_i^2 - F_{1,\nu2(\alpha)}V(\theta_i)} \tag{14}$$

The Correlated Case. When sample estimates of AUC_τ^i and AUC_τ^j come from the same subject on two different occasions in the course of chronic administration, the correlation between θ_i and θ_j must be taken into consideration. Hence, the explicit form for the variance contains a covariance term:

$$V(\theta_j - \rho\theta_i) = [\frac{\partial(\theta_j - \rho\theta_i)}{\partial\theta_j}]^2 V(\theta_j) + 2[\frac{\partial(\theta_j - \rho\theta_i)}{\partial\theta_i}]$$

$$[\frac{\partial(\theta_j - \rho\theta_i)}{\partial\theta_j}]Cov(\theta_i,\theta_j) + [\frac{\partial(\theta_j - \rho\theta_i)}{\partial\theta_i}]^2 V(\theta_i)$$

$$= V(\theta_j) - 2\rho\,Cov(\theta_i,\theta_j) + \rho^2 V(\theta_i) \tag{15}$$

where:

$$Cov\,(\theta_i,\theta_j) = r_{ij}\sigma_i\sigma_j$$

r_{ij} = the Pearson product-moment correlation coefficient

Substituting Equation (15) into Equation (10) and rearranging, we have:

$$[\theta_i^2 - V(\theta_i)F_{1,\nu2(\alpha)}]\rho^2 - 2[\theta_i\theta_j - Cov(\theta_i,\theta_j)F_{1,\nu2(\alpha)}]\rho$$

$$+ [\theta_j^2 - V(\theta_j)F_{1,\nu2(\alpha)}] = 0 \tag{16}$$

The solutions of Equation (16) represent the upper and lower $100(1-\alpha)\%$ confidence limits of ρ; they are:

$$\rho = [\theta_i^2 - V(\theta_i)F_{1,\nu2(\alpha)}]^{-1}\Big[\theta_i\theta_j - Cov(\theta_i,\theta_j)F_{1,\nu2(\alpha)} \pm$$

$$\{[\theta_i\theta_j - Cov(\theta_i,\theta_j)F_{1,\nu2(\alpha)}]^2 -$$

$$[\theta_i^2 - V(\theta_i)F_{1,\nu2(\alpha)}][\theta_j^2 - V(\theta_j)F_{1,\nu2(\alpha)}]\}^{\frac{1}{2}}\Big] \tag{17}$$

The Single-Dose Case. This is simply a correlated case in which there has been a specific designation of AUC_τ^i and AUC_τ^j as AUC_τ^1 and AUC_∞^1, respectively.

Joint Estimation of η. Suppose there are p independent estimates of θ_i and q independent estimates of θ_j. We now wish to use all of the available data to construct a joint estimate of η. Let θ_i^* denote a linear weighted combination of θ_i, and θ_j^* a linear weighted combination of θ_j. We require that:

$$\theta_i^* = \alpha_1 \theta_{i1} + \alpha_2 \theta_{i2} + \ldots + \alpha_p \theta_{ip} \tag{18}$$

and

$$V(\theta_i^*) = \alpha_1^2 \, V(\theta_{i1}) + \alpha_2^2 \, V(\theta_{i2}) + \ldots + \alpha_p^2 \, V(\theta_{ip}) \tag{19}$$

such that:

$$\sum_{k=1}^{P} \alpha_k = 1$$

Differentiating Equation (19) with respect to each of the α_k and setting the resulting derivatives to zero, we generate a set of (p-1) simultaneous equations which can be represented in matrix form as shown below.

$$
\begin{bmatrix} \alpha_1 \\ \alpha_2 \\ \cdot \\ \cdot \\ \cdot \\ \alpha_{p-1} \end{bmatrix}
=
\begin{bmatrix}
\{V(\theta_{i1}) + V(\theta_{ip})\} & V(\theta_{ip}) & \cdots & V(\theta_{ip}) \\
V(\theta_{ip}) & \{V(\theta_{i2}) + V(\theta_{ip})\} & \cdots & V(\theta_{ip}) \\
\cdot & \cdot & & \cdot \\
\cdot & \cdot & & \cdot \\
\cdot & \cdot & & \cdot \\
V(\theta_{ip}) & V(\theta_{ip}) & \cdots & \{V(\theta_{i,p-1}) + V(\theta_{ip})\}
\end{bmatrix}^{-1}
\begin{bmatrix} V(\theta_{ip}) \\ V(\theta_{ip}) \\ \cdot \\ \cdot \\ \cdot \\ V(\theta_{ip}) \end{bmatrix}
$$

or symbolically by:

$$A = M^{-1} P \tag{20}$$

Since M is a non-singular, positive definite, symmetric matrix, there exists a unique inverse and, therefore solutions exist for the coefficients α_k. Coefficients necessary for the determination of θ_j^* are obtained in the same manner.

Given values for θ_i^* and θ_j^*, they would be used instead of θ_i and θ_j for the determination of ρ and η in the usual manner.

EXPERIMENTAL

Materials and Methods

The experimental determination of an effective half-life will be illustrated with plasma concentration data from six studies of sulindac in healthy volunteers. Results on most of these have been reported elsewhere (3,7). The relevant parts of each are briefly as follows. In study A, 14 subjects received a single-dose (200 mg) of sulindac. Serial plasma samples were taken for 24 hours and urine samples for 96 hours. In study B, 12 subjects were given 200 mg of sulindac every 12 hours for ten days. Frequent plasma samples were taken from 0 to 12 hours after the first and the thirteenth dose. In studies C, D, E and F, 12 to 15 subjects in each study received 200 mg of sulindac every 12 hours for five days. Serial plasma samples were taken immediately before and for 12 hours after the morning dose on the sixth day. All plasma and urine samples were analyzed for sulindac and metabolite(s), but only sulindac concentrations will be used in this report.

The trapezoid approximation was used to calculate the area under the plasma concentration curve through 12 hours (AUC_{12}). Total areas after a single-dose (AUC_{∞}^l) were determined by Equation (5); i.e., the ratio of total urinary recovery to the individual renal clearance estimated from U_{12} and AUC_{12}^l.

Estimation Procedure

Equations (1), (3), (14) and (17) are the relevant expressions for the estimation of an effective half-life. Since the mean effective half-life is a function of the ratio of θ_j/θ_i, the quantities $AUC_{\tau}^j/AUC_{\tau}^i$ or $AUC_{\infty}^l/AUC_{\tau}^l$ in Equations (1) and (3) were used as sample estimates of the accumulation ratio ρ. The confidence limits for $t_{1/2,\eta}$ are those corresponding to the solutions for ρ from Equations (14) and (17). The best estimators of θ_i and θ_j are the arithmetic means of AUC_{τ}^i and AUC_{τ}^j, respectively. The best estimators of $V(\theta_i)$ and $V(\theta_j)$ depend on the sample variances s_i^2 and s_j^2. Under the assumption of homogeneity of variances, i.e.:

$$\sigma_i^2 = \sigma_j^2$$

the best linear unbiased pooled variances are:

$$s_p^2/N_i; \quad s_p^2/N_j$$

Tests of validity are applied to the raw data (i.e., AUC) for conformance to assumptions implicit in the construction of confidence limits. Normality is checked by the Wilk-Shapiro W-test (8). The method of Levene (9) is used to test homogeneity of variance in the independent case while that of Pitman (10) is used in the correlated case. Conservative statistical techniques have been proposed in situations when sample data do not conform. These include the consideration that:

$$s_i^2/N_i \text{ and } s_j^2/N_j \text{ are the best estimators of } V(\theta_i) \text{ and } V(\theta_j)$$

where:

$$\sigma_i^2 \neq \sigma_j^2$$

provided there is also an adjustment in the degrees of freedom (11, 12). Finally, the proposed procedures are uniformly robust to modest violations of the normality assumption.

RESULTS

Results from study A can be treated in two different ways. Individual estimates of η and, therefore, $t_{1/2,\eta}$ can be obtained with the aid of Equation (4). The mean and the confidence limits can be calculated directly. The results are summarized in Table I (Direct Method). Alternatively, the mean and confidence intervals can be estimated from the means of the individual AUC_{12}^1 and AUC_{∞}^1, with the recognition that θ_1 and θ_{∞} are correlated (Eq. (17)). For illustrative purposes only, these results are also shown in Table I under Indirect Method. Conceptually, the Direct Method is generally preferred in that it entails fewer assumptions, particularly when θ_i and θ_j appear to be highly correlated as in this case. A potential problem, which did not occur in this example, is when the individual ratios $AUC_{\infty}^1/AUC_{\tau}^1$ are unity within experimental error. Under these circumstances, the effective half-life is not necessarily zero ($\eta \simeq \infty$) as required by Equation (4). It simply means that the sample interval τ is too large and that no accumulation will occur. A shorter interval should have been chosen in order to obtain a valid estimation of $t_{1/2,\eta}$.

Results of study B are summarized in Table II. In theory, the Direct Method of estimation should be possible with the aid of Equation (1). However, given the stochastic nature of enterohepatic circulation, individual ratios of AUC_{12}^{13}/AUC_{12}^1 may be less than unity. This, in fact, occurred with one subject wherein $AUC_{12}^{13} = 22.4$ and $AUC_{12}^1 = 23.0$ µg-hr/ml. A negative accumulation in isolation has no physical meaning. On the other hand, by averaging the effects of accumulation among subjects (the same principle applies to multiple samples within a subject over time), the Indirect Method provides an overall estimate of the mean effective half-life wherein individual deviations are manifested in the observed confidence interval. Unlike the single-dose case, the

Table I. Estimates of effective half-life after a single dose of sulindac in man.

Variables or Parameters	Direct Method	Indirect Method
$N_i = N_j$	14	14
τ, hr	12	12
$\bar{\eta}$, hr^{-1}	0.122	--
SE $(\bar{\eta})$, hr^{-1}	0.0139	--
θ_i ($i = 1$), μg-hr-ml^{-1}	--	13.05
θ_j ($j = \infty$), μg-hr-ml^{-1}	--	19.91
s_i^2 ($i = 1$), μg^2-hr^2-ml^{-2}	--	16.63
s_j^2 ($j = \infty$), μg^2-hr^2-ml^{-2}	--	150.21
r_{ij}	--	0.833[b]
$F_{1,13}(0.05)$	--	4.67
$t_{1/2,\eta}$, hr[a]		
(C)	5.7	7.8
(L)	4.6	3.9
(H)	7.6	10.7
Tests of Validity		
Normality (8)	N.S.[c]	N.S.
Variability (10)	--	SIG.[d]

[a](C), (L) and (H) are the central value, and the lower and upper 95% confidence limits, respectively.
[b]Significantly different from zero, p. $\leqslant 0.05$.
[c]Not statistically significant, p > 0.05.
[d]Statistically significant, p $\leqslant 0.05$.

correlation coefficient r_{ij} is not significantly different from zero. Hence, the data could justifiably have been treated as in the Independent Case (vide infra) with a somewhat more favorable degree of freedom.

In the Independent Case, mean AUC_{12}^{11} from studies C, D, E and F are each compared with the mean AUC_{12}^{1} from study A. These results are summarized in Table III. The variability associated with θ_j from studies C, D, and E is significantly different from the variance associated with θ_i from study A. In each case, the determination of ν_2 is based on Welch's procedure (12). The downward adjustments in the degrees of freedom together with the uniformly high variability contribute to the length in the 95% confidence intervals. In some cases, the lower confidence limit for ρ is less than unity and, hence, no meaningful estimate of $t_{1/2,\eta}$ is given.

Finally, a joint estimate of the mean effective half-life is given in Table IV whereby a linear combination of θ_j from studies C, D, E and F is compared to that of θ_i from studies A and B. By pooling all of the data from the first and eleventh dosing intervals, the confidence limits associated with the overall mean effective half-life become much tighter, as expected.

DISCUSSION

The concept of an effective half-life evolves because there is a need for a practical solution to an experimentally difficult situation. The assumptions are that, on the average, drug will accumulate upon chronic usage and that the average rate of accumulation is approximately first-order. For best results, the choice of the dosage interval τ should be clinically relevant, while the sampling intervals i and j should be such as to maximize the difference between θ_i and θ_j.

Experimentally, equality between θ_i and θ_j signifies either that there is no accumulation or that both θ_j and θ_i represent estimates at steady state. On the other hand, both alternatives are compatible with the conclusion of a short effective half-life. Possible ambiguities can be avoided by judicious choices of τ, i and j.

The proposed strategy implicitly favors estimates of effective half-life that would primarily be accurate predictors of the extent of accumulation and only secondarily predictors of its time course. Thus, by maximizing the difference between θ_i and θ_j, effects of deviations from a monoexponential approach to steady state are minimized. In order to achieve a more accurate definition of the accumulation time course, additional sampling intervals should be

Table II. Estimates of effective half-life after multiple doses of sulindac[a].

Variables or Parameters	Study B
$N_i = N_j$	12
τ, hr	12
θ_i $(i = 1)$, μg-hr-ml^{-1}	13.54
θ_j $(j = 13)$, μg-hr-ml^{-1}	21.14
s_i^2 $(i = 1)$, μg^2-hr^2-ml^{-2}	18.78
s_j^2 $(j = 13)$, μg^2-hr^2-ml^{-2}	62.75
r_{ij}	0.181[c]
$F_{1,11}(0.05)$	4.84
$t_{1/2,n}$, hr[b]	
(C)	8.1
(L)	4.4
(H)	13.6
Tests of validity	
Normality (8)	N.S.[d]
Variability (10)	N.S.

[a]This study represents multiple doses of sulindac (200 mg every 12 hr) in the same subjects as in Table I.
[b](C), (L) and (H) are the central value, and the lower and upper 95% confidence limits, respectively.
[c]Not significantly different from zero, $p > 0.05$.
[d]Not statistically significant, $p > 0.05$.

Table III. Estimates of effective half-life after single and multiple doses of sulindac in different panels of subjects.

Variables or Parameters	Study				
	A	C	D	E	F
N_i	14	--	--	--	--
N_j	--	15	12	11	15
τ	12	12	12	12	12
θ_i $(i=1)$, $\mu g-hr^{-1}$	13.05	--	--	--	--
θ_j $(j=11)$, $\mu g-hr-ml^{-1}$	--	17.77	22.20	25.58	17.08
$s_i^2(i=1)$, $\mu g^2-hr^2-ml^{-2}$	16.63	--	--	--	--
$s_j^2(j=11)$, $\mu g^2-hr^2 ml^{-2}$	--	64.28	155.71	111.71	32.82
$F_{1,\nu_2(0.05)}$	--	4.32[a]	4.67[b]	4.75[c]	4.21[d]
$t_{1/2,\eta}$, hr[e]					
(C)	--	6.2	9.4	11.7	5.8
(L)	--	N.E.[f]	3.1	6.4	N.E.
(H)	--	10.4	15.9	18.0	10.3

Tests of Validity					
Normality	N.S.[g]	N.S.	N.S.	N.S.	N.S.
Variability	--	SIG[h]	SIG	SIG	N S.

[a] $\nu_2 = 21$;
[b] $\nu_2 = 13$;
[c] $\nu_2 = 12$;
[d] $\nu_2 = 27$.
[e] (C), (L), and (H) are the central value, and the lower and upper 95% confidence limits, respectively.
[f] No estimate ($\eta < 0$).
[g] Not statistically significant, $p > 0.05$.
[h] Statistically significant, $p \leq 0.05$.

Table IV. Joint estimation of effective half-life after single and multiple doses of sulindac in different panels of subjects.

Variables or Parameters	Study					
	A (i = 1)	B	C	D (j = 11)	E	F
N	15	14	12	15	12	11
θ, μ-hr-ml^{-1}	13.05	13.54	17.77	22.20	22.58	17.08
$V(\theta)$, μg^2-hr^2-ml^{-2}	1.19	1.56	4.29	12.98	10.16	3.16
$\theta*$, μg-hr-ml^{-1}	13.26			19.01		
$V(\theta*)$, μg^2-hr^2-ml^{-2}	0.675			1.385		
$F_{1,40}(0.05)$			4.08			
$t_{1/2,\eta}$, hr^a						
(C)			7.0			
(L)			4.6			
(H)			9.5			
Tests of Validity						
Normality (8)	N.S.^{b}			N.S.		
Variability (9)			SIG^c			

^{a}(C), (L) and (H) are the central value, and the lower and upper 95% confidence limits, respectively.
^{b}Not statistically significant, $p > 0.05$.
^{c}Statistically significant, $p < 0.05$.

included at intermediate times. The repeated application of Equation (1) should then result in estimates of the instantaneous rate of accumulation between contiguous sampling intervals.

The experimental determination of $t_{1/2,\eta}$ is not restricted to regimens where the same dose is administered at constant intervals. As long as linear kinetics prevail, estimates of η are possible from the observed area ratio for any two dosing intervals. The right-hand side of Equation (1) can be modified to accommodate any known regimen (13). An example involving unequal dosing intervals has been reported (2).

Finally, the concept of an effective half-life and the techniques for its determination should apply even to drugs that do not undergo enterohepatic circulation. Random variations in drug absorption and disposition and random deviations in the precise timing of a prescribed regimen tend to have a similar effect on the experimental attainment of a steady state. In essence, the effective half-life is a pharmacokinetic parameter that reflects the average tendency for a drug to accumulate. In this context, it serves the same purpose as the mean of half-lives estimated in the usual way. Differences in technique are born mainly out of necessity.

Acknowledgement. We thank Mr. N. Tonkonoh for providing most of the statistical computations.

REFERENCES

1. K.C. Kwan, G.O. Breault, E.R. Umbenhauer, F.G. McMahon and D.E. Duggan, Kinetics of indomethacin absorption, elimination, and enterohepatic circulation in man, J. Pharmacokin. Biopharm. 4:255-280 (1976).
2. K.C. Kwan, G.O. Breault, R.L. Davis, B.W. Lei, A.W. Czerwinski, G.H. Besselaar and D.E. Duggan, Effects of concomitant aspirin administration on the pharmacokinetics of indomethacin in man, J. Pharmacokin. Biopharm. 6:451-476 (1978).
3. K.C. Kwan and D.E. Duggan, Pharmacokinetics of sulindac, Acta Rheum. Belg. 1:168-178 (1977).
4. J.G. Wagner, J.I. Northam, C.D. Alway and D.S. Carpenter, Blood levels of drug at equilibrium state after multiple dosing, Nature 207:1301-1302 (1965).
5. J.M. van Rossum and A.H.M. Tomey, Rate of accumulation and plateau plasma concentrations of drug after chronic medication, J. Pharm. Pharmacol. 20:390-392 (1968).
6. J.M. van Rossum, Pharmacokinetics of accumulation, J. Pharm. Sci. 57:2162-2165 (1968).
7. D.E. Duggan, L.E. Hall, C.A. Ditzler, B.W. Lei and K.C. Kwan, The disposition of sulindac, Clin. Pharmacol. Ther. 21:326-335 (1977).
8. M.B. Wilk and S.S. Shapiro, The joint assessment of normality for several independent samples, Technometrics 10:825-839 (1968).

9. H. Levene, Robust tests for equality of variances, in: "Contributions to Probability and Statistics, Essays in Honor of Harold Hotelling," I. Olkin, S. Ghuaye, W. Hoeffding, W. Madow and H. Mann, eds., Stanford University Press, Stanford (1960), pp. 278-292.

10. E.J.G. Pitman, Test of homogeneity of two correlated variances, Biometrika 31:9-14 (1939).

11. W.G. Cochran, Testing a linear relationship among variances, Biometrics 7:17-32 (1951).

12. B.L. Welch, The generalization of Student's problem when several different populations are involved, Biometrika 37:28-35 (1947).

13. K.C. Yeh and K.C. Kwan, Bioavailability assessment under quasi- and nonsteady-state conditions II: Study designs, J. Pharm. Sci. 65:512-517 (1976).

Chapter 15

PHARMACOKINETIC ASPECTS OF NONLINEAR DRUG—PROTEIN BINDING

Milo Gibaldi

School of Pharmacy
University of Washington
Seattle, Washington

I have lived on the West Coast for about four years now and I have come to know what laid-back means. Although Sid Riegelman spent most of his professional career in the West, no one could ever accuse him of being laid-back. There are few if any among us who could match Sid in terms of unbounded energy, enthusiasm and intensity. Yet I know very well that occasionally Sid would stop to smell the flowers. From time to time, by note, or telephone or a tap on the shoulder Sid would tell me how much he enjoyed a particular paper or bit of work. The first time this occurred was many years ago. It concerned some studies on the role of bile salts in the dissolution of drugs in the gastrointestinal tract. The comment, the praise, were profoundly important; young assistant professors are not known for their high level of confidence. The last time this occurred was but a little while ago and it concerned some research we were doing in Buffalo on the consequences of nonlinear plasma protein binding. I have chosen to review this work, mostly because Sid thought it was very nice.

We have learned a great deal about plasma protein binding over the past decade. We now know that albumin is not the only important binding protein in plasma; we recognize that α_1-acid glycoprotein plays an important role in the binding of certain drugs, particularly basic compounds. We have an excellent fundamental understanding of the effect of plasma protein binding on drug kinetics and dynamics. The clearance of drugs with low extraction ratios is directly proportional to the fraction unbound in the plasma, whereas the clearance of drugs that are eliminated by a blood flow rate-limited process is rather independent of binding. Changes in free fraction of drugs with low extraction ratios may not provoke clinical consequences because they have no

163

effect on the steady-state concentration of unbound or free drug. On the other hand, there is a theoretical concern that displacement of high extraction ratio drugs from plasma protein binding sites will lead to elevated free drug concentrations at steady state and adverse effects.

Despite the progress in this area of pharmacokinetics, we have made little headway in understanding the consequences of nonlinear plasma protein binding. Nonlinear binding is observed after administration of therapeutic doses of certain drugs and commonly observed after overdoses of many drugs. Gerhard Levy, Patrick McNamara and I were mulling over this problem for a time and decided to study it in more detail. We were particularly interested in the effects of nonlinear binding on the time course of drug in plasma. The first theoretical treatment of this problem was presented by Kruger-Thiemer (1) in 1965. He concluded that the log concentration-time plot after bolus intravenous injection of a drug that rapidly distributed in the body (gave rise to a one-compartment model), but showed nonlinear plasma protein binding, would be concave and thereby resemble the concentration-time curve of a drug with multicompartment characteristics. However, a little later that year Martin (2) published a rather persuasive analysis of the same problem but concluded that the log concentration-time plot would be convex and thereby resemble the concentration-time curve of a drug that is eliminated by Michaelis-Menten kinetics.

Since this puzzlement had existed for more than a dozen years, we decided to investigate, by computer simulations, the effects of concentration-dependent plasma protein binding (with or without tissue binding) on the time course of free and total drug concentrations in plasma.

METHODS

Simulations were based on a model (Fig. 1) consisting of two physiological spaces. This model permits instantaneous distribution but preserves two distinct regions with different drug binding characteristics. The concentration-dependence of plasma protein binding was defined by the usual equation:

$$C_t = C_f + BPC_f/(K_d + C_f) \tag{1}$$

where C_t is the concentration of total drug in plasma, C_f is the concentration of free drug in plasma, B is the maximum binding capacity of plasma protein, P is the concentration of protein in plasma, and K_d is the dissociation constant of the drug-protein complex. The same type of equation was used to define concentration-dependent tissue binding. Linear plasma protein binding was defined by the equation:

$$C_t = sC_f \tag{2}$$

where s is the reciprocal of the free fraction in plasma. Linear tissue binding was defined by the equation:

$$C_t^T = rC_f \tag{3}$$

where C_t^T is the total drug concentration in the tissues and r is the reciprocal of the free fraction in tissues. Drug elimination was assumed to be proportional to either free drug concentration (simulating the case for a drug with a low extraction ratio) or total drug concentration (simulating the case for a drug with a very high extraction ratio).

Digital computer simulations of C_t and C_f were made with the MIMIC program (3) using differential equations that relate the change in drug concentration to the variables in the preceding equations (4). Since the apparent volume of distribution was concentration-dependent and therefore changed with time after drug administration, the instantaneous apparent volume of distribution (V) was determined from the relationship (5):

$$V = V_p + (f_p/f_T) (V_T) \tag{4}$$

where $f_p = C_f/C_t$, $f_T = C_f/C_t^T$, V_p is the volume of the vascular space and V_T is the volume of the extravascular space.

RESULTS AND DISCUSSION

Figure 2 shows simulations for drugs that have no tissue binding. The simulation shown in the left panel is for a drug that is extensively plasma protein bound and covers an f_p range from 0.05, initially, to 0.01. The simulation shown in the right panel is for

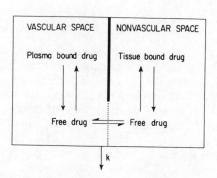

Figure 1. Pharmacokinetic model illustrating binding, distribution and elimination. Reprinted from (4), with permission.

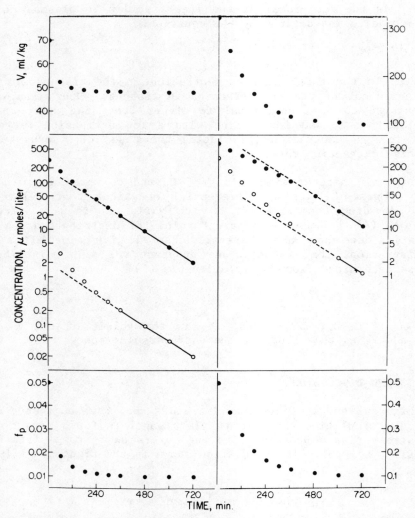

Figure 2. Effect of concentration-dependent plasma protein binding
with no tissue binding on the time course of free (open
circles) and total (filled circles) drug concentrations
in plasma. Also shown in this and the following figures
are instantaneous volume of distribution (V), the free
fraction in plasma (f_p), and, where appropriate, the
free fraction in tissue (f_T). The left panel shows
simulations for a high ratio of B to K_d whereas the
right panel applies to a low ratio. Reprinted from (4),
with permission.

a less extensively bound drug and covers an f_p range from 0.5 to
0.1. To span these respective ranges it was necessary to use
different doses in the two simulations. Concave log concentration-
time plots for both free and total drug were obtained when plasma
protein binding was extensive and, more specifically, when the
ratio of B/K_d in Equation (1) was high. As already noted, these
curves can be described quite well by a biexponential equation. On
the other hand, consistent with the findings of Martin (2), we also
found that log total concentration-time plots can be convex,
although the log C_f versus time curve is concave. This occurs when
the ratio of B/K_d is low. Kruger-Thiemer did not observe this
phenomenon because he used identical doses in his simulations.
Since his simulation of the potentially convex system was carried
out under conditions in which f_p had almost reached its limiting
value and was practically constant, he obtained only concave and
linear plots.

It is informative to compare the relative change of V and f_p
in the two sets of simulations shown in Figure 2. Considering only
the effect of f_p on the elimination rate (elimination rate being
proportional to the product of f_p and C_t), the slope of the log
concentration-time curve should decrease continuously with time
until f_p reaches a limiting value. However, f_p also affects V,
causing the latter to decrease with time until f_p reaches a limiting value. As a consequence of this effect, log concentration-time
plots will tend to be convex. It was found empirically that when
the ratio B to K_d is high the effect of changes in f_p on elimination rate predominates and when that ratio is low the effect of f_p
on V predominates. This is independent of the absolute values of
B, P, K_d, or k, according to our simulations. It should be noted
that both sets of simulations in Figure 2 involve a fivefold change
in f_p but that V decreased only by one-third in one case (concave
curve) and by about two-thirds in the other (convex curve).

In the next set of simulations (Fig. 3), we have examined the
effect of linear tissue binding on the time course of plasma
concentrations under conditions which, in the absence of tissue
binding, would result in a concave log concentration-time plot.
Thus, we have used the same plasma protein binding parameters as
were employed for the simulation shown in the left panel of
Figure 2. Relatively moderate tissue binding ($f_T = 0.5$) causes the
concavity of the log C_t versus time plot to almost disappear while
the log C_f versus time plot remains concave (Fig. 3, left panel).
When tissue binding is extensive ($f_T = 0.1$), the log C_t versus time
curve becomes convex and the log C_f versus time plot is less
concave (Fig. 3, right panel). Thus, linear tissue binding tends
to straighten the otherwise concave log concentration-time curves
resulting from nonlinear plasma protein binding. Tissue binding
may be largely responsible for the absence of significant curvature

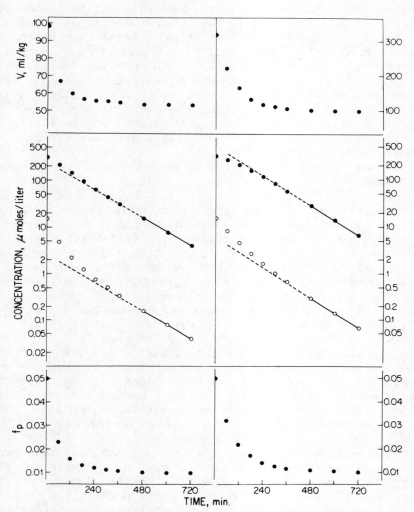

Figure 3. Effect of concentration–dependent plasma protein binding
on the time course of free (open circles) and total
(filled circles) drug concentrations in plasma.   Both
panels show simulations based on a high B/K_d value but
the one on the left has a constant tissue free fraction
of 0.5, whereas $f_T = 0.1$ for the panel on the right.
Reprinted from (4), with permission.

in log concentration-time plots of drugs with nonlinear plasma protein binding under clinical conditions.

The effect of nonlinear tissue binding on the elimination kinetics of a drug is examined in the simulations shown in Figure 4. The left panel illustrates a case of linear plasma protein binding (f_p = 0.1), while the right panel is a case of identical concentration-dependence for plasma protein and tissue binding, resulting in a concentration-independent V. As already shown by Wagner (6), nonlinear tissue binding causes concave log concentration-time plots. This concavity in the case of a concentration-independent V (Fig. 4, right panel) is a reflection of the direct relationship between f_p and elimination rate.

Finally, we have considered the special case of nonlinear plasma protein binding and linear tissue binding for a drug whose elimination rate is proportional to total, rather than free, drug concentration in plasma. This situation could occur if the drug is almost completely extracted from the blood in one pass through the liver, kidneys or other eliminating organs. Semilogarithmic plots of both free and total concentrations versus time are convex under the conditions used for this simulation (Fig. 5). This will always be the case because changes in f_p with concentration will affect the volume of distribution but not the elimination rate.

Nonlinear binding presents us with very complicated situations. Drugs with nonlinear plasma protein binding may be incorrectly assigned multicompartment characteristics even though rapid distribution occurs, or may be erroneously assumed to show Michaelis-Menten elimination even though the clearance of unbound drug is independent of dose. Out of this confusion arises one clear message: multicompartment pharmacokinetic analysis of data based on curve-fits of the time course of drug concentration in the plasma may be easily misinterpreted. Our findings provide a strong impetus for the further development of noncompartmental methods of analysis.

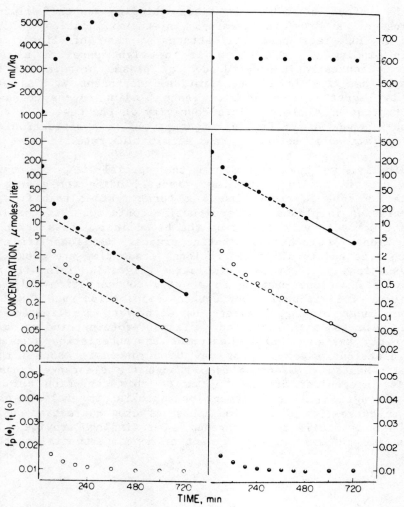

Figure 4. Effect of linear or concentration-dependent plasma
protein binding and concentration-dependent tissue
binding on the time course of free (open circles) and
total (filled circles) drug concentrations in plasma.
In the panel on the left, f_p = 0.1 and tissue binding is
nonlinear. In the panel on the right, both plasma and
tissue binding are nonlinear but BP = c and $K_d = K_d^T$.
Reprinted from (4), with permission.

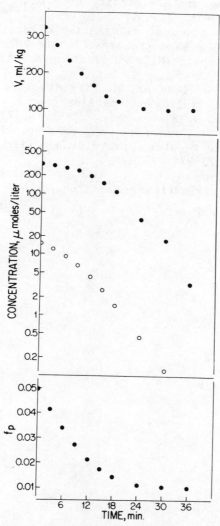

Figure 5. Effect of concentration-dependent plasma protein binding
and linear tissue binding (f_T = 0.1) on the time course
of free (open circles) and total (filled circles) drug
concentrations in plasma. A high value of B/K_d was used
and elimination was assumed to be proportional to C_t.
Reprinted from (4), with permission.

REFERENCES

1. E. Kruger-Thiemer, W. Diller and P. Bunger, Pharmacokinetic models regarding protein binding of drugs, Antimicrob. Agents Chemother. 5:183-191 (1965).
2. B.K. Martin, Kinetics of elimination of drugs possessing high affinity for the plasma proteins, Nature 207:959-960 (1965).
3. Control Data Corp., MIMIC, Publication No. 44610400, St. Paul, Minn. (1968).
4. P.J. McNamara, G. Levy and M. Gibaldi, Effect of plasma protein and tissue binding on the time course of drug concentrations in plasma, J. Pharmacokin. Biopharm. 7:195-206 (1979).
5. M. Gibaldi and P.J. McNamara, Apparent volumes of distribution and drug binding to plasma proteins and tissues, Eur. J. Clin. Pharmacol. 13:373-378 (1978).
6. J.G. Wagner, "Fundamentals of Clinical Pharmacokinetics," Drug Intelligence Publications, Hamilton, Ill., (1971), pp. 270-283.

Chapter 16

UNUSUAL PHARMACOKINETICS

John G. Wagner

College of Pharmacy and
Upjohn Center for Clinical Pharmacology
University of Michigan
Ann Arbor, Michigan

This chapter covers several items which are related only in that they are unusual; that explains the title. Two of these involve absorption kinetics, while the others involve disposition.

UNUSUAL ABSORPTION KINETICS

Penicillamine

Penicillamine or D-3-mercaptovaline is the most characteristic degradation product of the penicillin type antibiotics. It has been used as a medicinal agent since 1954 and recently has been shown to be effective for the treatment of rheumatoid arthritis. We have been studying the pharmacokinetics of penicillamine in both normal volunteers and in patients with rheumatoid arthritis for the past three years. To assay the compound in biological fluids, we use an HPLC cationic ion-exchange method with electrochemical detection (1). The drug is unusual in that it reacts with albumin, presumably forming covalent (-S-S-) bonds, and we have studied the kinetics of this reaction (2). To obtain appropriate pharmacokinetic data, we precipitate the plasma proteins as soon as the blood is withdrawn from the subject in order to terminate the albumin-penicillamine reaction.

Figure 1 shows penicillamine plasma concentration-time plots for subject M.V. following oral doses of 250, 500, 750 and 1000 mg of penicillamine. These data show representative examples of the double peaks we have observed on the ascending portions of plasma concentration-time plots (3). We have also observed that although

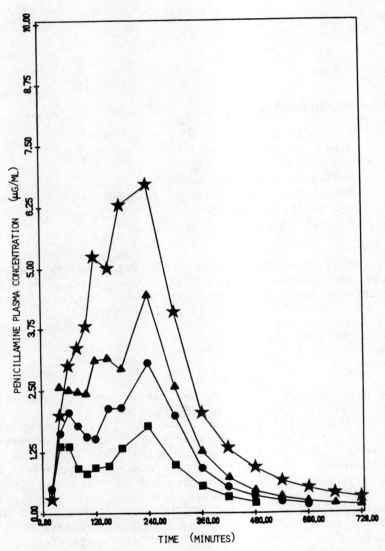

Figure 1. Penicillamine plasma concentrations after oral doses of 250 (squares), 500 (circles), 750 (triangles) and 1000 mg (asterisks) of the drug to fasting subject M.V. Reprinted from (3), with permission from Clinical Pharmacology and Therapeutics.

the times at which such double peaks occur vary from subject to subject, the times are relatively constant within the same subject. Such double peaks are readily explained by postulating two different absorption sites in the gastrointestinal tract. Simulations carried out with the model shown in Scheme I demonstrate that the double peaks and time courses may be represented by this model.

Theophylline

Plasma concentrations of theophylline were reported by Weinberger et al. (4) following intravenous infusion of theophylline (as aminophylline) over a 0.5 hr period, oral administration of an elixir, and oral administration of various sustained action formulations including Theo-Dur® (300 mg tablets). I have applied the Wagner-Nelson absorption equation (see reference 5) to the plasma concentration-time data following oral administration of the latter tablets, and obtained linear plots. I believe that Dr. Riegelman was the first person to report zero-order absorption with this particular dosage form, hence it is fitting for it to be described here.

In order to justify and validate the zero-order absorption interpretation, it is desirable to show that theophylline is essentially a one-compartment open model drug. To do this I chose to fit the post-infusion data of Weinberger et al. (4) with poly-exponential equations. There were data from seven subjects. Two of these required only one exponential term, four required two exponential terms and one required three exponential terms. The coefficients of these equations were corrected to those corresponding to a bolus intravenous injection (6). The coefficients and exponents of these latter equations were used in two ways to establish the essentially one-compartment character of theophylline. The biexponential equations may be written as:

$$C = A_1 e^{-\lambda_1 t} + A_2 e^{-\lambda_2 t}$$

$$(1)$$

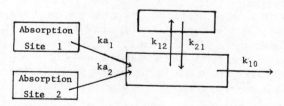

Scheme I. Model which can account for double peaks on the ascending portions of plasma concentration-time curves following oral administration of penicillamine.

The percent contribution of the λ_1 phase equals:

$$\frac{A_1/\lambda_1}{A_1/\lambda_1 + A_2/\lambda_2} \cdot 100 \tag{2}$$

Application of Equation (2) to the data for the four subjects and fitting to Equation (1) gave λ_1 phase contributions of only 0.3, 0.3, 6.6 and 2.8% (average 2.5%).

It may be readily shown that the percent error in the clearance (CL) and the volume of distribution (V) when the system is multicompartmental, but is treated as a one-compartment open model, is given by Equations (3A), (3B) and (3C):

$$\text{percent error in CL or V} = 100 \ [\frac{V_{ext}}{V} - 1] \tag{3A}$$

$$= 100 \ [\frac{\lambda_z (AUC_{0 \to \infty})}{A_z}] \tag{3B}$$

$$= 100 \ [\frac{\lambda_z}{A_z} \sum_{i=1}^{n} (A_i/\lambda_i)] \tag{3C}$$

where the terminal data are described by:

$$C = A_z e^{-\lambda_z t}$$

and:

$$V = CL/\lambda_z$$

$$V_{ext} = D/A_z$$

Equations (3A) and (3B) apply to both intravenous and oral data since bioavailability (FF*) cancels out in the ratio of volumes in Equation (3A); thus, $V_{ext}/FF*/V/FF* = V_{ext}/V$. When Equations (3A)-(3C) were applied to the seven theophylline polyexponential equations the error in CL or V was 0.4, 0.7, 0, 7.1, 0, 2.8 and 1.0% (average 1.7%). Thus, as a result of the very low percentage values given by both Equations (2) and (3A)-(3C) with theophylline intravenous data, one can conclude that theophylline is essentially a one-compartment open model drug.

Weinberger et al. (4) reported data on five subjects, each given one tablet of Theo-Dur® (300 mg, lot 6806). The Wagner-Nelson plots obtained from the plasma theophylline concentration-

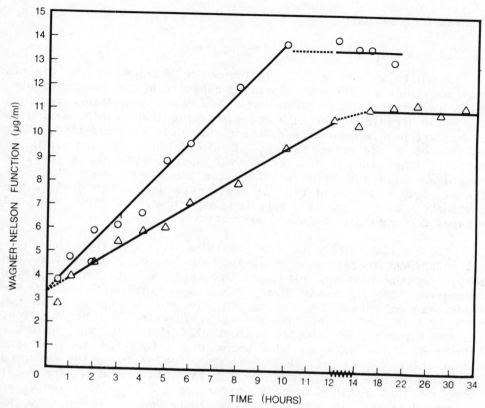

Figure 2. Plots of the Wagner-Nelson function $[C_T + k_e \int_0^T Cdt]$ versus time following single oral doses of theophylline as Theo-Dur® tablets, 300 mg to two subjects.

time data for two representative subjects are shown in Figure 2. These illustrate that absorption was <u>zero-order for the entire release period</u>, which was 10 hours for subject 3 (circles) and 12 hours for subject 2 (diamonds). The analysis of the data from five subjects in this group yielded an average zero time intercept of 2.43 µg/ml with a coefficient of variation (CV) of 37.7%. The average slope was 1.08 µg/ml/hr with a CV of 44.2% and the average asymptote was 11.9 µg/ml with a CV of 12.6%. The unusual nature of this data is that the absorption plot is linear over its entire length, and not for just a portion of the release, as has been observed with some other sustained release dosage forms. A considerable body of additional data, evaluated by the same method, yielded very similar results.

UNUSUAL DISPOSITION

<u>Digoxin</u>

Recently we reported (7) evidence of nonlinearity in digoxin pharmacokinetics. This is suprising considering the extent of previous investigations on this drug. Six normal volunteers received 0.5 mg of digoxin either as a bolus injection over 2 min, in 240 ml of 5% dextrose infused at a constant rate over a 1 hr period, or in 360 ml of 5% dextrose infused at a constant rate over a 3 hr period. The study had a cross-over design with all 6 possible treatment sequences being utilized for the 6 subjects. The same lot of ampules was used for all treatments and, after dosing, the residual solution in the infusion apparatus was blown out and assayed for digoxin, and the dose corrected.

The unusual nature of the resulting data was that the dose-corrected AUC increased with an increased rate of input into the body, and the nonrenal clearance increased as the rate of input decreased. The important averages are summarized in Table I. The dose-corrected areas per 0.5 mg digoxin, shown in the first two rows, are in the order: bolus > 1 hr infusion > 3 hr infusion. The AUC for the 3 hr infusion was only 72% of the AUC for the bolus injection. The AUC for the bolus was calculated in the most conservative manner possible by using the (0,0) point and the plasma concentration at 10 min as the first two points. The total clearance (CL) and the nonrenal clearance (CL-CL_R) both increased as the duration of administration increased. There were no significant differences amongst the mean renal clearances for the three intravenous treatments.

It is unlikely that the results were caused by the nonspecificity of the digoxin radioimmunoassay employed (8). This assay is sensitive to 0.05 ng/ml, and allows the digoxin concentrations to be measured for 99 hours after dosing. We have also developed a specific assay for digoxin employing HPLC separation and collection of the digoxin fraction followed by radioimmunoassay (9). Results on randomly selected samples of plasma and urine using this specific assay did not differ significantly from results obtained with the direct RIA (8), <u>in these normal volunteers</u>. However, in another study we carried out in adult cardiac patients with impaired renal function, the specific assay results were lower than those obtained by the conventional direct RIA procedure.

The nature of the results obtained in this study in which digoxin was administered intravenously at three different rates strongly suggests nonlinear pharmacokinetics and, specifically, some type of saturation phenomenon in the liver.

Table I. Summary of the average pharmacokinetic parameters for digoxin[a].

Parameter	Bolus i.v.	1-Hr Infusion	3-Hr Infusion
Dose-corrected AUC_{0-96} per 0.5 mg digoxin (ng/ml · hr)	32.85[b]	26.85	23.75
Dose-corrected $AUC_{0-\infty}$ per 0.5 mg digoxin (ng/ml · hr)	35.5	30.20	25.80
Percent of dose excreted in urine in 6 days	67.5	50.0	57.9
Percent of dose excreted in urine $0-\infty$	68.9	51.7	58.8
CL (ml/min)	239	300	366
CL_R (ml/min)	164	157	215
$CL - CL_R$ (ml/min)	75	143	151
Elimination rate constant (hr^{-1})	0.0252	0.0263	0.0313
V (L)	580	690	716

[a]Data from reference 7.
[b]There were significant differences amongst the underlined means in the same row when data were analyzed by analysis of variance for cross-over design.

Pentobarbital-Dexamethasone

Recently we reported profound effects of dexamethasone in normalizing the pharmacokinetics of pentobarbital in cats with acute focal cerebral ischemia induced by ligation of the left middle cerebral artery (LMCA) (10). Cats were assigned to one of three groups as follows: Group I underwent a sham operation with sodium pentobarbital administration; the LMCA in these cats was exposed but ligation was omitted; in Group II acute cerebral ischemia was produced by surgical ligation of the LMCA and sodium pentobarbital was administered; in Group III LMCA ligation was completed as for Group II, but 4 mg/kg dexamethasone was administered intravenously prior to the production of the stroke and every 6 hr for the 24-hr experimental period. Sodium pentobarbital was administered as for Groups I and II. It was known from previous work that pentobarbital was effective in reducing brain necrosis when administered 2 hr after the onset of ischemic stroke in cats, and that cats subjected to LMCA occlusion remained anesthetized much longer with pentobarbital anesthesia than cats given the same dose of pentobarbital but not subjected to LMCA occlusion. Figure 3 is a semi-logarithmic plot of plasma pentobarbital concentration versus time in selected representative cats from each of the experimental groups.

The numerical values of the pharmacokinetic parameters are summarized in Table II. Comparison of the averages in the first two rows in the top part of the table indicates that stroke had the effect of increasing the AUC and decreasing the clearance, elimination rate constant and volume of distribution of pentobarbital. The mean clearance decreased from 1.2 to 0.46 ml/min/kg, a decrease of 62%. The mean elimination rate constant decreased from 0.0596 to 0.0290, a decrease of 51%. The mean volume of distribution decreased from 1.22 to 0.955 L/kg, a decrease of 22%. Administration of dexamethasone prior to ligation (Group III) had the effect of essentially normalizing the pentobarbital pharmacokinetic parameters except that it did not totally correct the decrease in the volume of distribution of pentobarbital produced by the stroke. It is probable that dexamethasone acts by preventing the deleterious circulatory changes which may occur secondary to the combined effects of ischemic stroke and high dose pentobarbital treatment.

Bretylium Tosylate

This compound has the structure shown in Scheme II. It is a quaternary ammonium compound which exerts marked antifibrillatory effects. It is also an adrenergic blocking and antihypertensive agent. It was released in 1978 for life-threatening ventricular arrhythmias that failed to respond to conventional therapy. A group

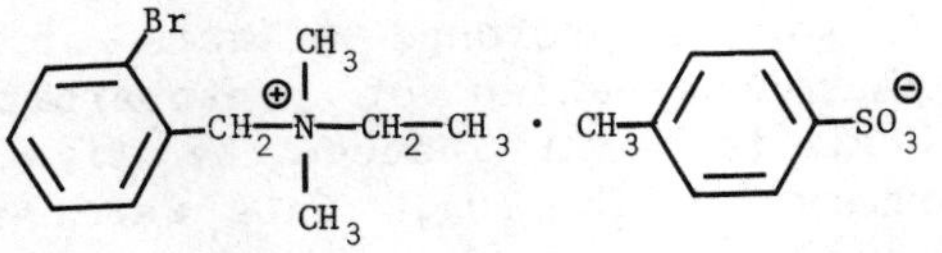

Scheme II. Structure of bretylium tosylate.

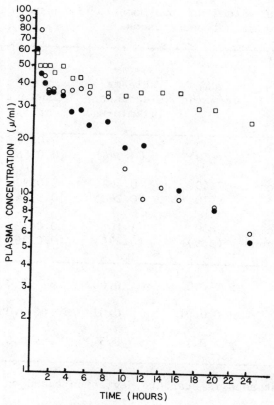

Figure 3. Semilogarithmic plot of pentobarbital plasma concentrations versus time in selected representative cats from
each of the three experimental groups: normals, group I
(filled circles); stroke and dexamethasone, group III
(open circles); stroke only, group II (squares).
Reprinted from (3) with permission.

at the University of Michigan has studied the pharmacokinetics of
this drug both in normal volunteers (11) and in survivors of
ventricular tachycardia or fibrillation (12).

We first studied the pharmacokinetics of bretylium tosylate in
normal volunteers. Each volunteer was administered a dose of
5 mg/kg by constant rate intravenous infusion in 5% dextrose over
0.5 hr and an oral dose of 5 mg/kg in solution in orange juice.
Treatments were given randomly. Blood was sampled and urine
collected over a 48 hr period. Unchanged drug was assayed using a
gas chromatographic method. Pharmacokinetic parameters were
estimated from individual subject data in the usual manner except
oral bioavailability (F_{po}) was calculated with Equation (4) after

Table II. Mean values of pharmacokinetic parameters for pento-barbital and statistical comparisons.

Group	AUC µg/ml·hr	Plasma Clearance (ml/min·kg)	Elimination Rate Constant (hr^{-1})	Volume of Distribution (L/kg)
I. Control	536 (50)[a]	1.20 (0.244)	0.0596 (0.0156)	1.22 (0.0830)
II. Stroke alone	2140 (910)	0.462 (0.260)	0.0290 (0.0126)	0.955 (0.244)
III. Stroke and dexamethasone	850 (369)	1.10 (0.435)	0.0682 (0.0336)	1.02 (0.157)
I and II	p < 0.01	p < 0.002	p < 0.01	p < 0.05
II and III	p < 0.01	p < 0.01	p < 0.05	p > 0.5
I and III	p > 0.1	p > 0.5	p > 0.5	p < 0.05

[a]Value in parentheses is standard deviation based on 6 cats.

Kwan and Till (13), which takes into account changing renal clearance, and the fraction of unchanged drug excreted in the urine (f) was calculated with Equation (5). In Equations (4) and (5):

$$F_{po} = \frac{D_{iv}(AUC)_{po}}{D_{po}(AUC)_{iv}} - \frac{[CL_R^{iv} - CL_R^{po}]}{D_{po}} \tag{4}$$

$$f = CL_R/CL \tag{5}$$

D_{iv} and D_{po} are the intravenous and oral doses, respectively, $(AUC)_{iv}$ and $(AUC)_{po}$ are the areas under the intravenous and oral serum concentration-time curves from zero to infinite time, CL_R^{iv} and CL_R^{po} are the renal clearances of bretylium tosylate following intravenous and oral administration, respectively, and CL is the total clearance.

The results are summarized in Table III. There were two unusual aspects. First, the drug is apparently not metabolized at

Table III. Summary of pharmacokinetic parameters of bretylium tosylate in ten normal volunteers.

Parameter	Mean	CV (%)	Range
Bioavailability (%)	22.6	40.2	11.6–36.6
f	1.01	8.7	0.88–1.19
CL^{iv} (ml/min)	299	31.9	160–475
CL_R^{iv} (ml/min)	300	27.8	163–417
CL_R^{po} (ml/min)	1,268	54.8	599–2642
V_{ss} (L/kg)	3.37	30.5	2.21–5.11
V (L/kg)	5.34	36.6	2.59–7.77
λ_z^{iv} (hr^{-1})	0.0510	12.8	0.0438–0.0638
λ_z^{po} (hr^{-1})	0.115	52.7	0.0367–0.199

all since, after intravenous administration, the total clearance was the same as the renal clearance ($CL^{iv} = CL_R^{iv}$). The coefficient of variation calculated from these paired values was only 6.9% and the ratio (Eq. (5)) averaged 1.01 with a coefficient of variation of only 8.4%. Secondly, both the renal clearance (CL_R^{po}) and elimination rate constant (λ_z^{po}), following oral administration were appreciably larger than the corresponding values after intravenous administration. Apparently the much higher concentrations attained after intravenous versus oral administration had an effect on the kidneys.

To evaluate drug efficacy and pharmacokinetics, we later studied 12 patients who were administered intravenous bretylium tosylate and/or who received chronic oral maintenance bretylium (12). The mean elimination rate constant in 7 patients who received intravenous drug was 0.0515 hr^{-1}, which did not differ significantly from the mean of 0.0510 hr^{-1} in normal volunteers (Table III). The mean value of f was 0.98 which did not differ significantly from the mean value of 1.01 obtained in normal volunteers (Table III). In seven patients chronically dosed with oral bretylium, minimum steady-state bretylium serum concentrations were measured (observed values), and also predicted, using Equation (6) and the mean population parameter values of the normal volunteers:

$$C_{ss}^{min} = \frac{F_{po} D_{po}}{V} \cdot \frac{\exp(-\lambda_z^{po}\tau)}{1-\exp(-\lambda_z^{po}\tau)} \tag{6}$$

shown in Table III. Predicted C_{ss}^{min} values were also estimated by an equation similar to Equation (6) except the mean λ_z^{iv} value of 0.0510 hr^{-1} replaced the λ_z^{po} mean value of 0.115 hr^{-1}. The results are summarized in Table IV.

The results support the concept that, to accurately predict the minimum steady-state bretylium serum concentration during oral therapy, one must use the apparent elimination rate constant for oral administration and not the one observed after intravenous administration. The standard deviation calculated from the paired observations in columns 5 and 6 of Table IV was 42 ng/ml, whereas the standard deviation calculated from values in columns 5 and 7 was 357 ng/ml. Linear least squares regression of the predicted C_{ss}^{min} values in column 6 with observed C_{ss}^{min} values in column 5 gave a slope of 1.12 and a correlation coefficient of 0.936.

Reversible Metabolism

Several examples of reversible metabolism have been reported in the literature. Examples given are the cortisone-cortisol and

Table IV. Predicted and observed minimum steady-state serum bretylium concentrations during oral therapy.

| | | | | | C_{ss}^{min} (ng/ml) | |
| | Creatinine | | | | Predicted | Predicted |
Pt	Clearance (ml/min)	Dose[a] (mg)	τ (hr)	Observed	(λ_z^{po}=0.115)	(λ_z^{iv}=0.0510)
6	86	416	8	105	173	518
7	82	104	6	140	66	182
8	104	208	8	72	87	260
9	35	312	6	159	200	547
10	57	416	6	170	264	728
11	33	312	6	196	200	547
12	70	832	6	461	533	1456

[a]Bretylium base equal to 0.52 x dose of bretylium tosylate given at intervals of τ hours.

prednisone-prednisolone pairs (14). The pharmacokinetic models for these systems look like the classical two-compartment open models but actually are quite different (Scheme III and Table V). In the classical models the two compartments contain the same entity, namely the drug. In cases of reversible metabolism, compartment 1 refers to the drug and compartment 2 refers to the metabolite. The symbolism is a bit more complicated too. The subscript on AUC refers to the compound measured in plasma, while the superscript refers to the compound that was administered. Thus, AUC_2^2 means the area under the metabolite concentration-time curve when the metabolite was administered. In such models we have to worry about six different clearances which may be symbolized by CL_{10}, CL_{20}, CL_{12}, CL_{21}, CL_{t1} and CL_{t2}. It must be emphasized that in such cases of reversible metabolism some of our cherished ideas of classical pharmacokinetics no longer apply. For example, the last area ratio in Table V indicates that one does not obtain the bioavailability if one makes a ratio of AUC_2^1/AUC_2^2 where the drug was given orally to obtain AUC_2^1 and the metabolite was given intravenously to obtain AUC_2^2. Also, time courses of both drug and metabolite concentrations are biexponential for these models, but the calculation of V_{ss} from the coefficients and exponents of the biexponential equations does not have the usual meaning.

IMPLICATIONS OF FINDINGS AND CONCLUSIONS FOR THE FUTURE

Penicillamine. As a result of the reaction of penicillamine with albumin, our investigations have shown that great care must be taken in appropriately processing blood as it is withdrawn from the subject or patient. Although the simulations we carried out indicate that the double peaks on the ascending part of penicillamine plasma concentration profiles may be explained by two different absorption sites, direct evidence for such sites will be necessary in the future to confirm the hypothesis.

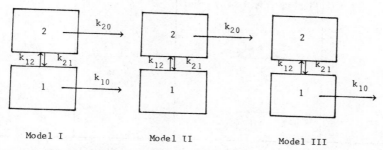

Model I   Model II   Model III

Scheme III. Pharmacokinetic models of reversible metabolism (1 = drug, 2 = metabolite.)

Table V. Pharmacokinetic parameters for model of reversible metabolism.

	Model I [a]	Model II	Model III
$CL_{10} = V_1 k_{10}$	$\dfrac{D_1\,AUC_2^2 - D_2\,AUC_2^1}{AUC_1^1\,AUC_2^2 - AUC_2^1\,AUC_1^2}$	0	$\dfrac{D_1}{AUC_1^1} = \dfrac{D_2}{AUC_1^2}$
$CL_{20} = V_2 k_{20}$	$\dfrac{D_2\,AUC_1^1 - D_1\,AUC_1^2}{AUC_1^1\,AUC_2^2 - AUC_2^1\,AUC_1^2}$	$\dfrac{D_1}{AUC_2^1} = \dfrac{D_2}{AUC_2^2}$	0
$CL_{12} = V_1 k_{12}$	$\dfrac{CL_{10}}{\dfrac{AUC_2^2}{AUC_2^1} - 1}$	$\dfrac{D_2}{AUC_1^1 - AUC_1^2}$	$\dfrac{CL_{10}}{\dfrac{AUC_2^2}{AUC_2^1} - 1}$
$CL_{21} = V_2 k_{21}$	$\dfrac{CL_{20}}{\dfrac{AUC_1^1}{AUC_1^2} - 1}$	$\dfrac{CL_{20}}{\dfrac{AUC_1^1}{AUC_1^2} - 1}$	$\dfrac{D_1}{AUC_2^2 - AUC_2^1}$
$CL_{t1} = \dfrac{D_1}{AUC_1^1}$	$CL_{10} + CL_{12}\left\{\dfrac{k_{20}}{k_{20}+k_{21}}\right\}$	$CL_{12}\left\{\dfrac{k_{20}}{k_{20}+k_{21}}\right\}$	CL_{10}
$CL_{t2} = \dfrac{D_2}{AUC_2^2}$	$CL_{20} + CL_{21}\left\{\dfrac{k_{10}}{k_{10}+k_{12}}\right\}$	CL_{20}	$CL_{21}\left\{\dfrac{k_{10}}{k_{10}+k_{12}}\right\}$
$\dfrac{D_2}{AUC_1^2}$	$CL_{10} + CL_{10} + CL_{12}\left\{\dfrac{k_{20}}{k_{21}}\right\}$	$CL_{12}\left\{\dfrac{k_{20}}{k_{21}}\right\}$	CL_{10}
$\dfrac{D_1}{AUC_2^1}$	$CL_{20} + CL_{20} + CL_{21}\left\{\dfrac{k_{10}}{k_{12}}\right\}$	CL_{20}	$CL_{21}\left\{\dfrac{k_{10}}{k_{12}}\right\}$
$\dfrac{AUC_1^1}{AUC_2^1}$	$\dfrac{CL_{20} + CL_{21}}{CL_{12}}$	$\dfrac{CL_{20} + CL_{21}}{CL_{12}}$	$\dfrac{CL_{21}}{CL_{12}}$
$\dfrac{AUC_2^1}{AUC_2^2}$	$\dfrac{k_{12}}{k_{10}+k_{12}}$	1	$\dfrac{k_{12}}{k_{10}+k_{12}}$

[a] See Scheme III.

Theophylline. By applying two different mathematical criteria to intravenous theophylline plasma concentration-time data, it was shown that theophylline exhibits minimal multicompartment character in humans, and the one-compartment open model is an adequate disposition model for the drug. Application of the Wagner-Nelson absorption method to theophylline plasma concentration-time data observed after oral administration of the sustained release product Theo-Dur® clearly shows that absorption is zero-order over essentially the entire drug release time period. The implications are, and others have clearly shown, that steady-state theophylline plasma concentrations during chronic therapy with this product may be predicted from either single dose data or in vitro release rate data.

Digoxin. We have found that upon intravenous administration both the total clearance and nonrenal clearance of digoxin increase as the input rate to the human body decreases. This implies some type of saturation phenomenon in the liver. The principal implication is that we are now left with no simple way of estimating the absolute bioavailability of digoxin. This deserves careful attention in the future. Also, it would be interesting to study other drugs by the same protocol.

Pentobarbital-Dexamethasone. We have shown in a feline stroke model that dexamethasone administered prior to left middle cerebral artery ligation essentially normalized the pentobarbital pharmacokinetic parameters that had been altered as a result of the stroke. Since adrenocortical steroids in relatively high doses are used concomitantly with other drugs for the treatment of cancer and some immune diseases, for prevention of rejection after organ transplantation, and for prevention of nausea and vomiting as a result of administration of anticancer agents, the effect of such steroids on the pharmacokinetics of the other drugs with which they may be administered should be studied.

Bretylium Tosylate. We have shown that the population average pharmacokinetic parameters of this drug in patients with life-threatening ventricular arrhythmias are very similar to those obtained in normal volunteers. We have also shown that when the drug is administered intravenously the average renal clearance is the same as the average total clearance indicating that the drug is not metabolized. Also, after oral administration the renal clearance is considerably greater than after intravenous administration. We have shown that when patients are given the drug orally on a chronic basis, useful clinical estimates of minimum steady-state plasma concentrations of the drug may be made from the population average parameters F_{po}, V and λ_z^{po}.

Reversible Metabolism. It was emphasized that in cases of reversible metabolism some of our traditional ideas of classical pharmacokinetics no longer apply and we must alter our approaches. Exactly how to do this in evaluating pharmacokinetic data is largely unknown at present, especially with respect to the systems cortisone-cortisol and prednisone-prednisolone. This deserves extensive study in the future.

REFERENCES

1. R.F. Bergstrom, D.R. Kay and J.G. Wagner, High-performance liquid chromatographic determination of penicillamine in whole blood, plasma and urine, J. Chromatogr. 222:445-452 (1981).
2. R.F. Bergstrom, D.R. Kay and J.G. Wagner, The in vitro loss of penicillamine in plasma, albumin solutions, and whole blood: Implications for pharmacokinetic studies of penicillamine, Life Sci. 27:189-198 (1980).
3. R.F. Bergstrom, D.R. Kay, T.M. Harkcom and J.G. Wagner, Penicillamine kinetics in normal subjects, Clin. Pharmacol. Ther. 30:404-413 (1981).
4. M. Weinberger, L. Hendeles and L. Bighley, The relation of product formulation to absorption of oral theophylline, N. Engl. J. Med. 299:852-857 (1978).
5. J.G. Wagner and E. Nelson, Percent absorbed time plots derived from blood level and/or urinary excretion data, J. Pharm. Sci. 52:610-611 (1963).
6. J.G. Wagner, Linear pharmacokinetic equations allowing direct calculation of many needed pharmacokinetic parameters from the coefficients and exponents of polyexponential equations which have been fitted to the data, J. Pharmacokin. Biopharm. 4:443-467 (1976).
7. J.G. Wagner, K.D. Popat, S.K. Das, E. Sakmar and H. Movahhed, Evidence of nonlinearity in digoxin pharmacokinetics, J. Pharmacokin. Biopharm. 9:147-166 (1981).
8. J.G. Wagner, M.R. Hallmark, E. Sakmar and J.W. Ayres, Sensitive radioimmunoassay for digoxin in plasma and urine, Steroids 29:787-807 (1977).
9. J.A. Morais, R.A. Zlotecki, E.Sakmar, P.L. Stetson and J.G. Wagner, Specific and sensitive assays for digoxin in plasma, urine and heart tissue, Res. Commun. Chem. Path. Pharmacol. 31:285-298 (1981).
10. D.J. Weidler, N.S. Jallad, K.L. Black and J.G. Wagner, Alteration of pharmacokinetic parameters for pentobarbital by ischemic stroke and reversion to normal by dexamethasone treatment, J. Clin. Pharmacol. 20:543-551 (1980).
11. J.L. Anderson, E. Patterson, J.G. Wagner, J.R. Stewart, H.L. Behm and B.R. Lucchesi, Oral and intravenous bretylium disposition, Clin. Pharmacol. Ther. 28:408-478 (1980).
12. J.L. Anderson, E.Patterson, J.G. Wagner, T.A. Johnson, B.R. Lucchesi and B. Pitt, Clinical pharmacokinetics of intravenous and oral bretylium tosylate in survivors of ventricular

tachycardia or fibrillation: Clinical application of a new assay for bretylium, J. Cardiovasc. Pharmacol. 3:485-499 (1981).

13. K.C. Kwan and A.E. Till, Novel method for bioavailability assessment, J. Pharm. Sci. 62:1494-1497 (1973).

14. J.G. Wagner, A.R. DiSanto, W.R. Gillespie and K.S. Albert, Reversible metabolism and pharmacokinetics: Application to prednisone-prednisolone, Res. Commun. Chem. Path. Pharmacol. 32:387-406 (1981).

Chapter 17

ASSESSMENT AND PREDICTION OF IN VIVO OXIDATIVE DRUG METABOLIZING ACTIVITY

Douwe D. Breimer, Nico P.E. Vermeulen, Meindert
Danhof, Michiel W.E. Teunissen, Rolf P. Joeres and
Martin van der Graaff

Department of Pharmacology
Subfaculty of Pharmacy
University of Leiden
Leiden, The Netherlands

INTRODUCTION

Enzymatic oxidation in the liver is one of the most important processes in the disposition of many drugs and other foreign chemicals in animals and humans. This process is often the rate-limiting step in the elimination of a compound from the body and/or in the formation of active (reactive) metabolites. Large differences have been shown to occur between different species, and among different individuals within one species, in their capacity to oxidize drugs and other xenobiotics. This interspecies and inter-individual variability is caused by genetic and environmental factors (1-3). In humans, for example, the in vivo metabolic clearance of an oxidized drug varies many-fold among different healthy subjects (4) and consequently there exist large differences in dose-effect relationships. As a result, individualization of drug dosage is required for drugs with a relatively narrow therapeutic concentration range. Also, the in vitro rate of bio-transformation of some carcinogens in liver samples obtained by surgical biopsy from different subjects was found to vary several-fold (5). It has been suggested that individuality in the metabolism of environmental carcinogens which require metabolic activation may help to explain individual differences in the sensitivity of people to the carcinogenic action of such chemicals (6).

In order to cope with the problems of interindividual differences in pharmacokinetics and individualization of drug dosage,

191

methods have been developed to predict dose requirements for individual patients on the basis of population pharmacokinetic data or from a limited number of concentration measurements in each patient after single dose administration (see references 7-9). Of course both approaches only have predictive value for the particular drug under study. A more general approach would be the quantitative assessment of drug metabolizing enzyme activity. This, at least theoretically, would make it possible to extrapolate or predict from one compound to another, and the term prediction is used in this sense herein unless stated otherwise. In this chapter, the methods currently used for the assessment of drug metabolizing capacity will be briefly reviewed; then some of the past attempts to predict oxidative drug metabolizing activity in vivo with the aid of model compounds will be evaluated (and possible reasons suggested for the low degree of success of this approach); finally a new approach with some promising results will be presented. The last section presents preliminary conclusions and perspectives.

METHODS FOR THE ASSESSMENT AND PREDICTION OF DRUG METABOLIZING ACTIVITY

The following methods are currently used to assess drug metabolizing activity in humans:

1. Measurement of parameters of endogenous compounds: γ-glutamyltranspeptidase (γ-GT) activity in plasma; D-glucaric acid excretion in urine; 6-β-hydroxycortisol excretion in urine.

2. Measurement of the rate of drug metabolism in vitro in liver samples (or samples obtained from other tissues) with a wide variety of substrates.

3. Measurement of pharmacokinetic parameters of marker drugs (probes) following single dose administration: antipyrine, aminopyrine, amobarbital, hexobarbital, diazepam, debrisoquine, sparteine, and so forth.

For all these methods it has become quite clear that their greatest potential is associated with the relative rather than the absolute assessment of drug metabolizing activity (that is, with changes in activity as established in longitudinal studies in the same panel of subjects). This has recently been discussed extensively with respect to the use of antipyrine as a marker drug in a semiquantitative determination of environmental factors influencing oxidative drug metabolizing activity (10). For predictive studies, however, the absolute values of certain parameters must be correlated, for example, the rates of metabolism of two drugs. It should further be realized that one of the preferred predictive indices of a certain parameter is not the correlation coefficient, but rather the square of the correlation coefficient (2,11). The correlation coefficient should, in principle, be at least 0.90 for the correlation to be of practical clinical usefulness. It is likely that parameters describing drug metabolizing activity will be correlated to such a strong degree only when they share a common biological mechanism.

The measurement of parameters of endogenous compounds (γ-GT, D-glucaric acid and 6-β-hydroxycortisol) has only been shown to be of value in the assessment of enzyme induction (12). No significant correlations between elimination kinetics of oxidized drugs and these parameters have been found (13,14). Studies of _in vitro_ drug metabolizing activity in liver biopsy samples as measured by benzo(a)pyrene, 7-ethoxycoumarin (0-deethylation), aminopyrine (demethylation) and aniline (hydroxylation), and _in vivo_ elimination (half-life or clearance) of antipyrine in the same subjects yielded only weak correlations (15-17). At present it seems that _in vitro_ measurements in human liver samples with commonly used substrates have little or no predictive value for the _in vivo_ situation. The difficulty of obtaining liver samples from human subjects also limits the general applicability of this approach. This does not imply that _in vitro_ studies with human liver microsomes or more purified drug metabolizing enzymes have little meaning; on the contrary, such studies, including the substrate selectivity of the enzymes involved, the regulation of their activity and so forth (18), are essential for a better understanding of drug metabolism in humans.

Several attempts have been made to correlate the elimination kinetics (half-life or clearance) of different oxidized drugs in the same group of healthy subjects. Some of the results obtained have been summarized in Table I. In most cases, the correlation coefficients are low and not significant; hence the predictive value of one compound for another is almost nonexistent. Very recently, Greenblatt et al. (21) studied the relationship between antipyrine and benzodiazepine clearance or half-life in young and elderly subjects (Table II). Correlations were quite strong with benzodiazepines that are oxidized, but absent with those that are eliminated by conjugation (lorazepam, oxazepam, temazepam). The authors concluded that antipyrine predicts reasonably well the capacity of healthy individuals to biotransform benzodiazepines metabolized by oxidative pathways.

POSSIBLE CAUSES OF POOR CORRELATIONS BETWEEN PHARMACOKINETIC PARAMETERS OF DIFFERENT DRUGS IN THE SAME SUBJECTS

Apart from the results obtained in the study by Greenblatt et al. (21) and a few other examples given in Table I, the correlation

Table I. Correlation of kinetic variables among different oxidized drugs in humans.

Drug Pairs	Number of Subjects	Kinetic Variable	Correlation Coefficient	Level of Significance
Antipyrine–phenylbutazone	14	$t_{\frac{1}{2}}$	0.58	$p < 0.05$
	12	$t_{\frac{1}{2}}$	0.35	N.S.[a]
	16	$t_{\frac{1}{2}}$	0.58	$p < 0.05$
" –phenytoin	16	$t_{\frac{1}{2}}$	0.07	N.S.
" –pentobarbital	6	$t_{\frac{1}{2}}$	0.12	N.S.
" –dicumarol	14	$t_{\frac{1}{2}}$	0.05	N.S.
" –glutethimide	10	$t_{\frac{1}{2}}$	0.02	N.S.
" –amobarbital	10	$t_{\frac{1}{2}}$	0.10	N.S.
" –carbamazepine	10	$t_{\frac{1}{2}}$	0.16	N.S.
		CL	0.08	N.S.
" –warfarin	16	$t_{\frac{1}{2}}$	0.38	N.S.
" –diazepam	17	CL	0.46	$p < 0.001$
" –aminoantipyrine	41	CL	0.33	$p < 0.005$
" –nortryptyline	7	Cl_{int}	0.20	N.S.
" –imipramine	7	CL_{int}	0.05	N.S.
Desmethylimipramine– nortriptyline	8	$t_{\frac{1}{2}}$	0.88	$p < 0.005$
		CL	0.90	$p < 0.005$

Data from references 1, 14, 19 and 20. [a]Not significant.

Table II. Correlation of kinetic variables among different drugs in humans.

Drug Pairs	Number of Subjects	Kinetic Variable	Correlation Coefficient	Level of Significance
Antipyrine-diazepam	26	$t_{1/2}$	0.73	$p < 0.001$
		CL	0.59	$p < 0.005$
" -lorazepam	17	$t_{1/2}$	-0.13	N.S.[a]
		CL	0.32	N.S.
" -oxazepam	25	$t_{1/2}$	-0.12	N.S.
		CL	0.10	N.S.
" -temazepam	29	$t_{1/2}$	-0.21	N.S.
		CL	-0.07	N.S.
" -desmethyl-diazepam	22	$t_{1/2}$	0.83	$p < 0.001$
" -desalkylflur-azepam	15	$t_{1/2}$	0.82	$p < 0.001$
Diazepam-desmethyldiazepam	22	$t_{1/2}$	0.77	$p < 0.001$
" -desalkylflurazepam	17	$t_{1/2}$	0.90	$p < 0.001$
Desmethyldiazepam-desalkyl-flurazepam	15	$t_{1/2}$	0.93	$p < 0.001$
Oxazepam-lorazepam	14	$t_{1/2}$	0.43	N.S.
		CL	0.60	$p < 0.025$
" -temazepam	21	$t_{1/2}$	0.18	N.S.
		CL	0.80	$p < 0.001$
Lorazepam-temazepam	11	$t_{1/2}$	0.13	N.S.
		CL	0.85	$p < 0.001$

Data from reference 21. [a]Not significant.

approach has not been satisfactory with regard to prediction from one compound to another. A number of possible causes of the poor correlations can be considered:

1. The use of inappropriate pharmacokinetic parameters; in many early studies elimination half-life was used rather than clearance. In principle the only parameter that will reflect enzyme activity in vivo is the intrinsic clearance, especially in studies with high clearance drugs.

2. The multiplicity of the cytochrome P-450 system; different drugs may be metabolized by different forms of cytochrome P-450 (intersubstrate selectivity). There is now overwhelming evidence that multiple forms of mammalian cytochrome P-450 exist, and that these have different substrate specificities and more or less different regulatory controls (22). This implies that only the rates of metabolism of compounds which are metabolized by the same form(s) can be expected to correlate.

3. In the oxidative metabolism of a single compound, several products are often formed. The formation of the individual products may be mediated by different forms of cytochrome P-450 (product or intrasubstrate selectivity). This is the case, for instance, for antipyrine (as will be outlined later), propranolol (23) and imipramine (24). The rate of metabolism of such compounds as measured by the (intrinsic) clearance of the parent drug is thus an overall index of oxidizing activity, but not an index of the activity of specific forms of cytochrome P-450. It is possible that despite equal total clearance values for a compound in two subjects, there are large differences in the activities of the individual metabolic pathways. For correlation studies it is therefore preferable to assess the activities of such individual pathways by measuring the rate of formation of metabolites in relation to substrate concentration.

4. The experimental design used previously in correlation studies may have been inappropriate; it does not exclude the influence of intraindividual variability in metabolizing activity. Generally, cross-over studies with two or more drugs are performed in the same panel of subjects, but at different points in time. Although oxidative drug metabolism seems to be primarily controlled by genetic factors, there still may be considerable influence by environmental factors which

potentially may cause intraindividual differences in
activity from one point in time to another (25,26).
Therefore, for correlation studies it would be desirable, in principle, to administer the different drugs
simultaneously.

An approach that would limit the number of drugs required to
assess the activity of the different forms of cytochrome P-450
would be the use of marker drugs which form several oxidized
metabolites (polyfunctional substrates). When these processes are
mediated by different forms of cytochrome P-450 (see reference 3),
the formation kinetics of metabolites can be used as an index of
differential drug oxidizing enzyme activity. It is this objective
that we (and other groups) have recently pursued with regard to
antipyrine.

ANTIPYRINE METABOLITE PROFILE TO ASSESS THE ACTIVITY OF DIFFERENT FORMS OF CYTOCHROME P-450

In Figure 1 the major metabolic pathways of antipyrine are
illustrated; these pathways are similar in humans and rats. Three
major primary metabolites have been identified: 3-hydroxymethyl-
antipyrine (HMA), norantipyrine (NORA) and 4-hydroxyantipyrine
(OHA); p-(4')-hydroxyantipyrine is quantitatively only a minor
metabolite in healthy humans and rats (27). The metabolites are
rapidly excreted into urine, predominantly in conjugated form.
HPLC techniques have been developed to measure the three major
metabolites in urine after hydrolysis of the conjugates (28,29).
The kinetics of metabolite formation (clearance for production:
CL_m) can quite simply be determined according to the following
general scheme when parallel primary pathways are followed:

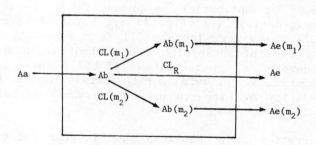

$$Ae_\infty + Ae(m_1)_\infty + Ae(m_2)_\infty = Ab \tag{1}$$

$$CL_R + CL(m_1) + CL(m_2) = CL = \frac{Ab}{AUC} \tag{2}$$

$$CL(m_1) = \frac{Ae(m_1)_\infty}{Ab} \cdot CL = \frac{Ae(m_1)_\infty}{AUC} \tag{3}$$

$$CL(m_2) = \frac{Ae(m_2)_\infty}{Ab} \cdot CL = \frac{Ae(m_2)_\infty}{AUC} \tag{4}$$

where Aa is the amount of parent drug at the site of absorption; Ab is the amount of drug in the body; CL is the total clearance of parent drug; CL_R is the renal clearance of parent drug; $CL(m_1)$ is the clearance for production of metabolite 1; $CL(m_2)$ is the clearance for production of metabolite 2; $Ab(m_1)$ is the amount of metabolite 1 formed; $Ab(m_2)$ is the amount of metabolite 2 formed; $Ae(m_1)$ is the amount of metabolite 1 excreted; $Ae(m_2)$ is the amount of metabolite 2 excreted; Ae is the amount of parent drug excreted unchanged; AUC is the area under the plasma concentration-time curve for the parent drug. In principle this means that for the experimental assessment of CL_m, only total urinary excretion of metabolite and AUC of parent compound have to be determined. For antipyrine in man the AUC in plasma is practically identical to the AUC in saliva (30) and, therefore, the CL_m of the different metabolites can be assessed entirely by noninvasive methods. In order for the urinary metabolite profile of antipyrine to reliably reflect enzyme activity in vivo, certain conditions must be met:

1. Linear kinetics should apply; this has been shown to be true for the 250-1000 mg dose range with antipyrine (31).

2. The metabolites should not be further metabolized except to conjugates which can be hydrolyzed. This is probably true for antipyrine, although the carboxy- and dihydroxy-derivatives (Fig. 1) are formed to a minor extent (32). However, there still is a substantial amount of the dose of antipyrine unaccounted for in humans (total recovery of metabolites 45-85%), despite complete absorption following oral administration (30). The identity of hitherto unknown metabolites has yet to be fully assessed.

3. Excretion of metabolites should occur entirely via the kidneys. There are no indications that this would not be true for antipyrine metabolites. It is essential that urine be collected for at least 36 hours following single dose administration in healthy subjects, otherwise extrapolation to $Ae(m)_\infty$ is not reliable (30).

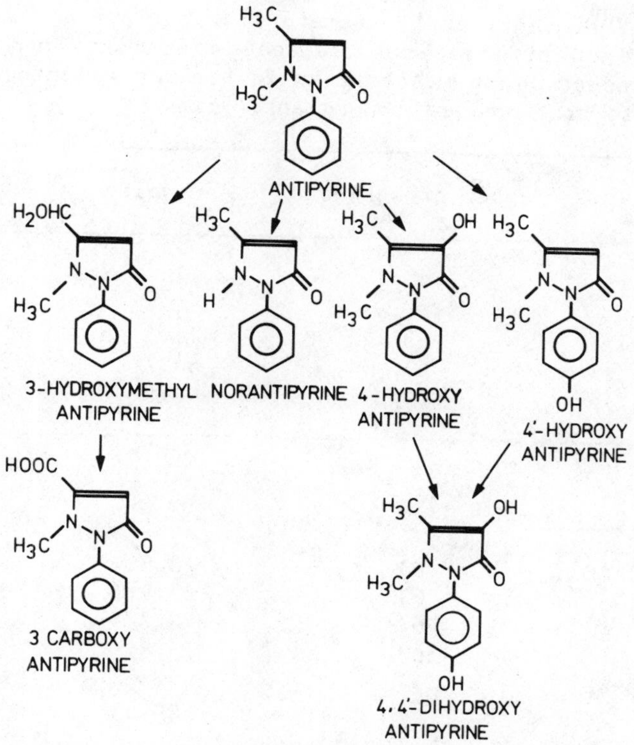

Figure 1. Metabolic pathways of antipyrine in healthy men and rats.

In Table III the pharmacokinetic parameters for antipyrine, the clearances for production of the three major metabolites and the percent dose excreted as parent drug and metabolites are given for 63 healthy volunteers (33). Total clearance of antipyrine varies almost 3-fold, but the clearances for production of metabolites vary 5 to 6-fold. Penno et al. (34) have shown in twin studies that the kinetics of formation of the metabolites are predominantly under genetic control. We came to a similar conclusion by comparing intra- and interindividual variability in the clearances for individual metabolite production in a group of 6 healthy subjects who participated on 5 different occasions in a single dose antipyrine experiment (33). The intraindividual coefficient of variation was 12-16% for the three metabolites, whereas the coefficient of variation was 28-44% interindividually.

Several studies have indicated that the three major oxidized metabolites of antipyrine are produced by different forms of cytochrome P-450 in humans, rats and pigs. In rats, a selective

Table III. Pharmacokinetic parameters of antipyrine (AP), percent dose excreted in urine as metabolites in 48 hours and the clearances for production of metabolites in healthy volunteers obtained after a single oral dose of 500 mg antipyrine.

Parameter	Number of subjects[a]	Mean value	Range
Saliva:			
$t_{1/2z}$ (hr)	63	11.3	6.2 – 15.8
V_d (L)	63	44.7	29.8 – 61.2
CL_{AP} (L/hr)	63	2.9	1.6 – 4.5
Excretion: **(percentage of dose)**			
unchanged AP	63	3.8	1.0 – 10.1
OHA	63	27.2	19.0 – 37.7
NORA	63	18.7	7.0 – 33.2
HMA	63	13.8	8.3 – 20.0
3-carboxy-AP	54	4.3	2.0 – 8.4
Total	54	68	45 – 85
Metabolite formation: **(L/hr)**			
$CL_{(OHA)}$	63	0.84	0.43 – 1.85
$CL_{(NORA)}$	63	0.57	0.20 – 1.29
$CL_{(HMA)}$	63	0.44	0.16 – 0.87

[a]Data from reference 33; 63 healthy volunteers (8 females, 55 males; ages 21-69 yr).

increase in the rate of OHA formation was obtained following 3-methylcholanthrene treatment (35,36). In pigs, OHA is the only known metabolite that is formed in appreciable quantities; HMA and NORA are almost totally absent (37). In humans, induction studies with pentobarbital, antipyrine and rifampicin showed a selective increase in NORA formation (38,39). Inhibition of antipyrine metabolism by propranolol appeared to be most prominent for HMA, although in some subjects clearances for production of NORA and OHA were decreased also (40). Oral contraceptive steroids inhibited antipyrine metabolism nonselectively (41). Boobis et al. (42)

compared the in vivo and in vitro rates of formation of antipyrine metabolites in subjects with normal hepatic function and in patients with suspected liver disease. They found that the rank order of the rate of formation (clearance for production) of the 3 metabolites of antipyrine was similar in vivo and in vitro (V_{max}/K_m). Also, there was no significant correlation between the relative rates of formation of any pair of antipyrine metabolites in vivo and in vitro. Furthermore, they found a significant correlation between in vivo and in vitro rates of formation of each of the three metabolites in the same group of patients. Although these studies are indicative of the involvement of different forms of cytochrome P-450 in the metabolism of antipyrine in humans, in vitro studies with purified forms are ultimately needed to assess the product selectivity of the different forms for antipyrine. A difficulty in human in vivo studies is the inability to study many different inducers and substrates which have proven to be very useful in the elucidation of the multiplicity of the cytochrome P-450 system in animals (22).

CORRELATION STUDIES WITH SIMULTANEOUSLY ADMINISTERED DRUGS

In considering the possible reasons why in vivo correlation studies have not been very successful in the past, it is clear that a more promising approach should contain certain essential features of experimental design. First, the design should be such that intrinsic clearances of parent compounds as well as clearances for production of metabolites are determined. The latter is particularly important when there is evidence that different enzymes are involved in the formation of primary metabolites; these enzymes could be quite different (for example, conjugation versus oxidation), but in the case of parallel oxidative pathways this is a far more subtle phenomenon. Clearance values, preferably of each pathway, should be used as the parameters to be correlated since they reflect enzyme activity, $CL_{int} = V_{max}/(K_m + C)$. Reliable data can be obtained by giving the drugs orally (complete absorption required) and measuring the area under the C_p versus time curve from time zero to infinity ($CL_{int} = D/AUC_{or}$). In addition, total urinary excretion of metabolite has to be measured for the assessment of clearance for production of metabolite (Eq. (3)). Second, the experimental design should require the different compounds to be administered simultaneously in order to assure that metabolizing activity is assessed under identical circumstances. However, in such experiments considerable problems at the enzyme-kinetic and analytical level may be encountered. In principle, the compounds should not significantly interact at the enzymatic level. This probably can only be excluded when relatively low doses are given so that concentrations substantially lower than K_m values are obtained. In general, such low concentrations are difficult to analyze and therefore this approach requires that sophisticated analytical methodology be developed to achieve a high degree of selectivity (several compounds to be analyzed) and sensitivity.

Using some model compounds such as antipyrine, hexobarbital and theophylline, we have recently started this approach in rats. To investigate the feasibility of the experimental design, one of the first studies was performed with two structurally closely related barbiturates: hexobarbital (HB; 1,5-dimethyl-5-(1'-cyclohexenyl) barbituric acid) and heptabarbital (HP; 5-ethyl-5-(1'-cycloheptenyl) barbituric acid).

Hexobarbital versus Heptabarbital. There are at least two important oxidative pathways involved in the biotransformation of HB and HP: hydroxylation at the 3'-position (allylic oxidation, which can be followed by dehydrogenation to the 3'-keto-derivatives); and epoxidation of the double bond in the 1',2'-position, which is almost quantitatively followed by side-chain cleavage via a retro-aldol reaction in intermediary diols (43,44). There is no evidence hitherto that different forms of cytochrome P-450 are involved in the two metabolic routes. Both compounds have comparable overall K_m values as determined in vitro with rat liver microsomes (50 µg/ml for HB and 67 µg/ml for HP), and their extraction ratios are about 0.7 (44). The two drugs were simultaneously administered orally to rats (25 mg/kg) and total blood concentrations were measured for 2 hours. The elimination half-lives in control rats were in the range of 13-28 minutes for HB and 8-21 minutes for HP. Peak concentrations were generally lower than 15 µg/ml and the descending phase of the C_p curves showed in all cases apparent first-order elimination kinetics. To increase the range of the data to be correlated, three groups of rats were studied: controls, phenobarbital (PB) pretreated and 3-methylchol-anthrene (MC) pretreated. The results are shown in Figure 2; a strong correlation exists between the intrinsic clearance values of the two compounds. Apparently induction by PB was mild and only occurred in some animals, whereas MC pretreatment inhibited the metabolism of the two barbiturates. In contrast to the clearance values, the correlation between the elimination half-lives of the two drugs was only weak (r = 0.46). This is quite understandable when one realizes that both compounds, particularly after induction, exhibit hepatic blood flow dependent elimination kinetics. The r^2 value for the in vivo kinetics of metabolism (intrinsic clearance) of HB and HP in rats is greater than 90%, suggesting a common enzyme (or enzymes) and regulatory control for the metabolism of the two drugs. The results of this feasibility study were encouraging and therefore experiments were continued with two drugs which do not show close structural similarity and which exhibit different oxidative metabolic pathways: hexobarbital (HB) and antipyrine (AP).

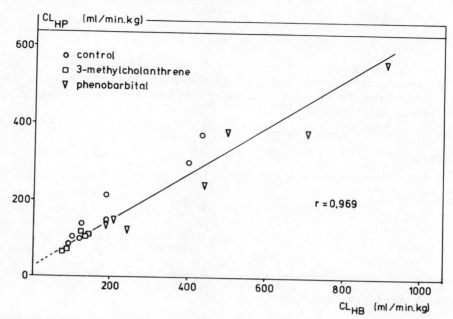

Figure 2. Correlation between the intrinsic clearances of hexobarbital (CL_{HB}) and heptabarbital (CL_{HP}) in control (circles), phenobarbital induced (triangles) and 3-methylcholanthrene induced (squares) rats. HB and HP were given simultaneously and orally (25 mg/kg each) as an aqueous solution of their sodium salts. Pretreatment with phenobarbital was once daily for one, two or three days (100 mg/kg; i.p.); pretreatment with 3-methylcholanthrene was for three days (18 mg/kg; orally).

<u>Antipyrine versus Hexobarbital</u>. The routes of metabolism of HB and AP have been discussed in previous sections. The overall K_m value for antipyrine as determined <u>in vitro</u> with rat liver microsomes is about 700 µg/ml; its <u>in vivo</u> hepatic extraction ratio is about 0.1. The two compounds were simultaneously administered orally to rats (50 mg/kg AP and 25 mg/kg HB). Plasma concentrations of unchanged drugs were measured for 4 hours and total urinary excretion of the following metabolites was determined: HMA, OHA and NORA as major primary metabolites of AP, and the sum of 3'-hydroxy- and 3'-keto-HB as the most important oxidative pathway for HB. Clearance values for production of metabolites were calculated according to Equation (3). Three groups of rats were used: controls, PB pretreated and MC pretreated. A representative example of the C_p curves obtained is shown in Figure 3 for one control rat. Both drugs are eliminated by apparent first-order elimination kinetics. After correlation of the intrinsic clearance

Table IV. Correlation between antipyrine (AP) and hexobarbital (HB) metabolism in the rat following simultaneous oral administration of the two drugs.[a]

Treatment	CL_{AP}^{b}	CL_{OHA}	CL_{NORA}	CL_{HMA}
Control (n = 7)				
CL_{HB}	0.10	0.51	0.41	0.70
$CL_{OH + KHB}$	0.03	0.55	0.50	0.66
Phenobarbital pretreated (n = 6)				
CL_{HB}	0.43	0.50	0.43	0.64
$CL_{OH + KHB}$	0.17	0.43	0.29	0.74
3-MC pretreated (n = 7)				
CL_{HB}	0.54	0.21	0.48	0.69
$CL_{OH + KHB}$	0.69	0.49	0.68	0.89
Total (n = 20)				
CL_{HB}	-0.07	-0.22	-0.26	0.92
$CL_{OH + KHB}$	-0.11	-0.25	-0.29	0.99

[a]Dose was 50 mg/kg antipyrine and 25 mg/kg hexobarbital; data represent correlation coefficients.
[b]CL = clearance; OHA = 4-hydroxyantipyrine; NORA = norantipyrine; HMA = 3-hydroxymethylantipyrine; OH + KHB = 3'-hydroxy- + 3'-keto-hexobarbital; 3-MC = 3-methylcholanthrene.

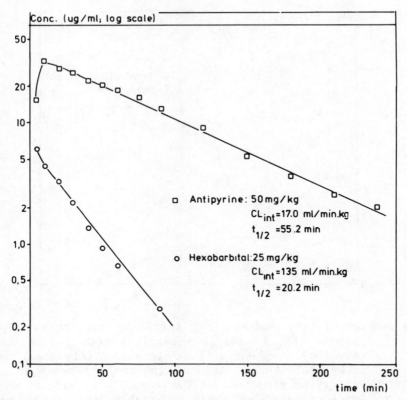

Figure 3. Plasma concentration curves of antipyrine and hexobarbital following simultaneous oral administration of the two drugs to one rat (antipyrine: 50 mg/kg; hexobarbital: 25 mg/kg).

values for all experiments, the results shown in Figure 4 were obtained. Apparently no correlation exists (r = 0.07). AP metabolism was clearly induced by both PB and MC, in agreement with previous findings (35). HB clearance was only increased by PB pretreatment. However, when intrinsic clearance of HB was compared to the clearance for production of the different metabolites of AP, a strong correlation was found with respect to HMA (Fig. 5). The overall correlation matrix is given in Table IV; it includes the correlation coefficients obtained in the three separate treatment groups. Rather poor or nonsignificant correlations were obtained between CL_{HB} and the clearances for production of OHA and NORA. In all cases, however, significant and relatively strong correlations were seen with HMA. Correlations were not much different when the clearance for production of 3'-hydroxy-HB instead of total clearance of HB was taken as the correlating parameter. Therefore, it is very likely that HB and AP have a form of cytochrome P-450 in

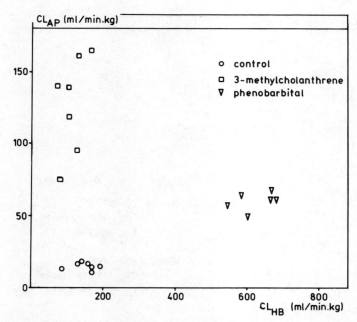

Figure 4. Correlation between the intrinsic clearances of antipyrine (CL_{AP}) and hexobarbital (CL_{HB}) in control
(circles), phenobarbital induced (triangles) and 3-
methylcholanthrene induced (squares) rats. AP and HB
were given simultaneously and orally in aqueous solution
(antipyrine: 50 mg/kg; hexobarbital: 25 mg/kg).
Pretreatment of the rats with phenobarbital and 3-
methylcholanthrene (see legend Figure 2) took place for
five and three days, respectively.

common which is responsible for the major part of HB metabolism and
for the formation of HMA in the metabolism of AP. It is also
likely that NORA and OHA are predominantly produced by other forms
of the oxidative enzyme system. However, some caution is needed
before definite conclusions can be drawn because in the present
study the problem of cluster formation of the data should not be
disregarded (Fig. 5). This may complicate the statistical evaluation of the results and also the interpretation. Further studies,
for instance with lower pretreatment doses of PB during shorter
periods of time, are required to see whether the gap between the
low and high clearance values can be randomly filled with experimental data around the present regression line.

In any case, the results of this study reveal that the differentiation of total clearance and clearance for production of
metabolites is a powerful tool in identifying pathways of metabolism which are mediated by the same enzyme.

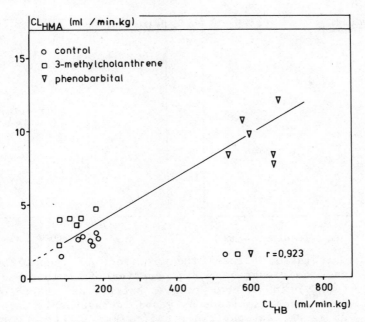

Figure 5. Correlation between the intrinsic clearances of hexo-barbital (CL_{HB}) and the clearances for production of 3-hydroxymethylantipyrine (CL_{HMA}); data obtained from the same experiments as were presented in Figure 4.

<u>Antipyrine versus Theophylline.</u> It was stated previously that MC pretreatment of rats gives rise to considerable acceleration of antipyrine metabolism and also that this induction is selective towards OHA formation. This suggests that this metabolite is formed by cytochrome P-448 or P_1-450. There is also evidence that theophylline (TP) is predominantly metabolized via cytochrome P-448 mediated pathways in different species (45-47). Therefore, as part of these correlation studies with simultaneously administered drugs, a third study was undertaken to challenge the hypothesis that there is a strong correlation between total metabolic clearance of TP and clearance for production of OHA. As has been found in humans (48), TP may exhibit nonlinear kinetics in rats at relatively low concentrations (49) and therefore only 6.5 mg/kg was given together with AP (25 mg/kg). Since both compounds have a low hepatic extraction ratio, they were administered intravenously to avoid possible absorption problems with TP. Plasma kinetics of TP and AP, as well as urinary excretion of unchanged TP and the three metabolites of AP, were determined. In Figure 6 it is shown that there was indeed a strong correlation between total TP clearance and clearance for production of OHA (r = 0.89). The correlation coefficient became slightly higher when total clearance of TP was

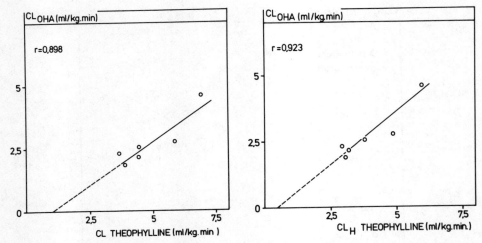

Figure 6. Correlation between the clearance of theophylline (CL) and the clearance for production of 4-hydroxyantipyrine (CL_{OHA}) in control rats. Antipyrine and theophylline were given simultaneously and intravenously (antipyrine: 25 mg/kg; theophylline: 6.5 mg/kg). Left: correlation with total clearance of theophylline. Right: correlation with metabolic clearance (CL_{H}) of theophylline (total clearance minus renal clearance).

corrected for renal clearance (Fig. 6). Upon inclusion of the data obtained after induction with MC, the correlation became even better, whereas the correlations between CL_{TP} and CL_{AP}, and CL_{HMA} and CL_{NORA} decreased. Both the strong correlation between CL_{TP} and CL_{OHA} and the far weaker correlations between CL_{TP} and the other AP metabolites suggest that total TP metabolism and the formation of OHA are mediated by the same enzyme (cytochrome P-448 or P_{1}-450).

    <u>Preliminary Conclusions.</u> Our findings of correlations between intrinsic clearance values and/or clearance values for production of metabolites of different compounds which are simultaneously administered indicate that this approach is interesting and worthwhile to pursue further. This surely holds for the <u>in vivo</u> recognition of metabolic pathways which are mediated by the same oxidative enzyme. The multiplicity of the cytochrome P-450 system requires that different model compounds be used to differentiate between the activity of the different forms of the enzyme system, or that a polyfunctional model compound be used which forms different oxidized metabolites as products of a single enzyme system. In this regard antipyrine has been shown to be a useful compound, at least in rats. For prediction of differential oxidative enzyme activity the presented approach also shows early promise. The fact

that no near perfect correlations ($r^2 > 0.9$) were as yet obtained can probably be explained by experimental errors and by the fact that the degree of differentiation between pathways is not maximal when, for instance, only total intrinsic clearance is determined (hexobarbital, theophylline). The present approach also has shown that the rational application of pharmacokinetic principles is of great value in elucidating and understanding important biological phenomena like drug oxidizing activity in vivo.

PERSPECTIVES IN HUMANS

In principle, the approach as suggested and experimentally elaborated in rats could also be applied in humans. As was outlined previously, there is evidence for multiplicity of the cytochrome P-450 system in humans also, but only very limited information is available about the substrate and product selectivity of the different enzyme forms. Only partial purification of some forms from human liver has been achieved and so far very few substrates have been used for in vitro characterization that can also be applied to humans in vivo (18,50). There are undoubtedly substantial differences between rats and humans with regard to the cytochrome P-450 system and its regulation, so that extrapolation from one species to the other is precarious. One of the most clear-cut proofs that different forms of cytochrome P-450 exists in humans is the genetically determined polymorphism in the oxidation of some drugs; the prototypic examples are debrisoquine and sparteine (reviews: 51-53). About 5-10% of the population appears to have a genetic deficiency in the oxidation of these drugs; this is generally determined by the ratio of the amount of parent drug to the amount of metabolite(s) excreted in urine. If this "metabolic ratio" in a group of healthy subjects is plotted as a frequency distribution histogram, it shows bimodal distribution. The assessment of this metabolic ratio for debrisoquine can be used to phenotype individuals as poor metabolizers and extensive metabolizers (54). By applying this approach it has been shown that the deficiency carries over to certain metabolic reactions of some other drugs (53). Among these is the E-10-hydroxylation of nortriptyline, but probably not hydroxylation in the Z-10-position (55). This indicates a certain degree of product selectivity for different forms of the oxidative enzyme system. In poor metabolizers, neither total antipyrine clearance (56) nor the clearance for production of any of the three primary metabolites were affected significantly (Fig. 7). Apparently, the forms of cytochrome P-450 involved in debrisoquine oxidation are different from those forms involved in antipyrine metabolism.

There is no doubt that it is clinically very important to identify individuals who exhibit the inability to hydroxylate drugs

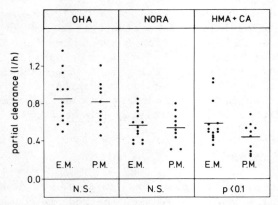

Figure 7. Individual values of the clearance for production (partial clearance) of 4-hydroxyantipyrine (OHA), norantipyrine (NORA) and 3-hydroxymethylantipyrine, including the formation of 3-carboxyantipyrine (HMA + CA) in extensive (EM) and poor (PM) metabolizers of debrisoquine, as determined following a single oral dose of 500 mg antipyrine (57).

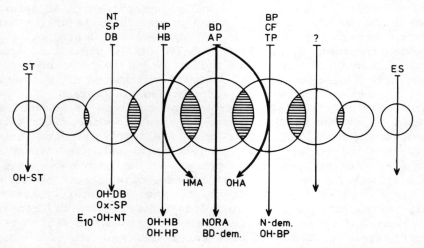

Figure 8. An artist's view of different forms of human cytochrome P-450 (circles) with different (but probably overlapping) substrate and product specificities. The arrows indicate single metabolic pathways. ST = endogenous steroids; NT = nortriptyline; SP = sparteine; DB = debrisoquine; HP = heptabarbital; HB = hexobarbital; BD = benzodiazepine; AP = antipyrine; BP = benzo(a)pyrene; CF = caffeine; TP = theophylline; ES = endogenous substrate.

like debrisoquine. The phenotype approach is very useful for this
purpose. However, that approach as presently applied must still be
regarded as qualitative; one that distinguishes between extensive
and poor metabolizers, but does not answer questions such as how
rapid is extensive? To answer that question a more quantitative
approach is required and for that purpose a parameter like
intrinsic clearance is required rather than the metabolic ratio.
Clinically, it should be regarded as equally relevant to distinguish between patients with respect to a drug that exhibits a
unimodal distribution histogram (or even within the modes of a bi-
or trimodal curve). When interindividual variablity is large
(severalfold difference in clearance), it is at least relevant to
identify patients at the extremes of the histogram, but it is, of
course, preferred that the metabolizing activities of any patient
be assessed quantitatively. It is possible that the lower total
clearance values are associated with a genetic deficiency of one
specific metabolic reaction in the total metabolism of the drug.
This can be investigated by measuring metabolites.

It is clear that for the assessment of in vivo drug oxidizing
activity in humans, as in rats, the multiplicity of cytochrome P-
450 must be taken into account. It is quite unlikely that it would
be possible with one model compound to differentiate between the
activities of the different forms, but rather a number of suitable
probes would be necessary. In Figure 8, an artist's view is given
of the presumed state of the art with regard to substrate and product selectivity of different forms of cytochrome P-450. A polyfunctional substrate like antipyrine offers the advantage that, by
measuring specific metabolites, information can be obtained on the
activity of different enzyme forms. It is possible that the relatively high correlation coefficients between total antipyrine
clearance and the clearance or half-life of oxidized benzodiazepines (reference 12; Table II) can be explained by the fact that
the total metabolism of such benzodiazepines (in which parallel
oxidative pathways are also involved), is mediated by the same
forms of cytochrome P-450 as act on antipyrine. Of course, the
whole picture awaits further substantiation and completion.
Several cross-over studies with different drugs have to be performed. Preferably the different compounds should be given
simultaneously and intrinsic clearance plus clearance for production of the major metabolites should be measured. Only on the
basis of such studies can the predictive value of a certain
parameter of a certain compound towards the rate of metabolism of
another oxidized drug be assessed. Once cross-correlations have
been established, the question of whether the assessment of differential enzyme activity (with a combination of probes) as determined
at a certain point in time has any predictive value can be
answered. This will largely depend on the sensitivity of the
different forms of cytochrome P-450 in vivo towards changes in
environmental factors.

Acknowledgements. These studies were supported in part by the Dutch Prevention Fund, Ministry of Health and Enviromental Protection, The Hague, The Netherlands. R.P. Joeres was a visiting scientist of the University of Wurzburg (G.F.R.), Department of Internal Medicine and he was supported by a grant from the Deutsche Forschungsgemeinschaft.

REFERENCES

1. F. Sjöqvist and C. von Bahr, Interindividual differences in drug oxidation, Drug Metab. Disp. 1:469–482 (1973).
2. E.S. Vesell, Genetic and environmental factors affecting drug disposition in man, Clin. Pharmacol. Ther. 22:659–679 (1977).
3. D.D. Breimer and M. Danhof, Interindividual differences in pharmacokinetics and drug metabolism, in: "Towards Better Safety of Drugs and Pharmaceutical Products," D.D. Breimer, ed., Elsevier/North–Holland, Biomedical Press, Amsterdam (1980), pp. 117–141.
4. G. Alván, Individual differences in the disposition of drugs metabolized in the body, Clin. Pharmacokin. 3:155–175 (1978).
5. A.H. Conney, E.J. Pantuck, C.B. Pantuck, J.G. Fortner, A.P. Alvares, K.E. Anderson and A. Kappas, Variability in human drug metabolism, in: "Clinical Pharmacology and Therapeutics," P. Turner, ed., Macmillan, London (1980), pp. 51–62.
6. A.H. Conney, Microsomes and drug oxidations: perspectives and challenges, in: "Microsomes, Drug Oxidations and Chemical Carcinogenesis," M.J. Coon, A.H. Conney, R.W. Estabrook, H.V. Gelboin, J.R. Gillette and P.J. O'Brien, eds., Academic Press, New York (1980), pp. 1103–1118.
7. L.B. Sheiner, S. Beal, B. Rosenberg and V. Marathe, The statistical basis for forecasting individual pharmacokinetics, in: "Methods in Clinical Pharmacology," N. Rietbrock, B.G. Woodcock and G. Neuhaus, eds., Vieweg, Braunschweig/Wiesbaden (1980), pp. 136–139.
8. J.T. Slattery, M. Gibaldi and J.R. Koup, Prediction of maintenance dose required to attain a desired drug concentration at steady state from a single determination of concentration after an initial dose, Clin. Pharmacokin. 5:377–385 (1980).
9. L.B. Sheiner, S. Beal, B. Rosenberg and V.V. Marathe, Forecasting individual pharmacokinetics, Clin. Pharmacol. Ther. 26:294–305 (1979).
10. E.S. Vesell, The antipyrine test in clinical pharmacology: conceptions and misconceptions, Clin. Pharmacol. Ther. 26:275–286 (1979).
11. J. Kapitulnik, P.J. Popper and A.H. Conney, Comparative metabolism of benzo(a)pyrene and drugs in human liver, Clin. Pharmacol. Ther. 21:166–176 (1977).

12. B.K. Park and A.M. Breckenridge, Clinical implications of enzyme induction and inhibition, Clin. Pharmacokin. 6:1-24 (1981).

13. S.E. Smith and M.D. Rawlins, Prediction of drug oxidation rates in man: lack of correlation with serum γ-glutamyl transpeptidase and urinary excretion of D-glucaric acid and 6β-hydroxycortisol, Eur. J. Clin. Pharmacol. 7:71-75 (1974).

14. D. Kadar, T. Inaba, L. Endrenyi, G.E. Johnson and W. Kalow, Comparative drug elimination capacity in man - glutethimide, amobarbital, antipyrine, sulfinpyrazone, Clin. Pharmacol. Ther. 14:552-560 (1973).

15. O. Pelkonen, E. Sotaniemi, O. Tokola and J.T. Ahokas, Correlations between cytochrome P-450 and oxidative metabolism of benzo(a)pyrene and 7-ethoxycoumarin in human liver in vitro and antipyrine elimination in vivo, Drug Metab. Disp. 8:218-222 (1980).

16. R. Kalamegham, K. Krishnaswamy, S. Krishnamurthy and R.N.K. Bhargava, Metabolism of drugs and carcinogens in man: antipyrine elimination as an indicator, Clin. Pharmacol. Ther. 25:67-73 (1979).

17. D. Vuitton, J.P. Miguet, G. Camelot, C. Delafin, C. Joanne, P. Bechtel, M. Gillet and P. Carayon, Relationship between metabolic clearance rate of antipyrine and hepatic microsomal drug-oxidizing enzyme activities in humans without liver disease, Gastroenterology 80:112-118 (1981).

18. R. Kato and T. Kamataki, Importance of purification of hepatic cytochrome P-450 for studying drug metabolism in man, in: "Clinical Pharmacology and Therapeutics," P. Turner, ed., Macmillan, London (1980), pp. 80-85.

19. L.F. Gram, P. Buch Andreasen, K. Fredericson Overø and J. Christiansen, Comparison of single dose kinetics of imipramine, nortriptyline and antipyrine in man, Psychopharmacology 50:21-27 (1976).

20. C.J. van Boxtel, J.T. Wilson, P. Collste and F. Sjöqvist, A cross-over study of antipyrine and carbamazepine kinetics in human volunteers after single oral doses, personal communication.

21. D.J. Greenblatt, M. Divoll, D.R. Abernethy, J.S. Harmatz and R.I. Shader, Antipyrine kinetics in the elderly: prediction of age-related changes in benzodiazepine oxidizing capacity, J. Pharmacol. Exp. Ther. 220:120-126 (1982).

22. A.Y.H. Lu and S.B. West, Multiplicity of mammalian cytochromes P-450, Pharmac. Rev. 31:277-295 (1980).

23. B. Silber, B.A. Mico, P.R. Ortiz de Montellano, D.M. Dols and S. Riegelman, In vivo effects of the cytochrome P-450 suicide substrate 2-isopropyl-4-pentenamide (allylisopropylacetamide) on the disposition and metabolic pattern of propranolol, J. Pharmacol. Exp. Ther. 219:125-133 (1981).

24. K. Nakazawa, Studies on the demethylation, hydroxylation and N-oxidation of imipramine in rat liver, Biochem. Pharmacol.

19:1363-1369 (1970).

25. A.P. Alvares, A. Kappas, J.L. Eiseman, K.E. Anderson, C.B. Pantuck, E.J. Pantuck, K.C. Hsiao, W.A. Garland and A.H. Conney, Intraindividual variation in drug disposition, Clin. Pharmacol. Ther. 26:407-419 (1979).

26. M. Rowland, Intraindividual variability in pharmacokinetics, in: "Towards Better Safety of Drugs and Pharmaceutical Products," D.D. Breimer, ed., Elsevier/North-Holland Biomedical Press, Amsterdam (1980), pp. 143-151.

27. T. Inaba, H. Uchino and W. Kalow, Identification of p(4')-hydroxy-antipyrine as a metabolite of antipyrine in man, Res. Commun. Chem. Pathol. Pharmacol. 33:3-8 (1981).

28. M. Danhof, E. de Groot-van der Vis and D.D. Breimer, Assay of antipyrine and its primary metabolites in plasma, saliva and urine by HPLC with some preliminary results in man, Pharmacology 18:210-223 (1979).

29. M. Danhof, M.W.E. Teunissen and D.D. Breimer, 3-Hydroxymethyl-antipyrine excretion in urine after an oral dose of antipyrine: A reconsideration of previously published data and synthesis of a pure reference substance, Pharmacology 24:181-184 (1982).

30. M. Danhof, A. van Zuilen, J.K. Boeijinga and D.D. Breimer, Studies of the different metabolic pathways of antipyrine in man. Oral versus i.v. administration and the influence of urinary collection time, Eur. J. Clin. Pharmacol. 21:433-441 (1982).

31. M. Danhof and D.D. Breimer, Studies on the different metabolic pathways of antipyrine in man I. Oral administration of 250, 500 and 1000 mg to healthy volunteers, Br. J. Clin. Pharmacol. 8:529-537 (1979).

32. H. Bässmann, J. Böttcher and R. Schüppel, Dihydroxyphenazone as a urinary metabolite of phenazone in different species including man, Naunyn-Schmiedeberg's Arch. Pharmacol. 309:203-205 (1979).

33. M. Danhof, Antipyrine metabolite profile as a tool in the assessment of the activity of different drug oxidizing enzymes in man, Ph.D. thesis, University of Leiden (1980).

34. M.B. Penno, B.H. Dvorchik and E.S. Vesell, Genetic variation in rates of antipyrine metabolite formation: a study in uninduced twins, Proc. Natl. Acad. Sci. 78:5193-5196 (1981).

35. M. Danhof, D.P. Krom and D.D. Breimer, Studies on the different metabolic pathways of antipyrine in rats: influence of phenobarbital and 3-methylcholanthrene treatment, Xenobiotica 9:695-702 (1979).

36. T. Inaba, M. Lucassen and W. Kalow, Antipyrine metabolism in the rat by three hepatic monooxygenases, Life Sci. 26:1977-1983 (1980).

37. J.M. van den Broek, M.W.E. Teunissen and D.D. Breimer, Induction of hexobarbital and antipyrine metabolism by rifampicin treatment in the pig, Drug Metab. Disp. 9:541-544 (1981).

38. M. Danhof, R.M.A. Verbeek, C.J. van Boxtel, J.K. Boeijinga
     and D.D. Breimer, Differential effects of enzyme induction on
     antipyrine metabolite formation, Br. J. Clin. Pharmacol.
     13:379-386 (1982).

39. E.L. Toverud, A.R. Boobis, M.J. Brodie, S. Murray, P.N.
     Bennett, V. Whitmarsh and D.S. Davies, Differential induction
     of antipyrine metabolism by rifampicin, Eur. J. Clin. Pharma-
     col. 21:155-160 (1981).

40. N.D.S. Bax, M.S. Lennard and G.T. Tucker, Inhibition of
     antipyrine metabolism by β-adrenoreceptor antagonists, Br. J.
     Clin. Pharmacol. 12:779-784 (1981).

41. M.W.E. Teunissen, A.K. Srivastava and D.D. Breimer, The
     influence of sex and oral contraceptive steroids on antipy-
     rine metabolite formation in man, Clin. Pharmacol. Ther.,
     32:240-246 (1982).

42. A.R. Boobis, M.J. Brodie, G.C. Kahn, E.L. Toverud, I.A.
     Blair, S. Murray and D.S. Davies, Comparism of the in vivo
     and in vitro rates of formation of the three main oxidative
     metabolites of antipyrine in man, Br. J. Clin. Pharmacol.
     12:771-777 (1981).

43. N.P.E. Vermeulen, B.H. Bakker, J. Schultink, A. van der Gen
     and D.D. Breimer, The epoxide-diol pathways in the metabolism
     of hexobarbital in rat and man, Xenobiotica 9:289-299 (1979).

44. N.P.E. Vermeulen, The epoxide-diol pathway in the metabolism
     of hexobarbital and related barbiturates, Ph.D. thesis,
     University of Leiden (1980).

45. J.F. Williams, S. Lowitt and A. Szentivanyi, Effects of
     phenobarbital and 3-methylcholanthrene pretreatment on the
     plasma half-life and urinary excretion profile of theophyl-
     line and its metabolites in rats, Biochem. Pharmacol.
     28:2935-2940 (1979).

46. C.J. Betlach and T.N. Tozer, Biodisposition of theophylline.
     II. Effect of aromatic hydrocarbon treatment in mice, Drug
     Metab. Disp. 8:271-273 (1980).

47. J.R. Powell, J.F. Thiercelin, S. Vozeh, L. Sansom and S.
     Riegelman, The influence of cigarette smoking and sex on
     theophylline disposition, Am. Rev. Respir. Dis. 116:17-23
     (1977).

48. D. Dan-Shya Tang Liu, R.L. Williams and S. Riegelman.
     Nonlinear theophylline elimination, Clin. Pharmacol. Ther.
     31:358-369 (1982).

49. M.W.E. Teunissen, I.O.N. Brorens, and D.D. Breimer, Dose-
     dependent pharmacokinetics of theophylline in rats, in:
     "Abstracts of the 41st International Congress of Pharmaceu-
     tical Sciences of F.I.P.," Vienna (1981), p. 179.

50. Ph. Beaune, P. Kremers, P.M. Dansette, J.P. Flinois and J.P.
     Leroux, Mono-oxygenease activities of partially purified
     cytochromes P-450 from human liver microsomes, in: "Micro-
     somes, Drug Oxidations and Chemical Carcinogenesis," M.J.
     Coon, A.H. Conney, R.W. Estabrook, H.V. Gelboin, J.R.

Gillette and P.J. O'Brien, eds., Academic Press, New York (1980), pp. 107-110.

51. J.R. Idle and R.L. Smith, Polymorphism of oxidation at carbon centres of drugs and their clinical significance, Drug Metab. Rev. 9:301-317 (1979).

52. R.L. Smith and J.R. Idle, Genetic polymorphism in drug oxidation, in: "Drug Reactions and the Liver," M. Davis, J.M. Tredger and R. Williams, eds., Pitman Medical, London (1981), pp. 95-104.

53. M. Eichelbaum, Defective oxidation of drugs: pharmacokinetic and therapeutic implications, Clin. Pharmacokin. 7:1-22 (1982).

54. T.P. Sloan, A. Mahgoub, R. Lancaster, J.R. Idle and R.L. Smith, Polymorphism of carbon oxidation of drugs and clinical implications, Br. Med. J. 2:655-657 (1978).

55. B. Mellström, L. Bertilsson, J. Säwe, H.-U. Schultz and F. Sjöqvist, E- and Z-10-hydroxylation of nortriptyline: relationship to polymorphic debrisoquine hydroxylation, Clin. Pharmacol. Ther. 30:189-193 (1981).

56. L. Bertilsson, M. Eichelbaum, B. Mellström, J. Säwe, H.-U. Schultz and F. Sjöqvist, Nortriptyline and antipyrine clearance in relation to debrisoquine hydroxylation in man, Life Sci. 27:1673-1677 (1980).

57. M. Danhof, J.R. Idle, M.W.E. Teunissen, T.P. Sloan, D.D. Breimer and R.L. Smith, Influence of the genetically controlled deficiency in debrisoquine hydroxylation on antipyrine metabolite formation, Pharmacology 22:349-358 (1981).

Chapter 18

PHARMACOKINETIC AND PHARMACOLOGICAL ASPECTS OF POLYMORPHIC DRUG OXIDATION IN MAN

D.M. Roden, T. Wang, R.L. Woosley, A.J.J. Wood,
R.A. Branch, A. Küpfer and G.R. Wilkinson

Departments of Pharmacology and Medicine
Vanderbilt University
Nashville, Tennessee

INTRODUCTION

Variability in drug responsiveness between individuals is well established and considerable insight into its causes has been obtained in recent years. Much of the focus has been upon factors affecting drug disposition, and pharmacokinetic principles and concepts have made an important contribution in this area. The extension of similar modeling approaches to the analysis of the pharmacodynamic determinant has also been of value (1). In general, it is thought that the often pronounced differences in drug sensitivity result from environmental factors, including concomitant drug use, and disease state considerations interacting at many levels with an individual's genetic characteristics. A plethora of clinical studies has demonstrated the importance of the first two components, but only limited investigation has been made of the role of genetic constitution in humans. The major reason for this is that most disposition processes, in particular drug metabolism, appear to be determined by several genes. Such polygenic control results in a continuous (unimodal) frequency distribution of the process within the population. Although considerable interindividual variation may be present, it is difficult, except by twin studies, to assess the role of genetic constitution (2,3). A major exception to this situation is the polymodally distributed ability to N-acetylate certain arylamines, for example, isoniazid, dapsone, hydralazine, procainamide and certain sulfonamides (4). This discontinuous distribution arises because N-acetylation is controlled by only two alleles at a single gene locus. Furthermore, inheritance of the deficiency exhibits classical autosomal recessive

Mendelian characteristics with approximately half of Caucasians and Negroes being phenotypically "slow" acetylators. The other half are "rapid" acetylators and comprise the homozygous dominant and heterozygous genotypes; considerable interethnic variability is also present (4). Similar polymorphism occurs in the hydrolysis of paraoxon by arylesterase (EC3.1.1.2) to form p-nitrophenol and ethyl phosphate (5). Another well-recognized hereditary situation affecting drug metabolism is the occurrence in about 1 in 2500 individuals of an atypical pseudocholinesterase (EC3.1.1.8); administration of succinylcholine results in prolonged apnea due to impaired hydrolysis of the drug (6). A number of other variants of drug metabolism have also been attributed to a genetic causation including phenytoin, bishydroxycoumarin, phenacetin and amobarbital, but their frequency has been thought to be rare (2,3). However, recent evidence is beginning to indicate that monogenically determined polymorphism of drug metabolism is more common than previously considered, especially with regard to oxidative biotransformation, and that the deficient traits have relatively high frequencies of expression affecting a significant proportion of the population.

In 1977, evidence began to accumulate indicating that the alicyclic oxidation of the antihypertensive agent, debrisoquine, to its major metabolite, 4-hydroxydebrisoquine, exhibited a discontinuous distribution (7,8). On the basis of an 8 hour urinary excretion profile following a single 10 mg oral dose, a "metabolic ratio" (percent dose excreted as debrisoquine/percent dose excreted as 4-hydroxydebrisoquine) discriminated between two distinct phenotypes. Individuals with a ratio of greater than 12.6 were defined as "poor metabolizers" whereas a value less than this antimode indicated the capacity to extensively metabolize debrisoquine. Family studies indicated that the deficient trait is inherited as an autosomal recessive character, and hence the "extensive metabolizers" represent both the homozygous dominant and the heterozygous genotypes (9). In the British Caucasian population the frequency of the deficient trait was found to be about 8.9% (9). However, interethnic variability has subsequently been demonstrated. For example, in Saudi Arabians the incidence of defective hydroxylation is only 1.0% (10), in Egyptians 1.5% (11), in Ghanaians 6.3% (12), and in Nigerians 8.6% (13).

Independent of these investigations were studies showing that N-oxidation of sparteine was polymorphically distributed and that a metabolic ratio based on a 12-hour urinary excretion profile could characterize the population into "metabolizers" and "non-metabolizers" (14,15). Conventional pharmacokinetic studies following intravenous administration demonstrated additional differences between these two phenotypes (15). In particular, threefold differences in elimination half-life and total clearance were present, and for the latter this was accounted for by the presence or absence of metabolism since renal clearance was the same in both groups. Subsequently, a close relationship was demonstrated between an individual's ability to oxidize sparteine and debriso-quine, suggesting that the two processes are regulated by the same pair of alleles (16,17).

The control of the oxidative metabolism of other drugs has been indirectly linked to the same alleles as those involved in the N-oxidation of sparteine and 4-hydroxylation of debrisoquine. The approach generally taken has been to use two groups of subjects of known debrisoquine phenotype and to examine the disposition of a test drug in such phenotype panels (18). Aromatic hydroxylation of guanoxan (19), O-deethylation of phenacetin (19), formation of the E-10-hydroxy metabolite of nortriptyline (20,21), hydroxylation of phenformin (22), perhexilene (23) and phenytoin (24) have been shown to be related to the alicyclic hydroxylation of debrisoquine. In certain instances, such as with phenytoin (24), the relationship is not so robust as with other drugs, which probably reflects an involvement of metabolic enzymes not controlled by the "debriso-quine" alleles. The existence of other isozymes of cytochrome P-450 is also implied by the complete absence of any relationship between the hydroxylation of antipyrine (20,23), acetanilide (18) and tolbutamide (25).

The role and importance of defective drug oxidation in the therapeutic and toxicological effects of drugs is only slowly beginning to emerge. The defect's relatively high incidence (about 5-10%) in Caucasian populations suggests that it may be quite important in interpatient variability in drug responsiveness, especially in so-called idiosyncratic effects. With debrisoquine, the hypotensive effect is much more pronounced following adminis-tration of a standard dose to poor metabolizers than to individuals able to metabolize the drug more effectively (26). Individuals who developed side effects following sparteine administration were subsequently found to be non-metabolizers (14), and it has been speculated that the 2-3% of patients who developed tetanic contrac-tions of the uterus when the drug first underwent clinical trial in the 1950's were deficient metabolizers (14). The generation of the methemoglobin-forming toxic metabolite of phenacetin, 2-hydroxy-phenetidine, is two to three times greater and methemoglobin concentrations are significantly higher in poor metabolizers of debrisoquine than in extensive metabolizers (23,27). Deficient drug oxidation has also been linked to the development of lactic acidosis following phenformin administration (22), to neuropathy associated with perhexilene use (28), and to an increased risk of side effects after administration of the β-adrenergic blocker, bufuralol (29). A possible involvement of defective oxidative biotransformation has also been suggested in chemically induced carcinogenesis (27).

It is clear then that a significant proportion of the population exhibits a pronounced deficiency in oxidative drug metabolism. Moreover, this defect, typified by a relative inability to 4-hydroxylate debrisoquine, is involved in a number of different oxidative pathways and affects a wide spectrum of drugs. However, not all routes of metabolism are equally affected and this is consistent with the existence of multiple forms of cytochrome P-450. Because of such multiplicity it is possible that additional forms of oxidative polymorphism are present in humans. Studies of the clinical consequences and implications of such discontinuously distributed deficient biotransformations have mainly focused on the therapeutic and adverse effects of the parent drug. However, many metabolites are pharmacologically active and such activity may significantly contribute to the drug's overall action. A genetic impairment in the formation of such metabolites may profoundly alter the drug's effects. This chapter will describe initial findings from ongoing studies to explore new forms of polymorphic drug oxidation and the pharmacological consequences of impaired metabolism.

POLYMORPHIC METABOLISM AND PHARMACOLOGICAL ACTIVITY OF ENCAINIDE

The antiarrhythmic agent encainide was developed about 10 years ago; however, it is only recently that controlled clinical trials have been undertaken to evaluate its efficacy and toxicity. In patients with chronic, high frequency ventricular arrhythmias, encainide was found to be a highly effective and well-tolerated antiarrhythmic agent (30). However, in one of the eleven patients in this initial study no antiarrhythmic effect was observed. The patient also exhibited distinctly different disposition character-istics of encainide compared to the responders. Using a radio-immunoassay (31), the elimination half-life of encainide after a single 25 mg oral dose was 2.7 ± 0.2 hr (mean $\pm$ SEM, range 1.9 to 3.8 hr) in the responders but in the nonresponder this value was 7.8 hr (Fig. 1). Steady-state plasma concentrations were also 20 to 100 times higher than the mean concentrations in the other ten patients. These and other observations raised the question of whether the nonresponder represented the extreme of a continuously distributed population or whether a discontinuity was present. They also suggested the involvement of metabolites in encainide's overall clinical pharmacology.

Encainide (4-methoxy-[2'-[N-methyl-2-piperidyl]ethyl]benzani-lide) is extensively metabolized in humans (Fig. 2). Demethylation can occur at both the 4-methoxy and the N-positions, and the 3-methoxy-O-desmethyl metabolite may also be formed along with addi-tional minor metabolites. Extraction followed by high performance liquid chromatography permits accurate and specific determinations of each of these metabolites and unchanged encainide in plasma from

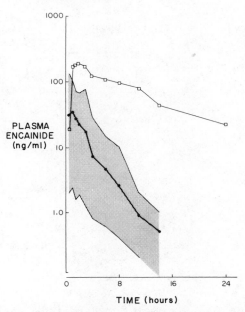

Figure 1. Plasma concentrations of encainide following a single 25
mg oral dose. The shaded area represents the mean
(circles) and range for the 10 patients who exhibited an
antiarrhythmic response, and the square symbols indicate
the single patient who did not respond. Reprinted by
permission of the New England Journal of Medicine (30).

subjects receiving both single and multiple doses of the antiarrhythmic (31,32). This methodological approach also permits
determination of the radioactivity of an eluted peak by liquid
scintillation spectrometry. Thus, in studies to fully characterize
encainide's disposition and pharmacokinetics in young (18–38 years)
normal subjects, it was possible to simultaneously give a radiolabeled dose of drug (54 µCi) intravenously along with orally
administered drug (50 mg every 8 hr) in order to determine conventional disposition parameters and metabolite patterns without the
problems of intrasubject variability (33).

In eight of the subjects encainide had a high systemic plasma
clearance (1.8 ± 0.16 L/min, mean ± SD) and short half-life (2.67 ±
0.93 hr). Oral plasma clearance was also very high but exhibited
considerable interindividual variability (12.4 ± 4.3 L/min), and as
a result, oral bioavailability was low (26.3 ± 6.7%). No differences were apparent in encainide's pharmacokinetics between acute
drug administration and following 3 days of chronic dosing at which
time steady state had been achieved (Fig. 3). In contrast, four
subjects exhibited completely different pharmacokinetics. The rate

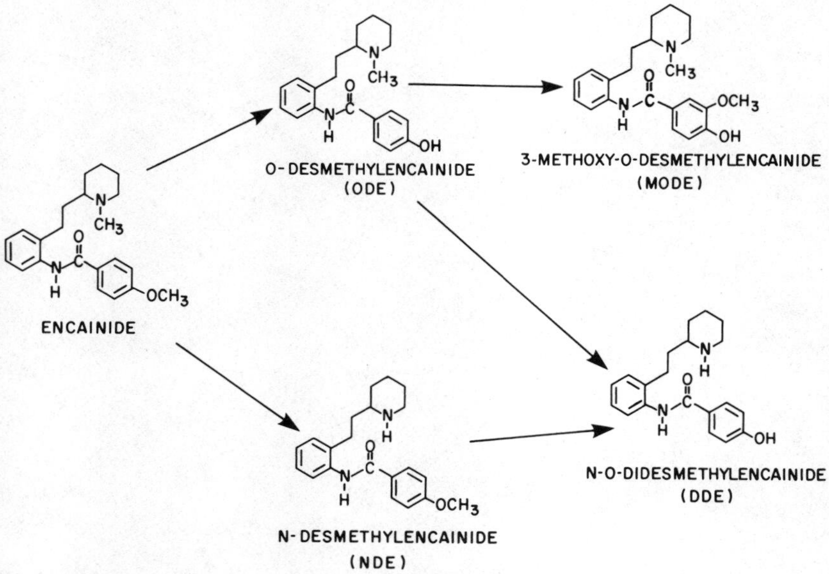

Figure 2. Encainide and its major metabolites in man. Reprinted from (33) with permission.

of encainide elimination was much slower than in the other subjects (half-life, 8.09 ± 1.08 hr), with values similar to those observed for the nonresponder in the clinical study. This slower elimination was caused by an almost tenfold smaller systemic plasma clearance (0.21 ± 0.02 L/min), associated with a fifteen to one hundredfold lower oral clearance. As a result, the oral bioavailability of encainide was almost complete in these subjects (Fig. 3). Again, there were no changes in pharmacokinetics following three days of dosing, but significant accumulation of encainide occurred during chronic dosing and plasma concentrations were twenty to fiftyfold higher than in the group of rapid metabolizers (Fig. 4).

Considerable differences were also noted in the disposition of encainide's metabolites in the rapid and slow metabolizers. The metabolites were found to have significantly longer apparent half-lives of elimination than the parent drug, and they accumulated during chronic dosing (Fig. 4). The plasma levels of O-desmethyl-encainide were about tenfold higher in the group of eight subjects who rapidly eliminated encainide compared to the slow metabolizers (Fig. 4). The 3-methoxy-O-desmethyl metabolite was also formed in these eight subjects, whereas none of this metabolite was detectable in the slow metabolizers. Instead, these two subjects

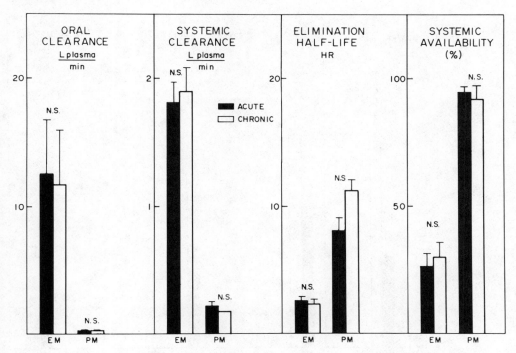

Figure 3. Pharmacokinetic parameters of encainide following acute
and chronic oral dosing in 8 fast metabolizers and 4
slow metabolizers.

generated significant amounts of N-desmethylencainide which was not
detected in the eight rapid metabolizers (Fig. 4).

The profoundly different pharmacokinetic behavior of encainide
and its metabolic profile in the two groups of subjects suggests
that the antiarrhythmic's disposition is discontinuously distributed and strongly influenced by genetic constitution. Initial
studies based on the family of the clinical index case indicated
that the oxidative metabolism of encainide by O-demethylation was
related to an individual's ability to 4-hydroxylate debrisoquine
(34). This finding was confirmed in the pharmacokinetic study; the
four "slow metabolizers" were also "poor metabolizers" of debrisoquine and vice versa for the "rapid metabolizers." Additional
studies also support the fact that the two traits are co-inherited
and are probably controlled by the same alleles.

The observation of high encainide plasma concentrations but no
O-desmethyl metabolite in the nonresponder (30), and the pronounced
differences in metabolite plasma concentrations, especially after
chronic dosing, in the extensive and poor metabolizers obviously

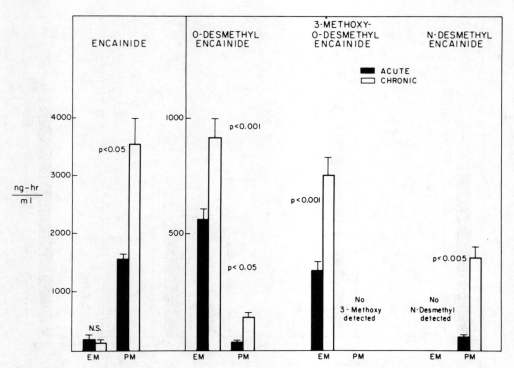

Figure 4. Areas under plasma concentration-time curves (0-8 hr)
for encainide and metabolites following acute and
chronic oral dosing in 8 fast metabolizers and 4 slow
metabolizers. Reprinted from (33) with permission.

suggests a role for pharmacologically active metabolites in encainide's overall activity.   Initial studies in animal models of
arrhythmia have indeed shown that the O-desmethyl and 3-methoxy-O-
desmethyl metabolites have antiarrhythmic activity at comparable or
lower doses than encainide (35,36).   For example, the slow intravenous infusion of aconitine to rats produces premature ventricular
contractions that ultimately develop into sustained tachycardia and
fibrillation.   Pretreatment with an antiarrhythmic agent prolongs
the time taken to achieve sustained ventricular tachycardia and
also the survival time.   In this model, encainide administration
appeared to be more efficacious than its O-desmethyl metabolite but
considerably less potent (Fig. 5).   The in vivo production of
metabolites complicates the interpretation of these types of
studies. However, it is noteworthy that when the blood flow to
the splanchnic organs, including the liver, was interrupted, encainide's potency increased (36).   Thus, while O-desmethylencainide

and also 3-methoxy-0-desmethylencainide exhibit antiarrhythmic
activity, the parent compound also produces similar effects,
although at higher dosages. Extrapolation of these findings to the
situation in humans must, however, be made cautiously prior to
clinical evaluation of the metabolites themselves. It would
presently appear that in rapid metabolizers encainide itself may
briefly exert some effects, but most of the overall activity,
especially following chronic dosing, is attributable to active
metabolites that accumulate, particularly the 0-desmethyl and 3-
methoxy-0-desmethyl metabolites. This would account for the
qualitatively different electrophysiological effects of single and
chronic oral doses of the drug (37). On the other hand, patients
unable to 0-demethylate encainide may exhibit antiarrhythmic
effects due to the unchanged drug, but high plasma concentrations
are required (30,38).

STEREOSELECTIVE AND POLYMORPHIC DISPOSITION OF MEPHENYTOIN

The anticonvulsant, mephenytoin, has been used clinically for
many years, however, relatively little is known of its disposition

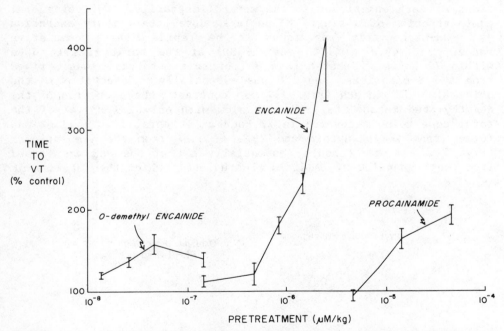

Figure 5. Dose-response relationships for 0-desmethylencainide,
encainide and procainamide for prolongation of the time
to aconitine induced ventricular tachycardia in the rat.
Reprinted from (36), with permission.

as it relates to the drug's therapeutic and adverse effects. Two
major routes of metabolism have been described in humans (Fig. 6).
These are aromatic hydroxylation to 4-OH-mephenytoin (3-methyl-5-
(4-hydroxyphenyl)-5-ethylhydantoin) which is subsequently conjugated with glucuronic acid and rapidly excreted in the urine; and
demethylation to PEH (5-phenyl-5-ethylhydantoin), a metabolite with
similar anticonvulsant activity and potency as the parent drug.
However, the 5-position of the hydantoin ring is chirally active
and previous studies in dogs based on the urinary excretion of
metabolites of the enantiomers indicated a modest degree of stereoselectivity of hydroxylation but not of demethylation (39).
Accordingly, these studies were extended in order to determine the
extent of stereoselectivity of metabolism in humans (40).

The experimental approach taken was to use a differentially
radiolabeled pseudo-racemate of mephenytoin wherein the S-enantiomer was specifically labeled with carbon-14 and the R-enantiomer
with tritium. After administration of the pseudo-racemate to seven
normal volunteers, the urinary excretion of the 4-OH-mephenytoin
and PEH metabolites was determined by a high performance liquid
chromatographic procedure following acid hydrolysis. Double
isotope liquid scintillation counting of the appropriate eluant
fractions then permitted determination of the relative contributions of each enantiomer to the metabolic profile. Following oral
administration of a single 23 μmole/kg dose, the urinary excretion
of 4-OH-mephenytoin was found to be rapid with a cumulative
recovery of 45.8 ± 4.7% (mean ± SD) of the total racemic dose
within 72 hours. Greater than 90% of this metabolite was derived
from the S-enantiomer and ^{14}C was essentially undetectable in the
urine after 72 hours (Fig. 7). In contrast, the excretion of the
demethylated metabolite, PEH, was slow with only 2.9 ± 1.4% of the
total dose being recovered in 72 hours. Of this, 71.0 ± 11.6% was
formed from R-mephenytoin and 29.0 ± 11.6% from the S-enantiomer
(Fig. 7). After 72 hours, essentially all of the PEH was formed
from the R-enantiomer. Additional studies in which the labeling of

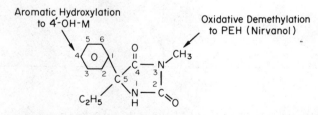

Figure 6. Major metabolic pathways of mephenytoin in humans. The
5-position of the hydantoin ring is chirally active.
Reproduced from (40), with permission.

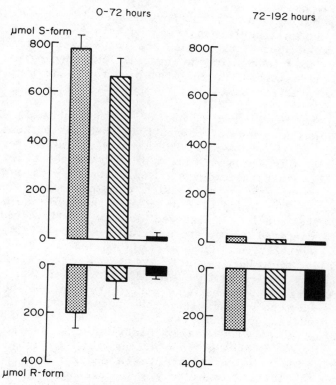

Figure 7. The relative contributions (mean ± SD) of S- and R-enantiomers of mephenytoin to the 72 hr urinary recovery of radioactivity (stippled bars), 4-OH-mephenytoin (hatched bars) and PEH (solid bars) following single dose administration of a radiolabeled pseudo-racemate of mephenytoin in 7 subjects, and the 72-192 hr contributions in two of these subjects. Reprinted from (40), with permission.

the enantiomers of the pseudo-racemate was reversed provided similar data, indicating the absence of any isotope effect. Also, tritium originally present at the 4-position of S-mephenytoin was still present in the hydroxylated metabolite, strongly suggesting the involvement of an NIH shift and epoxide formation in the oxidation reaction.

These studies clearly demonstrated a marked stereoselectivity in the metabolism of mephenytoin. Essentially all of the S-enantiomer is hydroxylated and rapidly removed from the body with a half-life of about four hours. However, R-mephenytoin is slowly but extensively metabolized by N-demethylation and the half-life of elimination of the generated R-PEH is greater than 80 hours.

Accordingly, during chronic therapy neither S-mephenytoin nor its metabolites accumulate whereas R-mephenytoin and its metabolite R-PEH would be expected to accumulate and significantly, if not exclusively, contribute to the overall pharmacological effects. Subsequent disposition studies under chronic dosing conditions support these predictions (41).

During the above studies one of the subjects developed mild sedation following a dose of mephenytoin that was without effect in the remainder of the subjects. Further investigation revealed that this subject's plasma concentration of PEH was about twice as high as that in the other individuals. Administration of a dose of the radiolabeled pseudo-racemate revealed that the reason for this was a deficiency in the hydroxylation of S-mephenytoin such that less than 5% of the total administered dose was eliminated as 4-OH-mephenytoin, compared to the normal value of 35-45% (42). Almost all of the administered dose was eliminated as PEH, which was formed equally from both enantiomers (Fig. 8). Studies of the proband's family indicated that two of his brothers were also deficient hydroxylators whereas the other brother and both parents eliminated 4-OH-mephenytoin within the normal range (42). Initial population studies (43,44) suggest that the ability to hydroxylate S-mephenytoin is polymorphically distributed and that a defect occurs in about 5% of the populations that have been studied. Moreover, this deficiency appears to be under a different genetic control than the ability to hydroxylate debrisoquine.

The observed urinary excretion kinetics would suggest profoundly dissimilar plasma disposition profiles for mephenytoin's enantiomers and metabolites. In "extensive metabolizers," R- and S-mephenytoin will have completely different pharmacokinetics. The R-enantiomer, because of a low total intrinsic clearance, should have a high oral bioavailability and will be eliminated slowly by demethylation to R-PEH which will accumulate and exert a major pharmacological effect during chronic dosing. In contrast, S-mephenytoin will exhibit a high first-pass effect following oral administration and it will have a short half-life. The predominant metabolite will be S-4-OH-mephenytoin which will be rapidly eliminated and will not accumulate and S-PEH formation will be minimal. However, in individuals with an impaired ability to hydroxylate S-mephenytoin the disposition of the two enantiomers and metabolites will be comparable and similar to that of R-mephenytoin in extensive metabolizers. That is, S-mephenytoin will no longer be a high clearance drug and, therefore, its oral bioavailability will be high, its elimination slow and S-PEH will be formed in considerable amounts and will accumulate in a similar fashion to R-PEH. Studies to confirm these predictions are presently being pursued (45).

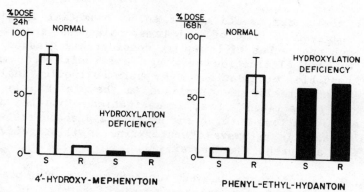

Figure 8. Comparison of the enantiomeric urinary excretion of mephenytoin metabolites in normal (extensive) metabolizers (mean ± SE) and in a subject with impaired hydroxylation (poor metabolizer) following a single dose of a radiolabeled pseudo-racemate of mephenytoin.

PERSPECTIVES

It has been a longstanding hope that the metabolic elimination of a drug could be predicted in some fashion by use of a marker compound(s). In this fashion, the problems of interpatient variability in drug disposition could be reduced since knowledge of the handling of one drug could be extrapolated to others. However, the involvement of multiple drug metabolizing enzymes, including the several isozymes of cytochrome P-450, has made this goal extremely difficult to achieve, and there are few practically useful relationships between the qualitative and/or quantitative elimination of different drugs. Accordingly, the discovery of discrete populations with markedly different disposition characteristics for certain index drugs such as debrisoquine and mephenytoin, and the correlation between these and the pharmacokinetic and pharmacodynamic behavior of other drugs is very exciting. It is, however, surprising, considering the relatively high incidence of these defects in drug oxidation and their apparent involvement in severe side effects, that this discovery did not occur earlier. Moreover, pharmacokinetics made a negligible contribution to the initial and seminal findings. Several reasons may account for these situations. Previously, the major emphasis on interindividual differences in drug disposition was upon the pharmacokinetic characteristics of the parent drug, especially in plasma. Elegant mathematical approaches were developed and applied for this purpose. However, the formation and elimination of metabolites, regardless of their pharmacological activity, has largely been neglected, at least by most pharmacokineticists. Consideration of the clearance processes of individual metabolic processes, such as fractional clearances, would appear to be essential if additional insights into variability of drug responsiveness are to be obtained. Such approaches will require considerably greater emphasis upon the urinary elimination of drugs and their metabolites, as well as possible elucidation and pharmacokinetic analysis of metabolite concentration-time profiles in the plasma. In addition to the studies described above, investigations into the differential effects of various interacting drugs and disease states on the individual metabolic pathways of antipyrine is illustrative of the value of this approach (see Chapter 17).

Another factor that delayed recognition of the presence of polymorphic drug oxidation relates to the frequency of defective metabolism. Although a large number of individuals are affected, (possibly between 10 and 20 million people in the U.S. may be deficient in the metabolism of debrisoquine), within the relatively small groups of subjects in whom various studies are performed during the initial development of a drug only a small number of these deficient individuals will be present. There is, therefore, a danger of overlooking the findings from such subjects and regarding them as "outliers." This attitude and approach discards the very information that provides the entrée to the elucidation of the critical mechanisms that are responsible for interindividual variability. It is to be hoped, therefore, that greater emphasis will be placed on in-depth studies of apparently aberrant pharmacokinetic and/or pharmacological findings.

The implications of the recent studies concerning the genetics of drug oxidation are only in the early stages of recognition. What is the biochemical mechanism of defective metabolism, how many different types of polymorphism exist, what effect do environmental factors and disease states have on the polymorphism, what is the relationship of polymorphism to therapeutic and adverse effects, especially those previously considered to be idiosyncratic? Such questions will require contributions from many different aspects of the pharmacological sciences, including pharmacokinetics, and hopefully the knowledge developed will permit more rational and safer drug use.

Acknowledgements. This research was supported in part by U.S. P.H.S. grants GM-15431 and GM-31304.

REFERENCES

1. N.H.G. Holford and L.B. Sheiner, Pharmacokinetic and pharmacodynamic modeling in vivo, CRC Critical Reviews in Bioengineering 5:273-322 (1981).
2. E.S. Vesell, Pharmacogenetics, Biochem. Pharmacol. 24:445-450 (1975).

3. E.S. Vesell, Intraspecies differences in frequency of genes directly affecting drug disposition: The individual factor in drug response, Pharmacol. Rev. 30:555-563 (1979).

4. W.W. Weber, Acetylation of drugs, in: "Metabolic Conjugations and Metabolic Hydrolysis," (Vol. 3), W.H. Fishman, ed., Academic Press, New York (1973), pp. 249-296.

5. J.R. Playfer, L.C. Eze, M.F. Bullen and D.A.P. Evans, Genetic polymorphism and interethnic variability of plasma paraoxonase activity, J. Med. Gen. 13:337-342 (1976).

6. W. Kalow and N. Staron, On distribution and inheritance of atypical forms of human serum cholinesterase as indicated by dibucaine numbers, Can. J. Biochem. Physiol. 35:1305-1320 (1957).

7. A. Mahgoub, J.R. Idle, L.G. Dring, R. Lancaster and R.L. Smith, Polymorphic hydroxylation of debrisoquine in man, Lancet II:584-586 (1977).

8. G.T. Tucker, J.H. Silas, A.O. Iyun, M.S. Lennard and A.J. Smith, Polymorphic hydroxylation of debrisoquine, Lancet II:718 (1977).

9. D.A. Price-Evans, A. Mahgoub, T.P. Sloan, J.R. Idle and R.L. Smith, A family and population study of the genetic polymorphism of debrisoquine oxidation in a white British population, J. Med. Gen. 17:102-105 (1980).

10. S.I. Islam, J.R. Idle and R.L. Smith, The polymorphic 4-hydroxylation of debrisoquine in a Saudi arab population, Xenobiotica 10:819-825 (1980).

11. A. Mahgoub, J.R. Idle and R.L. Smith, A population and familial study of the defective alicylic hydroxylation of debrisoquine among Egyptians, Xenobiotica 9:51-56 (1979).

12. N.M. Woolhouse, B. Andoh, A. Mahgoub, T.P Sloan, J.R. Idle and R.L. Smith, Debrisoquine hydroxylation polymorphism among Ghanaians and Caucasians, Clin. Pharmacol. Ther. 26:584-591 (1979).

13. C. Mbanefo, E.A. Bababunmi, A. Mahgoub, T.P. Sloan, J.R. Idle and R.L. Smith, A study of the debrisoquine hydroxylation polymorphism in a Nigerian population, Xenobiotica 10:811-818 (1980).

14. M. Eichelbaum, N. Spannbrucker, B. Steincke and H.J. Dengler, Defective N-oxidation of sparteine in man: A new pharmacogenetic defect, Europ. J. Clin. Pharmacol. 16:183-187 (1979).

15. M. Eichelbaum, N. Spannbrucker and H.J. Dengler, Influence of defective metabolism of sparteine on its pharmacokinetics, Europ. J. Clin. Pharmacol. 16:189-194 (1979).

16. T. Inaba, S.V. Otton and W. Kalow, Deficient metabolism of debrisoquine and sparteine, Clin. Pharmacol. Ther. 27:547-549 (1980).

17. M. Eichelbaum, L. Bertilsson, J. Säwe and C. Zekorn, Polymorphic oxidation of sparteine and debrisoquine: Related pharmacogenetic entities, Clin. Pharmacol. Ther. 31:184-186 (1982).

18. J.R. Idle and R.L. Smith, Polymorphism of oxidation at carbon centers and their clinical significance, Drug Metab. Rev. 9:301-317 (1979).

19. T.P. Sloan, A. Mahgoub, R. Lancaster, J.R. Idle and R.L. Smith, Polymorphism of carbon oxidation of drugs and clinical implications, Brit. Med. J. 2:655-657 (1978).

20. L. Bertilsson, M. Eichelbaum, B. Mellström, J. Säwe, H.U. Schulz and F. Sjöqvist, Nortriptyline and antipyrine clearance in relation to debrisoquine hydroxylation in man, Life Sci. 27:1673-1677 (1980).

21. B. Mellström, L. Bertilsson, J. Säwe, H. U. Schulz and F. Sjöqvist, E- and Z-10-hydroxylation of nortriptyline: relationship to polymorphic debrisoquine hydroxylation, Clin. Pharmacol. Ther. 30:189-193 (1981).

22. N.S. Oates, R.R. Shah, J.R. Idle and R.L. Smith, Genetic polymorphism of phenformin 4-hydroxylation, Clin. Pharmacol. Ther. 32:81-89 (1982).

23. M. Eichelbaum, Defective oxidation of drugs: pharmacokinetic and therapeutic implications, Clin. Pharmacokin. 7:1-22 (1982).

24. T.P. Sloan, J.R. Idle and R.L. Smith, Influence of D^H/D^L alleles regulating debrisoquine oxidation on phenytoin hydroxylation, Clin. Pharmacol. Ther. 29:493-497 (1981).

25. L.A. Wakile, T.P. Sloan, J.R. Idle and R.L. Smith, Genetic evidence for the involvement of different mechanisms in drug oxidation, J. Pharm. Pharmacol. 31:350-351 (1979).

26. J.R. Idle, A. Mahgoub, R. Lancaster and R.L. Smith, Hypotensive response to debrisoquine and hydroxylation phenotype, Life Sci. 22:979-984 (1978).

27. J.C. Ritchie, T.P. Sloan, J.R. Idle and R.L. Smith, Toxicological implications of polymorphic drug metabolism, in: "Environmental Chemicals, Enzyme Function and Human Disease," (CIBA Foundation Symposium 76), Excerpta Medica, Amsterdam (1980); pp. 219-244.

28. R.R. Shah, N.S. Oates, J.R. Idle, R.L. Smith and J.D.F. Lockhart, Impaired oxidation of debrisoquine in patients with perhexilene neuropathy, Brit. Med. J. 284:295-299 (1982).

29. P. Dayer, A. Kubli, A. Küpfer, F. Courvosier, L. Balant and J. Fabre, Defective hydroxylation of bufuralol associated with side effects of the drug in poor metabolisers, Brit. J. Clin. Pharmacol. 13:750-752 (1982).

30. D.M. Roden, S.B. Reele, S.B. Higgins, R.F. Mayol, R.E. Gammans, J.A. Oates and R.L. Ooosley, Total suppression of ventricular arrhythmias by encainide: pharmacokinetic and electrocardiographic characteristics, New Engl. J. Med. 302:877-882 (1981).

31. R.F. Mayol and R.E. Gammans, Analysis of encainide in plasma by radioimmunoassay and high pressure liquid chromatography, Therap. Drug Monitor. 1:507-524 (1979).

32. R.F. Mayol, R.E. Gammans and I.A. LaBudde, Analysis of encain-
     ide and its metabolites in man using a new high pressure
     liquid chromatographic method, Clin. Pharmacol. Ther. 29:265-
     266 (1981).
33. T. Wang, D.M. Roden, H.T. Wolfenden, R.L. Woosley, A.J.J. Wood
     and G.R. Wilkinson, Influence of genetic polymorphism on the
     metabolism and disposition of encainide in man, J. Pharmacol.
     Exp. Ther. 228:605-611 (1984).
34. R.L. Woosley, D.M. Roden, H.J. Duff, E.L. Carey, A.J.J. Wood
     and G.R. Wilkinson, Co-inheritance of deficient oxidative
     metabolism of encainide and debrisoquine, Clin. Res. 29:501A
     (1981).
35. A.W. Gomoll, J.E. Byrne and R.F. Mayol, Comparative anti-
     arrhythmic (AA) and local anesthetic actions of encainide (E)
     and its two major metabolites, Pharmacologist 23:209 (1981).
36. D.M. Roden, H.J. Duff, D. Altenbern and R.L. Woosley, Anti-
     arrhythmic activity of the O-demethyl metabolite of encainide,
     J. Pharmacol. Exp. Ther. 221:552-557 (1982).
37. R.A. Winkle, F. Peters, R.E. Kates, C. Tucker and D.C.
     Harrison, Clinical pharmacology and antiarrhythmic efficacy of
     encainide in patients with chronic ventricular arrhythmias,
     Circulation 64:290-296 (1981).
38. E.L. Carey, H.J. Duff, D.M. Roden, R.K. Primm, G.R. Wilkinson,
     T. Wang, J.A. Oates and R.L. Woosley, Encainide and its
     metabolites: comparative effects in man on ventricular
     arrhythmia and electrocardiographic intervals, J. Clin.
     Invest. 73:539-547 (1984).
39. A. Küpfer and J. Bircher, Stereoselectivity of differential
     routes of drug metabolism: The fate of the enantiomers of
     (^{14}C) mephenytoin in the dog, J. Pharmacol. Exp. Ther.
     209:190-195 (1979).
40. A. Küpfer, R.K. Roberts, S. Schenker and R.A. Branch, Stereo-
     selective metabolism of mephenytoin in man, J. Pharmacol. Exp.
     Ther. 218:193-199 (1981).
41. A. Küpfer, P.V. Desmond, S. Schenker and R.A. Branch, Stereo-
     selective metabolism and disposition of the enantiomers of
     mephenytoin during chronic oral administration of the racemic
     drug in man, J. Pharmacol. Exp. Ther. 221:590-597 (1982).
42. A. Küpfer, P. Desmond, S. Schenker and R. Branch, Family study
     of a genetically determined deficiency of mephenytoin hydrox-
     ylation in man, Pharmacologist, 21:173 (1979).
43. A. Küpfer, B. Dick and R. Preisig, Polymorphic mephenytoin
     hydroxylation in man: A new phenotype in the genetic control
     of hepatic drug metabolism, Hepatology 1:524 (1981).
44. W. Aslanian, P.J. Wedlund, C.B. McAllister, G.R. Wilkinson and
     R.A. Branch, Polymorphic hydroxylation of S-mephenytoin and
     its relationship to debrisoquine phenotype, Pharmacologist
     25:606 (1983).

45. P.J. Wedlund, B.J. Sweetman, C.B. McAllister, R.A. Branch and
    G.R. Wilkinson, Direct enantiomeric resolution of mephenytoin
    and N-demethylated metabolite in plasma and blood using chiral
    capillary gas chromatography, J. Chromatogr. 307:121-127
    (1984).

Chapter 19

PROBLEMS IN CORRELATING IN VITRO AND IN VIVO STUDIES OF DRUG METABOLISM

James R. Gillette

Laboratory of Chemical Pharmacology
National Heart, Lung and Blood Institute
National Institutes of Health
Bethesda, Maryland

No single approach for studying drug metabolism provides all the necessary information required for a complete understanding of the factors that govern the time courses of the concentrations of drugs and other foreign compounds and their metabolites in tissues of the body. Some of the factors are best studied with pure enzymes, while others are best studied with subcellular organelles, intact cells, intact organs or living animals. Well integrated programs encompassing all of these approaches are required if we are ever going to understand fully the metabolism of drugs by living animals and the ways by which pharmacokinetic characteristics may be altered. In order to make extrapolations between approaches, however, it is necessary to test data obtained by various approaches for consistency. Only in this way can we gain confidence that the conclusions derived from in vitro experiments do indeed account for the events that occur in vivo.

Although pharmacokinetics provides ways of comparing the results of different kinds of experiments, all too frequently the parameters required for making these comparisons are either not determined or not reported in research communications. Occasionally there are practical reasons for this failure to report relevant parameters, but more often than not, there is a lack of understanding between the biochemists, who perform in vitro experiments, and the pharmacokineticists, who attempt to extrapolate the information to living animals. The purpose of the present paper is to point out the kinds of information that theoretically can be obtained from each of the approaches to drug metabolism and the theoretical and practical limitations of each approach.

235

STUDIES WITH SINGLE ENZYMES

There are many reasons for purifying the enzymes that catalyze the metabolism of drugs. Some investigators purify enzymes as a requisite step in the production of antibodies. These antibodies are useful in identifying the contribution of the enzyme to the total metabolism of drugs in complex systems, in determining the location of the enzymes in tissues and organs, and in estimating the amounts of the enzyme in these organs. The primary objectives, however, are to determine the substrate specificity of the enzymes, the mechanisms of the enzymes and the kinetic relationships that govern the combinations between the enzymes and the substrates, cosubstrates, activators, products and inhibitors. The importance of determining the mechanisms of the enzymes, however, has been largely ignored by pharmacokineticists.

One of the major problems in making extrapolations from in vitro to in vivo is the lack of universally accepted nomenclature. Nearly everyone is aware of the Michaelis-Menten mechanism in which:

$$[E] + [S] \underset{k_2}{\overset{k_1}{\rightleftharpoons}} [ES] \overset{k_3}{\rightarrow} [E] + [P] \tag{1}$$

The steady-state equation derived for this mechanism is:

$$-\frac{d[S]}{dt} = \frac{[E]k_3[S]}{K_m + [S]} = \frac{[V_{max}][S]}{K_m + [S]} \tag{2}$$

and the integrated form of the equation is:

$$[V_{max}] t = [S]_o - [S] + K_m \ln [S]_o/[S] \tag{3}$$

where $[S]_o$ is the initial substrate concentration and $[S]$ is the concentration at time (t).

Because the rate of metabolism $(- d[S]/dt)$ in Equation (2) and $[V_{max}]$ in Equations (2) and (3) have dimensions of concentration per time, the values obtained will vary with the volume of the system and therefore are virtually useless not only to the biochemist, who is interested in obtaining parameters that characterize the kinetics of an enzyme, but also to those pharmacokineticists who are interested in extrapolating results from one kind of system to another.

As used by biochemists, V_{max} means the maximum rate of metabolism (expressed as amount of substrate metabolized per time) per mole of enzyme that would theoretically be achieved at infinite concentrations of substrate, cosubstrate and obligatory activators.

It thus does not have the same meaning as the $[V_{max}]$ in Equation (2), but should equal the terms represented by k_3. To achieve the same meaning, the "$k_{(cat)}$" of the biochemist (see Higuchi, Chapter 9) should be multiplied by the number of moles of enzyme in the assay system, whereas both sides of Equation (2) must be multiplied by the volume of the system, V_d. The K_m in the equation is expressed as the concentration of unbound substrate in the system. When the substrate is reversibly bound to macromolecules other than the enzyme in the system, the relationship between the total and unbound concentration must be known, i.e., $[S]_{free}/[S]_{total} = f_f$. With these modifications, Equation (2) may be expressed as:

$$-V_d(d[S]/dt) = \text{Rate} = \frac{V_d[E]k_3f_f[S]_{total}}{K_m + f_f[S]_{total}} = \frac{V_{max}f_f[S]_{total}}{K_m + f_f[S]_{total}}$$

$$= \frac{V_{max}[S]_{total}}{(K_m/f_f) + [S]_{total}} \tag{4}$$

The ratio of V_{max}/K_m has become a useful parameter to both biochemists and pharmacokineticists, although for different reasons. For biochemists, it is useful in evaluating the relative contributions of k_2 and k_3 to the value of K_m, whereas for pharmacokineticists it is useful as an "enzyme intrinsic clearance" or $CL_{int(enz)}$. With these relationships in mind, Equation (3) may be converted to more useful forms as follows:

$$V_{max}t/V_d = [S]_o - [S] + (K_m/f_f)\ln[S]_o/[S] \tag{5}$$

$$f_fCL_{int(enz)}t/V_d = [f_f([S]_o - [S])/K_m] + \ln[S]_o/[S] \tag{6}$$

$$\frac{Vd([S]_o - [S])}{t} = \frac{CL_{int(enz)}}{\dfrac{1}{K_m} + \dfrac{1}{f_f[\hat{S}]}} \tag{7}$$

where $[\hat{S}] = ([S]_o - [S])/\ln[S_o]/[S]$; $[S]_o$ is the initial total concentration and $[S]$ is the total concentration at time (t).

Another parameter that is useful under steady-state conditions is the ratio of the rate of metabolism to the concentration of unbound substrate, i.e.:

$$\frac{\text{Rate}}{f_f[S]_{total}} = \frac{V_{max}}{K_m + f_f[S]_{total}} = CL_{int(ss)} \tag{8}$$

Although its value varies with the concentration of the substrate, this ratio will be constant under steady-state conditions and thus will be called a "steady-state intrinsic clearance" ($CL_{int(ss)}$) in this chapter.

It should be kept in mind that the Michaelis-Menten equation almost always is a degenerate form of far more complex equations that describe many different kinds of enzymatic mechanisms. In these equations the V_{max} and the K_m values represent complex relationships which may be modified by changing not only the concentration of cosubstrates or activators but also the products formed from the substrate and the cosubstrate. The extent of the changes in the apparent V_{max} and K_m values, however, depends on the mechanism.

To illustrate why it is necessary to know the mechanism of the enzyme reaction, let us consider two rather common general mechanisms. In the first mechanism, the cosubstrate and substrate combine with two independent sites on the enzyme to form a ternary complex. If the products of the reaction have a low affinity for the enzyme and there is no interaction between the sites, the various forms of the enzyme and the equations for the steady-state intrinsic clearance may be illustrated as in Figure 1.

Inspection of the equation shown in Figure 1 reveals that the value of the apparent V_{max} will be directly related to the concentration of the cosubstrate, whereas the value of K_s will be independent of the concentration of the cosubstrate. Thus, the

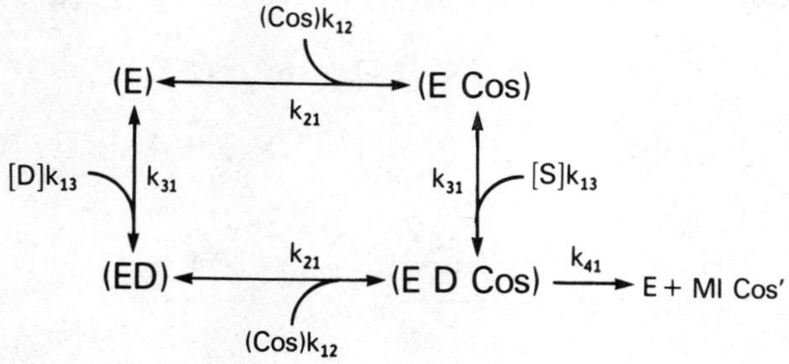

$$Ks = \frac{k_{21}}{k_{12}} \qquad Kc = \frac{k_{31}}{k_{13}}$$

$$CL_{int\ (ss)(D \to MI)} = Rate/[D] = V_{max(D \to MI)}/(Ks + [D])$$

$$V_{max\ (D \to MI)} = E_t\,k_{41}/(1 + (Kc/[Cos]))$$

Figure 1. A simple random equilibrium mechanism.

concentration of substrate at which the system leaves first-order kinetics will be independent of the concentration of the cosubstrate. Both the enzyme intrinsic clearance and the steady-state enzyme intrinsic clearance will be smaller at lower concentrations of cosubstrate than at higher concentrations. Studies by Banerjee and Roy (1) indicated that the initial rates of formation of phenyl sulfates by guinea pig liver sulfotransferase were consistent with this mechanism. However, recent studies have shown that the mechanism of rat liver aryl sulfotransferase IV is somewhat more complex. With 2-chloro-4-nitrophenol as the substrate, the apparent K_m will decrease from a maximum of 15 µM to a minimum of 4 µM as the 3'-phosphoadenosine 5'-phosphosulfate (PAPS) concentration is increased (2). Unfortunately, the mechanisms of the other sulfotransferases in rat liver, including those known to form acetaminophen sulfate, have not been studied.

In another mechanism, an enzyme initially combines only with the cosubstrate to form an activated species of the enzyme. The substrate then reacts with the activated species to form a complex that decomposes to the product. The acetylation of aromatic amines is thought to occur by this mechanism; acetyl-CoA acetylates the enzyme with the release of CoA and the amine then reacts with the acylated enzyme (3). If the products of the reaction have a low affinity for the enzyme, the various intermediate complexes and the

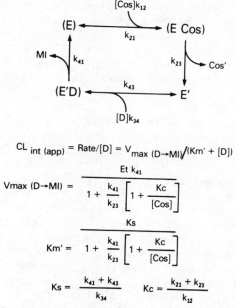

$$CL_{int\,(app)} = Rate/[D] = V_{max\,(D \to MI)}/(Km' + [D])$$

$$V_{max\,(D \to MI)} = \cfrac{Et\,k_{41}}{1 + \cfrac{k_{41}}{k_{23}}\left[1 + \cfrac{Kc}{[Cos]}\right]}$$

$$Km' = \cfrac{Ks}{1 + \cfrac{k_{41}}{k_{23}}\left[1 + \cfrac{Kc}{[Cos]}\right]}$$

$$Ks = \frac{k_{41} + k_{43}}{k_{34}} \qquad Kc = \frac{k_{21} + k_{23}}{k_{12}}$$

Figure 2. A simple ping-pong mechanism.

equations for the steady-state enzyme intrinsic clearance will be those shown in Figure 2. Inspection of the equations reveals that both the apparent V_{max} and the apparent K_m depend on the concentration of the cosubstrate. Thus the concentration of drug at which the system will no longer follow first-order kinetics will vary with the concentration of the cosubstrate. But notice that the terms representing the concentration of the cosubstrate appear in the equations for both the apparent V_{max} and the apparent K_m. Thus the equation predicts that as long as the system follows first-order kinetics, the enzyme intrinsic clearance should be independent of the concentration of the cosubstrate.

There are, of course, enzyme mechanisms that are far more complex than the ones described here. The mechanisms of the cytochromes P-450, which catalyze the metabolism of many drugs, still remain incompletely understood. In the commonly accepted general mechanism, oxidized cytochrome P-450 combines with a substrate to form a complex that is reduced by NADPH cytochrome P-450 reductase. The reduced complex is then oxygenated to form a complex that accepts another electron from either NADPH cytochrome P-450 reductase or cytochrome b_5 to form an "active oxygen" complex that decomposes to the products. The equation for a general model in which each of the intermediate complexes dissociate would be very complex and would contain terms in which the substrate concentration is raised to powers ranging from 1 to 4 (4). A Lineweaver-Burk plot of the equation should thus be curved rather than straight. The fact that most Lineweaver-Burk plots of the rate of metabolism are virtually straight rather than curved indicates that most of the endogenous NADPH oxidation observed with liver microsomes is associated with forms of cytochrome P-450 that do not catalyze the metabolism of the drug. The apparent K_m of such reactions is also complex and usually is larger than the dissociation constant of the complex between the oxidized cytochrome P-450 and the drug.

Because each of the various cytochromes P-450 may give rise to several different metabolites, the equations for the relationships between the apparent V_{max} and apparent K_m values would become obscure even if we were to accept the simple Michaelis-Menten mechanism for these enzymes. There are, of course, several hypothetical mechanisms which could lead to the formation of different metabolites. For example, a single chemically unstable intermediate could be formed by the enzyme; this intermediate might then dissociate from the enzyme and decompose to several different products. In this mechanism the K_m for the formation of each of the products would appear to be the same and the apparent V_{max} values would be a fraction of the V_{max} for the formation of the chemically reactive metabolite. Methods for estimating the V_{max} for the formation of the chemically unstable intermediate have been described elsewhere (5,6). It is also possible, however, that the substrate may fit onto the active site of the enzyme in several different ways resulting in different enzyme–substrate complexes, which might be visualized as having different dissociation constants. Because all of the complexes would be formed simultaneously, however, K_m values for all of the reactions would appear to be the same (Fig. 3) (7). It follows from this relationship that the ratio of the rates of formation of the various metabolites of the substrate by any given isozyme of cytochrome P–450 should be independent of the substrate concentration. Moreover, according to this mechanism, the enzyme intrinsic clearance for the formation of any given product obtained at low substrate concentrations should be the amount of enzyme times the rate constant for the conversion of the specific complex leading to the product divided by the K_s of that complex, i.e., $E_t\ k_1/K_1$.

Similar equations may be derived for the metabolism of two drugs by the same enzyme under conditions in which the relative concentrations of the two drugs are held constant (Fig. 4), as would occur, for example, with racemic mixtures. Thus, the relative rates at which the various products of the two drugs would be formed from a given mixture of drugs should be independent of the

$$E + D \rightleftharpoons (ED)_1 \rightarrow MIA + E$$

$$E + D \rightleftharpoons (ED)_2 \rightarrow MIB + E$$

$$E + D \rightleftharpoons (ED)_3 \rightarrow MIC + E$$

$$CL_{int(ss)\ (D \rightarrow MIA)} = Rate_{D \rightarrow MIA}/[D]$$

$$= V_{max(D \rightarrow MIA)}/(K_m' + [D]$$

$$V_{max(D \rightarrow MIA)} = \left[\frac{E_t k_{D \rightarrow MIA}}{K_{MIA}} \right] \left[\frac{1}{\dfrac{1}{K_{MIA}} + \dfrac{1}{K_{MIB}} + \dfrac{1}{K_{MIC}}} \right]$$

$$K_m' = \frac{1}{\dfrac{1}{K_{MIA}} + \dfrac{1}{K_{MIB}} + \dfrac{1}{K_{MIC}}}$$

or

$$CL_{int\ (ss)\ (D \rightarrow MIA)} = \frac{(E_t\ k_{D \rightarrow MIA}/K_{MIA})\ K_m'}{K_m' + [D]}$$

Figure 3. Equation for the formation of several products catalyzed by a single enzyme.

$$\frac{V_{D_1} \rightarrow MI_1}{[D_1]} = \frac{\left[\dfrac{(Enz)\, k_{D_1} - MI_1}{K_{D_1} \rightarrow MI_1}\right]\left[\left(\sum \dfrac{1}{K_{D_1}}\right) + \left(\sum \dfrac{[D_2]/[D_1]}{K_{D_2}}\right)\right]}{\left[\dfrac{1}{\left(\sum \dfrac{1}{K_{D_1}}\right) + \left(\sum \dfrac{[D_2]/[D_1]}{K_{D_2}}\right)}\right] + [D_1]}$$

$$\frac{V_{D_2} \rightarrow MI_2}{[D_2]} = \frac{\left[\dfrac{(Enz)\, k_{D_2} \rightarrow MI_2}{K_{D_2} \rightarrow MI_2}\right]\left[\left(\sum \dfrac{1}{K_{D_1}}\right) + \left(\sum \dfrac{[D_2]/[D_1]}{K_{D_2}}\right)\right]}{\left[\dfrac{1}{\left(\sum \dfrac{1}{K_{D_1}}\right) + \left(\sum \dfrac{[D_2]/[D_1]}{K_{D_2}}\right)}\right] + [D_1]}$$

Therefore

$V_{D_1} \rightarrow MI_1/V_{D_2} \rightarrow MI_2$ should be constant at any given $[D_2]/[D_1]$.

Figure 4. Equation for the metabolism of constant mixtures by a single enzyme.

total concentration of the mixture. Nevertheless, the enzyme intrinsic clearance for the formation of a product formed from one of the drugs should be the same as the enzyme intrinsic clearance obtained in an assay system containing that drug alone.

The inhibitory effects of products of an enzymatic reaction are also markedly dependent on the mechanism of the enzyme. Indeed, studies revealing whether the product derived from the cosubstrate inhibits competitively, noncompetitively, uncompetitively or mixed with respect to the cosubstrate and to the substrate provide valuable clues to the mechanism of the enzyme. For example, in the random equilibrium mechanism shown in Figure 1 representing an enzyme that requires NAD for the oxidation of a drug, NADH may be a competitive inhibitor with respect to NAD and a noncompetitive inhibitor with respect to the substrate. By contrast, the oxidation product of the drug may inhibit the reaction competitively with respect to the drug and noncompetitively with respect to NAD. Both products, therefore, would be expected to decrease the enzyme intrinsic clearance.

In the irreversible ping-pong mechanism shown in Figure 2, however, the cosubstrate reaction product (Cos') would be expected to inhibit the reaction only by combining with the unactivated form of the enzyme (E), whereas the metabolite of the drug would be expected to inhibit the reaction only by combining with the activated form of the enzyme (E'). In this kind of mechanism, therefore, the cosubstrate reaction product (Cos') would be expected to inhibit the reaction competitively with respect to the cosubstrate and uncompetitively with respect to the drug. Thus Cos' would not be expected to affect the enzyme intrinsic clearance of the drug if the concentration of the drug were below the K_m value in the uninhibited system because both the V_{max} and the K_m would be decreased to the same extent. By contrast, the metabolite of the drug would be expected to inhibit the reaction competitively with respect to the drug and noncompetitively with respect to the cosubstrate. Thus, the metabolite of the drug should decrease the enzyme intrinsic clearance by increasing the apparent K_m value.

If the cosubstrate reaction product combined with E' rather than with E and if the metabolite of the drug combined with E rather than with E', the ping-pong mechanism would be reversible rather than irreversible. In the absence of the Cos', however, the metabolite of the drug should then inhibit the reaction competitively with respect to the cosubstrate and uncompetitively with respect to the drug. In this reversible mechanism, therefore, the metabolite should not affect the enzyme intrinsic clearance, because it should decrease the apparent V_{max} and K_m values to the same extent.

There are, of course, more complex enzymatic mechanisms than the ones I have discussed here. The effects of the concentrations of the cosubstrates and the products derived from the cosubstrates and the drugs on the steady-state enzyme intrinsic clearances may in turn be complex. What should be evident from the simple enzyme mechanisms discussed here is the difficulty in extrapolating the effects from one kind of preparation to another unless the mechanism of the enzyme is known.

STUDIES WITH CELL-FREE PREPARATIONS

Although studies with purified enzymes provide information about the mechanism of an enzyme, its substrate specificity and the "k_{cat}/K_m" (the V_{max}/K_m per mole of enzyme) with any given drug, such studies cannot provide information concerning the amount of enzyme present in an organ and the occurrence of other enzymes that metabolize the drug.

Studies with cell-free preparations, properly performed and interpreted, could conceivably provide information that would facilitate the extrapolation of information obtained with pure enzymes to more highly integrated systems. As frequently performed and reported in the literature, however, the information gained from such studies is largely useless to the pharmacokineticist.

All too often a cell-free preparation, such as liver microsomes, is incubated with a single initial concentration of a drug and a single set of concentrations of cofactors for an arbitrary length of time and the metabolites of the drug are assayed. Such studies can be grossly misleading especially with drugs that are rapidly metabolized by the preparation.

To illustrate how such studies may be misleading, let us consider a hypothetical drug (D, in Figure 5) that undergoes both N-demethylation to MIA and hydroxylation to MIB. Let us also consider that MIA undergoes hydroxylation and MIB undergoes N-demethylation to form MIIA. Let us further consider that both hydroxylated metabolites MIB and MIIA undergo glucuronidation to form metabolites MIIB and MIII, respectively. With the first-order rate constants (microsomal intrinsic clearances divided by the volume of the incubation mixture) assumed for this system, we can simulate the expected concentrations of drug and the metabolites at various times in the absence (Fig. 6) and presence (Fig. 7) of UDP-glucuronic acid (UDPGA), the cosubstrate required for glucuronidation. As shown in Figure 6, the pattern of metabolites that the experimenter would find would depend on when he or she stopped the experiment. In Figure 6 the ratio of MIB to MIA would be greater at the shorter times than at the longer times, because the intrinsic clearance for the conversion of MIB to MIIA is greater than the intrinsic clearance for the conversion of MIA to MIIA. Moreover, at 15 minutes nearly all of the MIIA in the incubation mixture would have been formed from MIB. If the investigator had stopped the incubation at this time, he or she might have been led to the mistaken conclusion that the conversion of MIA to MIIA was of trivial importance. The simulation reveals, however, that ultimately the conversion of MIA to MIIA would have accounted for a third of the amount of MIIA formed in the absence of UDPGA. In the presence of UDPGA (Fig. 7), part of MIB would be converted to MIIB. Consequently, the t_{max} for MIB would be shortened and the maximum concentration of MIB decreased. Moreover, the amounts of MIIA and MIII formed from MIB would be decreased, but at 15 minutes it might still appear to be the predominant pathway. The simulation shows,

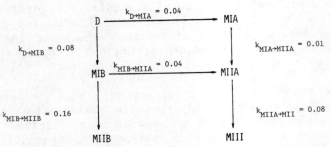

Figure 5. Metabolic pathways of a hypothetical drug.

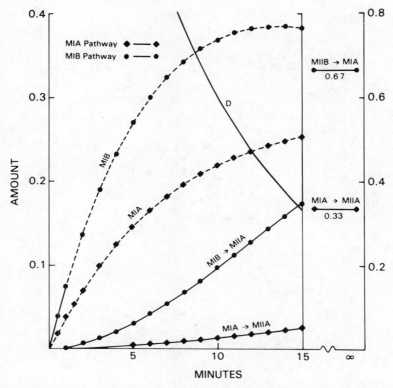

Figure 6. A simulation of the concentration of a drug and its metabolites in the absence of UDPGA. The rate constants are those shown in Figure 5.

however, that ultimately the major pathway for the formation of MIIA and MIII would be by way of MIA.

Seldom do experimenters choose drug concentrations that follow first-order kinetics. Instead, they frequently use concentrations that would saturate the enzyme or enzymes that metabolize the drug. If the drug and all the first generation metabolites were metabolized by the same enzyme, the high concentration of the substrate would inhibit the metabolism of the first generation metabolite. As shown in Figure 3, the relative rates of formation of the first generation metabolites formed at high concentrations of the parent drug could reflect the relative enzyme intrinsic clearances for the formation of the metabolites. However, drugs are rarely metabolized by only one enzyme. Thus, the relative rates obtained with high concentrations of the drug merely reflect the relative V_{max} values and the pattern of metabolism may appear to be different at low substrate concentrations.

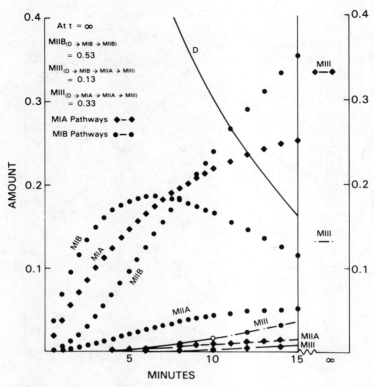

Figure 7. A simulation of the concentration of the drug and its
metabolites in the presence of UDPGA. The rate
constants are those shown in Figure 5.

Clearly, initial rates of metabolism of the drug over a wide
range of concentrations would be needed to determine whether the
drug is likely to be metabolized by different enzymes, and to estimate the K_m and V_{max} values for each of the enzymes. Such studies
should be repeated with each of the drug's metabolites. Only in
this way can one estimate the enzyme intrinsic clearances with
cell-free preparations, estimate the concentrations of drug above
which the system no longer follows first-order kinetics, and
determine the concentrations of metabolites above which mutual
inhibition might be expected.

STUDIES WITH INTACT CELLS

After the appropriate dilution and recovery factors have been
taken into account, the V_{max} and the K_m values obtained with intact
cells ideally should be the same as those obtained with cell-free

preparations. Indeed, if studies with cell-free preparations are to be useful in making quantitative extrapolations to living animals, these relationships should be confirmed.

In making these comparisons, however, the experimenter should be aware of the differences between the two kinds of experiments and the implications of these differences. Studies with cell-free preparations are usually performed at the optimum pH and with "maximal" concentrations of cofactors, including cosubstrates as well as "maximal" concentrations of substrates. However, the intracellular concentrations of these cofactors and the intracellular pH values in the biophase of the enzymes are seldom known in studies with intact cells. The intracellular concentrations of cosubstrates may be considerably below those required for maximal activity. Thus, depending on the enzyme mechanism, either the V_{max} alone or both the V_{max} and the K_m values may differ from those obtained with cell-free preparations. As pointed out in Figure 1, a less than maximal concentration of cosubstrate intracellularly would result in a decrease in the apparent V_{max}, but little or no change in the K_m value if the enzyme acts by an irreversible random equilibrium mechanism. By contrast, a less than maximal concentration of cosubstrate intracellularly would result in a decrease in both the V_{max} and K_m values, but little or no change in the enzyme intrinsic clearance if the mechanism of the enzyme is an irreversible ping-pong mechanism (Fig. 2). Because the drug may be metabolized by different enzymes acting through different mechanisms, the relative rates at which the drug metabolites are formed by the two enzymes may differ even when the same cosubstrate is metabolized by the enzymes.

Because intact cells are surrounded by lipoidal membranes, the entrance and exit of the drug, its metabolites and the precursors and products of the cosubstrates are governed in part by the diffusional clearances of the substances across the lipoidal membranes. Thus, studies with intact cells should be visualized as multicompartmental systems for each of these substances. Products of the cosubstrates may accumulate within the cells until a steady state is reached and thereby cause competitive, uncompetitive, noncompetitive or mixed inhibition with regard to either the cosubstrate or the drug depending on the mechanism of the enzyme. Indeed, it is quite probable that when the rate of metabolism of a drug in intact cell systems is increased by addition of precursors of the cosubstrate, the rate is governed primarily by the ratio of the intracellular concentrations of the cosubstrate and its product rather than by the absolute concentration of the cosubstrate.

If the diffusional clearance of the drug metabolite out of the cells is sufficiently slow, other effects may occur. The pseudo-steady state of intracellular concentration of the metabolite may become high enough to inhibit the metabolism of the drug. But again the mechanism of inhibition may be competitive, uncompetitive, noncompetitive or mixed depending on the enzyme mechanism. On the other hand, the metabolite may be further metabolized within the cells.   Thus, second generation metabolites may appear in the medium very shortly after the start of the incubation.   In this case, the rate of release of the second generation metabolites may appear to parallel the release of the first generation metabolites as the concentration of drug is increased, when the first generation metabolites are formed and eliminated by different enzymes. But if the first generation metabolites are metabolized by the same enzyme that catalyzes their formation, the rates of appearance of the second generation metabolites should increase to a maximum and then decrease as the concentration of the parent drug is increased.

If the diffusional clearance of the drug into and out of the cells is slow, the apparent K_m value, but presumably not the V_{max} value, for the formation of the first generation metabolites may differ from that observed with cell-free preparations.   If the passage of the drug into and out of cells is solely by passive diffusion, the K_m of the reaction will appear to be higher than that obtained with cell-free preparations.   If the drug enters cells by active transport systems, however, the K_m value will appear to be less than that obtained with cell-free preparations.

There are, of course, other reasons for discrepancies between the values obtained with cell-free systems and intact cells; perhaps the drug is metabolized within cells by enzymes that require cofactors not added to the cell-free systems; perhaps proteolytic enzymes are released during homogenization that inactivate enzymes that metabolize the drug.   In any case, studies to elucidate the reasons for the differences between cell-free and intact cell preparations should broaden our understanding of drug metabolism and facilitate extrapolation of the results obtained with cell-free systems to intact cells.

STUDIES WITH INTACT ORGANS

When the organ clearance of a drug is considerably smaller than the blood flow rate through the organ, the organ clearance should approach the sum of the individual clearances of all the cells within the organ.   Under these conditions the results obtained with intact cells may be compared to those obtained in organ perfusion experiments to determine whether the results obtained with the two kinds of preparations are consistent.

When the   organ clearance   of a drug approaches   the blood flow rate through the organ, the relationships between the blood flow rate and the cellular intrinsic clearances become obscure, because the steady-state concentrations of the unbound drug in the immediate environment of any given cell within the organ is unknown. Two simplistic models have been proposed to relate blood flow rates and the sum of the cellular intrinsic clearances when the concentrations are well below the K_m values of the enzymes, namely the "well-stirred" and "parallel tube" models. The problems of establishing the validity of these models have been beautifully summarized in this book by Rowland (see Chapter 13). Both of these models assume that the drug is metabolized by first-order kinetics, or by a single enzyme or by several enzymes having nearly identical K_m values. If the drug is metabolized by two enzymes with widely different K_m values, however, the concentration of drug may approach or exceed the K_m value of one enzyme but may still be much less than the other K_m value. In this situation, the well-stirred model predicts that the organ clearance will be:

$$CL_{(organ)} = \frac{Q\, f_f\, [CL_{int(2)} + \frac{V_{max(1)}}{K_{m(1)} + f_f(C_{out})}]}{Q + f_f\, [CL_{int(2)} + \frac{V_{max(1)}}{K_{m(1)} + f_f(C_{out})}]} \qquad (9)$$

The clearance predicted by the parallel tube model would be:

$$\frac{C_{out}}{C_{in}} \left[\frac{1 + f_f C_{out} F_2/K_{m(1)}}{1 + f_f C_{in} F_2/K_{m(1)}} \right]^{\frac{CL_{int(1)}}{CL_{int(2)}}} = e^{-f_f\left(CL_{int(1)} + CL_{int(2)}\right)/Q} \qquad (10)$$

where: $K_{m(1)}$ = smaller Michaelis constant

$CL_{int(1)}$ and $CL_{int(2)}$ = the enzyme instrinsic clearances

$F_2 = CL_{int(2)}/(CL_{int(1)} + CL_{int(2)})$

Useful though these simple models may be, they probably are not sufficiently sophisticated to predict accurately the relationships between the enzyme intrinsic clearances within cells and the microcirculation of blood within organs such as the liver. Neither model considers the following:

1.   Neither the intrinsic clearance nor perhaps even the apparent K_m of any given enzyme is exactly the same in all cells within the liver.

2. The relative amounts of the enzymes that metabolize a drug are also not the same for all cells of the liver.

3. The cellular intrinsic clearances are more apt to be governed by diffusional clearances when the intracellular intrinsic clearances are large than when they are small.

4. The blood entering a lobule probably follows a random drift through the sinusoids and thus a set of distances rather than a single distance would describe the blood flow through the lobule.

5. After the administration of a dye that is completely sequestered by hepatocytes during a single pass, the liver appears mottled, indicating a considerable variation in the flow rates of blood perfusing the lobules at any given time.

6. It is likely that the blood flow rate through any given lobule varies with time according to a sine function.

Therefore, the concentration of drug leaving the liver probably should be visualized as the average of a set of blood flow rates through a nearly infinite set of parallel tubes of various lengths and thus of various intrinsic clearances. According to this view, the kinetics of diseased liver may be even more complex because a part of the blood may pass through functional shunts in which the intrinsic clearances are small or absent, or because there are functional blocks in which a part of the organ intrinsic clearance does not contribute significantly to the extraction ratio. For these reasons, the relationships between the intrinsic clearance of an organ and the blood flow through the organ may be more accurately visualized as a partially mixed model, which includes characteristics of both the well-stirred and the parallel tube models (8).

STUDIES IN VIVO

When the total body clearance of a drug is considerably smaller than the blood flow rate through any organ participating in the elimination of the drug, the total body metabolic clearance calculated from the concentration of unbound drug should equal the sum of the cellular intrinsic clearances of all cells in the body (sometimes modified when a polar drug is metabolized by cells separated from blood by diffusional barriers such as the blood-brain barrier). When the extraction ratio by several organs becomes appreciable, however, the total body clearance should equal the sum of the effective organ clearances, each of which is calculated from the equation for the poly-input organ clearance

$(CL_{pin(organ)})$ as described by Gillette (9):

$$CL_{pin(organ)} = E_{(organ)} \sum (Q_i \Pi F_{pre(i)}) \qquad (11)$$

where Q_i represents the partitioned blood flow rate through a sequential set of organs through which the blood has flowed before it reaches the organ under consideration, and $\Pi F_{pre(i)}$ is the mathematical product of the availabilities for each of the sets of preorgans, and $E_{(organ)}$ is the extraction ratio for the organ under consideration.

FINAL COMMENTS

Because studies with purified enzymes, subcellular organelles, intact cells or intact organs cannot predict the volume of distribution of the drug in either the central or the peripheral compartments, studies with such preparations cannot predict the rate constants for the passage of the drug between compartments, or for the elimination of the drug from the body via the compartments. It follows therefore that any pharmacokinetic parameter such as biological half-life, the maximum concentration achieved after rapid injection or oral absorption of a drug, or the time required to achieve a steady state cannot be predicted solely from the results of in vitro studies. Only those relationships that are governed solely by clearances, such as the relationships that are achieved under steady-state conditions during constant infusion, are theoretically predictable. On the other hand, the in vivo rate constants can be the result of many different interrelated factors governed by many different mechanisms that are impossible to differentiate solely from the results of in vivo studies.

Thus, the purpose of in vitro experiments in combination with in vivo studies is to aid the investigator in separating plausible from implausible explanations of the results of the in vivo studies. For example, it is not possible to predict from in vitro experiments alone whether a given dose of drug will result in non-linear kinetics in vivo. But knowledge of the apparent K_m value of an enzyme, and the factors that affect it, aids in determining whether a given concentration of unbound drug in blood is likely to result in nonlinear kinetics, especially for the formation of the metabolites by reactions catalyzed by the enzyme. Moreover, the knowledge of the substrate specificity and the kinetic character-istics associated with each substrate should aid in predicting the concentrations at which drug interactions due to competitive and noncompetitive inhibition should be manifested. Such knowledge should also be valuable in predicting the relative steady-state concentrations of two or more drugs when they all are eliminated from the body solely by a single enzyme. Although pharmacokinetics cannot prove the validity of plausible mechanisms, it can aid in differentiating the plausible from the implausible.

REFERENCES

1. R.W. Banerjee and A.B. Roy, Kinetic studies of the phenol sul-photransferase, Biochim. Biophys. Acta 151:573-586 (1968).
2. M.W. Duffel and W.B. Jakoby, On the mechanism of aryl sulfo-transferase, J. Biol. Chem. 256:11123-11127 (1981).
3. W.W. Weber and S.N. Cohen, N-Acetylation of drugs: Isolation and properties of an N-acetyltransferase from rabbit liver, Mol. Pharmacol. 3:266-273 (1967).
4. J.R. Gillette, H. Sasame and B. Stripp, Mechanisms of inhibi-tion of drug metabolic reactions, in: "Microsomes and Drug Oxi-dations," R.W. Estabrook, J.R. Gillette and K.C. Leibman, eds., Williams and Wilkins, Baltimore (1973), pp. 164-175.
5. J.R. Gillette, Kinetics of decomposition of chemically unstable metabolites in the presence of nucleophiles: Derivation of equations used in graphical analyses, Pharmacology 20:64-86 (1980).
6. J.R. Gillette, S.D. Nelson, G.J. Mulder, D.J. Jollow, J.R. Mitchell, L.R. Pohl and J.A. Hinson, Formation of chemically reactive metabolites of phenacetin and acetaminophen, in: "Biological Reactive Intermediates - II. Part B," R. Snyder, D.V. Parke, J.J. Kocsis, D.J. Jollow, C.G. Gibson and C.M. Witmer, eds., Plenum Press, New York (1982), pp. 931-950.
7. W.R. Porter, R.V. Branchflower and W.F. Trager, A kinetic method for the determination of the multiple forms of micro-somal cytochrome P-450, Biochem. Pharmacol. 26:549-550 (1977).
8. K.S. Pang and J.R. Gillette, Kinetics of metabolite formation and elimination in the perfused rat liver preparation: Dif-ferences between the elimination of preformed acetaminophen and acetaminophen formed from phenacetin, J. Pharmacol. Exp. Ther. 207:178-194 (1978).
9. J.R. Gillette, Sequential organ first-pass effects: Simple methods for constructing compartmental pharmacokinetic models from physiological models or drug disposition by several organs, J. Pharm. Sci. 71:673-677 (1982).

Chapter 20

INTEGRAL PROCEDURES IN PHARMACOKINETICS AND THEIR APPLICATION TO THE PARAMETER DETERMINATION OF APPEARING METABOLITES

Edward R. Garrett

The Beehive
College of Pharmacy
J. Hillis Miller Health Center
University of Florida
Gainesville, Florida

The pharmacokinetics of a substance are studied best by the simultaneous measurement of the drug and all of its possible metabolites, especially if they possess similar pharmacological activities, in all monitorable tissues of the animal (1,2). The mathematical delineation of the plasma concentration-time course of the administered drug yields only an equation. Thus, it is difficult to predict the time course of drug and metabolites in plasma and urine under selected conditions of dose and administration. An integrated model, that quantitatively describes the tissue concentrations, interconversions, transformations, and excretory patterns of the drug and its metabolites as functions of the dose, may permit correlations with pharmacodynamic activities and give insight into the mechanisms of action.

These approaches demand novel methods of data manipulation to determine the pharmacokinetic parameters, and levels of abstraction above the mere statement or plotting of the numbers obtained from tissues monitored as a function of time. Such methods may permit the deduction of pharmacokinetic parameters for metabolites after administration of the precursor drug, without performing specific studies involving direct metabolite administration.

With the advent of elegant analytical methodology, such as HPLC, and the ability to simultaneously monitor a drug and its manifold metabolites in body fluids and excreta, there is no reason to conduct future pharmacokinetic studies without such simultaneous monitoring. Thus all modern pharmacokinetic studies

253

of drugs should be expected to provide pharmacokinetic parameters for all metabolites and all in vivo transformations.

The concepts of clearance have been revitalized (3-5). These concepts can be utilized further to describe the integral pharmacokinetics of a drug and its metabolites. In this chapter, the utility and power of such integral methods for characterization and prediction will be stressed and examples given.

CLEARANCE CONCEPTS

If the rate of total transformation and elimination, dA_{el}/dt of a drug to amounts of metabolites (M) and amounts in urine (U) can be formulated as proportional to the amount of drug (P) in the body, where $A_{el} = M + U$, then:

$$dA_{el}/dt = kP = kV_p C_p = CL \cdot C_p \tag{1}$$

where k is the first-order rate constant for the elimination, V_p is the apparent overall volume of distribution of the drug referenced to the plasma concentration and the product kV_p, which is the proportionality constant between the rate of elimination of amounts and the plasma concentration (C_p), is termed the total (body) clearance of the drug (CL). The integral expression which implicitly defines clearance can be obtained by integrating Equation (1) with respect to time:

$$A_{el,t} = CL \cdot AUC_t \tag{2}$$

where the cumulative amount of drug eliminated at any time (t) is the constant clearance (CL) multiplied by the area under the plasma concentration-time curve to that time. The cumulative amount of drug excreted at infinite time ($A_{el\infty}$) is equal to the systemically available dose (FD) and is related by the total clearance to the total or infinite area under the plasma concentration-time curve (AUC_∞):

$$FD = A_{el\infty} = CL \cdot AUC_\infty \tag{3}$$

If the rate of formation of an amount of a metabolite (M) or the rate of elimination of an amount of unchanged drug into the urine (U) can be formulated similarly as proportional to the amount of drug (P) in the body, then the metabolic and renal clearances can be implicitly defined in an analogous manner. That is:

$$dU/dt = CL_R C_p; \quad U_t = CL_R AUC_t \tag{4}$$

$$dM/dt = CL_{met} C_p; \quad M_t = CL_{met} AUC_t \tag{5}$$

where U_t and M_t, respectively, are the cumulative amounts of drug excreted into the urine and transformed into metabolite at time (t). If a rate of elimination or the cumulative amount eliminated can be monitored, the clearance can be obtained from the slope of appropriate plots in accordance with Equations (1),(2),(4) and (5).

COMPARTMENTAL PHARMACOKINETIC MODELS

Pharmacokinetic parameters can be determined from compartmental body models where the time course of amounts or concentrations in observable tissues can be constructed in terms of their kinetics of transport or transformation to another compartment. Such compartments are defined as those hypothetical volumes in the body wherein the drug is homogeneously and instantaneously dispersed and within which there is no barrier to free diffusion. The evaluated rate constants are those invariant proportionality factors that relate rates of tranfer to amounts of material in compartments. An example is the two-compartment body model with first-order transfers between amounts in plasma, tissue and excreta (6,7). Such a model is described by linear pharmacokinetics.

The term "linear" is used because the equations comprise a set of linear homogeneous differential equations (a terminology of analytical mathematics) and plasma concentration-time or compartmental concentration-time equations can be constructed from the solutions of such linear differential equations. Such systems have definite properties: transfers are first-order; multiples of the dose give the same multiple of amount or concentration of drug in any compartment for the same time; the plasma concentration-time curve for such systems can be characterized by a linear sum of exponentials:

$$C_p = A_1 e^{-\lambda_1 t} + A_2 e^{-\lambda_2 t} + \ldots + A_z e^{-\lambda_z t} \qquad (6)$$

where $C_p = P/V_p$ for an amount of drug P in an apparent volume of distribution V_p. This volume V_p can be operationally defined as the proportionality constant that relates the amount of material in the central or sampled compartment to the observed concentration therein (8). Compartmental analysis in pharmacokinetics demands the postulation of the minimum number of compartments necessary to quantitatively describe the pharmacokinetic model consistent with physiological reality. The simplest compartmental model that fits the data is chosen and is then challenged by proper experimental design for validation. The terminal slope of a semilogarithmic plot of such plasma concentrations (ln C_p versus t) approaches linearity where the slope is $-\lambda_z$ since:

$$\lambda_z \ll \ldots \lambda_2 \ll \lambda_1$$

and:

$$e^{-\lambda_1 t} + e^{-\lambda_2 t} + \ldots$$

vanish or approach zero values with increasing time so that the terminal plasma concentration is ultimately characterized solely by the final exponential, $e^{-\lambda_z t}$, in Equation (6).

A nonlinear model does not have the above properties. It is "nonlinear" because linear differential equations cannot describe the processes. A rate of transference or elimination is not simply proportional to amount or concentration. A simple example is the Michaelis-Menten formulation of the saturable rate of elimination of a uniquely metabolized drug from a one-compartment body model, $P \overset{sat}{\rightarrow} M$, where the numbers of enzyme molecules in the clearing organ are limited and finite (9). The rate of elimination can be described in terms of amounts (P) in plasma by:

$$dA_{el}/dt = V_{max} \ P/(K_m + P) \tag{7}$$

or in terms of concentrations (C_p) in plasma by:

$$dA_{el}/dt = V_{max} \ V_p C_p/(K_m + V_p C_p) \tag{8}$$

where K_m is the Michaelis-Menten apparent dissociation constant of the enzyme-substrate complex and V_{max} is the theoretical maximal rate of metabolism of the drug. In general, the clearance is not constant but varies with the plasma concentration: $V_{max} \ V_p/(K_m + V_p C_p) = CL$.

NONCOMPARTMENTAL BODY MODELS

Many pharmacokinetic parameters can be estimated without recourse to compartmental models. Although frequently termed "model-free" parameters, actually, they are not. Implicit in their determination are the underlying postulates that all transfers are first-order and that the pharmacokinetics are dose-independent or "linear". The experimental verification of such assumptions is obtained when plots of plasma concentrations of drug and metabolites, and urinary amounts of drug and metabolites divided by the available dose are superimposable when plotted against time. Also implicit in the determination of these model-free parameters is the postulation that the clearance occurs from the central compartment so that equations of the form of Equations (1-5) are operationally valid. The calculable model-free parameters (10) include:

terminal half-life, $t_{1/2} = 0.693/\lambda_z$

total clearance, $CL = Dose/AUC_\infty$

renal clearance, $CL_R = U_t/AUC_t$

metabolic clearance, $CL_{met} = CL - CL_R$

steady-state volume of distribution (V_{ss})

the apparent pseudo-steady-state volume of distribution,
        V (often designated V_{area})

The area under the plasma concentration-time curve can be obtained
from the application of the trapezoidal rule or by use of integral
expressions derived from a sum of exponentials (Eq. (6)) fitted to
such curves:

$$AUC_\infty = \frac{A_1}{\lambda_1} + \frac{A_2}{\lambda_2} + \ldots + \frac{A_z}{\lambda_z} \tag{9}$$

The area under the curve at any time (t) is:

$$AUC_t = \frac{A_1}{\lambda_1}(1-e^{-\lambda_1 t}) + \frac{A_2}{\lambda_2}(1-e^{-\lambda_2 t}) + \ldots + \frac{A_z}{\lambda_z}(1-e^{-\lambda_z t}) \tag{10}$$

The apparent pseudo-steady-state volume of distribution (V) can be
calculated as:

$$V = CL/\lambda_z \tag{11}$$

INTEGRAL APPROACHES TO THE DETERMINATION OF COMPARTMENTAL MODEL-FREE PHARMACOKINETIC PARAMETERS

Clearances are implicitly defined in the integral expressions
(Eqs. (2)-(5)) obtained from simple first-order dependencies of
rates of formation and elimination on plasma concentrations. Such
integral expressions merely state that the cumulative amount of
drug transformed, metabolized or excreted at any time is directly
proportional to the area under the plasma concentration-time curve
up to that time. The clearance (CL) is the proportionality
constant.

The simplest example of the application of the integral method
is the estimation of renal clearance from the slope of a plot of
the cumulative amount of drug excreted into the urine against the
area of the plasma concentration-time curve so that this cumulative
amount can be predicted for any time (t) in accordance with Equation (4). The ability of this equation to fit the experimentally

determined cumulative amounts of heroin and its metabolites
excreted into the urine as a function of time is illustrated in
Figure 1 (2).

An example of the power of these simple procedures (Eqs. (1)–
(5)) is the determination of the rate constants for the sequential
first-order kinetics of the degradation of an amount of reactant
(A) in a solution of volume (V) (11):

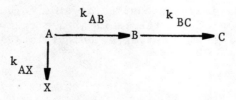

where the concentrations [A], [B] and [C] are monitored with time.
The reactant (A) may or may not degrade by other simultaneous processes (k_{AX}) to other products (X). The stoichiometric expression

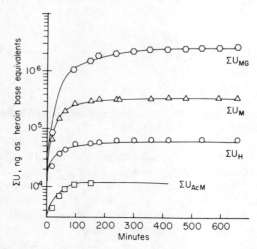

Figure 1. Plots of experimental values of cumulative heroin, $\Sigma\ U_H$,
monoacetylmorphine, $\Sigma\ U_{AcM}$, morphine $\Sigma\ U_M$ and morphine
conjugate, $\Sigma\ U_{MG}$, in urine against time for an i.v.
0.337 mg/kg dose of heroin in the dog. The solid lines
through the data were calculated from $\Sigma\ U = CL_R AUC$ where
$CL_R^H = 48$, $CL^{AcM} = 22$, $CL_R^M = 67$ and $CL_R^{MG} = 50$ ml/min.
Reprinted from (2) with permission of the Journal of
Pharmaceutical Sciences, the copyright owner.

for (B) at any time (t) can be constructed from the appropriate
integral expressions:

$$B_t = \text{(Total amount A} \rightarrow \text{B)} - \text{(Amount B} \rightarrow \text{C)}$$

$$= V_B[B] = CL_{AB}AUC_t^A - CL_{BC}AUC_t^B \tag{12}$$

where:

CL_{AB} and CL_{BC} are the clearances of A to B and B to C

AUC_t^A and AUC_t^B are the respective areas under the A and B
concentration-time curves at time (t)

$$CL_{AB} = k_{AB}V$$

$$CL_{BC} = k_{BC}V$$

$$V_A = V_B = V_C = V$$

Equation (12) can be rearranged to:

$$\frac{[B]}{AUC_t^A} = \frac{CL_{AB}}{V} - \frac{CL_{BC}}{V} \frac{AUC_t^B}{AUC_t^A} = k_{AB} - k_{BC} \frac{AUC_t^B}{AUC_t^A} \tag{13}$$

or:

$$\frac{[B]}{AUC_t^B} = \frac{CL_{AB}}{V} \frac{AUC_t^A}{AUC_t^B} - \frac{CL_{BC}}{V} = k_{AB}\frac{AUC_t^A}{AUC_t^B} - k_{BC} \tag{14}$$

where the rate constants k_{AB} and k_{BC} can be estimated from the
slope and intercept of appropriate plots in accordance with these
equations. The total clearance of A is:

$$CL_{tot}^A = k_{tot}^A V = CL_{AB} + CL_{AX} = A_0/AUC_\infty^A \tag{15}$$

where AUC_∞^A is the total area under the concentration versus time
plot for an initial amount of reactant (A_0) and $k_{tot}^A = k_{AB} + k_{AX}$.
Thus, the rate constant k_{AX} can be estimated from:

$$k_{AX} = \frac{CL_{tot}^A - CL_{AB}}{V} = CL_{tot}/V - k_{AB} \tag{16}$$

If the concentration of C, [C], is monitored, $V[C]$ can be
substituted into Equation (12) for $CL_{BC}AUC_t^B$, and the
stoichiometry can be established as:

$$V[B] = CL_{AB}AUC_t^A - V[C] \tag{17}$$

which can be rearranged to:

$$\frac{[C]}{[B]} = \frac{CL_{AB}}{V} \frac{AUC_t^A}{[B]} - 1 = k_{AB} \frac{AUC_t^A}{[B]} - 1 \tag{18}$$

or:

$$\frac{[C]}{AUC_t^A} = \frac{CL_{AB}}{V} - \frac{[B]}{AUC_t^A} = k_{AB} - \frac{[B]}{AUC_t^A} \tag{19}$$

where the rate constant k_{AB} can be estimated from the slope or intercept of appropriate plots in accordance with Equations (18) and
(19), respectively.

EXAMPLES AND APPLICATIONS OF INTEGRAL METHODS FOR THE DETERMINATION OF THE METABOLIC CLEARANCE OF A DRUG AND THE APPARENT OVERALL VOLUME OF ITS METABOLITE(S)

Metabolite(s) Renally Excreted Unchanged

The stoichiometry for the cumulative amount of a metabolite
formed at any time (M_t) can be formulated as:

$$M_t = CL_{met} AUC_t = U_M + V_m C_m \tag{20}$$

when it can be assumed that the metabolite is instantaneously
equilibrated among the body tissues of apparent volume V_m (apparent
overall volume of metabolite). The cumulative amount of metabolite
in the urine (U_M) and the concentration of drug (C_p) and metabolite
(C_m) in the plasma are monitored with time. This equation can be
rearranged to:

$$U_M/C_m = -V_m + CL_{met}(AUC_t/C_m) \tag{21}$$

or:

$$U_M/AUC_t = -V_m(C_m/AUC_t) + CL_{met} \tag{22}$$

where CL_{met} and V_m can be estimated from the slope and intercept of
appropriate plots in accordance with Equations (21) and (22), respectively. The concentration of metabolite in the plasma can be
calculated at various times (t) by:

$$C_m = (CL_{met} AUC_t - \Sigma U_M)/V_m \tag{23}$$

The determination of these parameters demands no explicit
knowledge of the compartmental model for the drug or the fraction
of drug transformed to metabolite, or the bioavailability of the
systemically acting drug. It is independent of the mode or rate of

administration.   Complete monitoring of plasma concentrations and
urinary amounts to infinite time may not be necessary.   The elimination of the metabolite into the urine does not have to be a
linear process; its pharmacokinetics need not be dose-independent.
The CL_{met} and V_m values can be determined for each of multiple
metabolites.   The requirements are concentration-independent metabolic clearances for the drug and the assumption of relatively
instantaneous equilibration of the metabolite in the overall volume
of distribution in the body.

This method has been applied to the determination of the metabolic clearance of sulfisoxazole to its N^4-acetylsulfisoxazole
metabolite and the determination of the latter's overall volume of
distribution in humans (12) where:

$CL_{S \to N^4}^{met}$ is the metabolic clearance of sulfisoxazole to its
             N^4-acetyl metabolite

$V_d^{N^4}$ is the N^4-acetylsulfisoxazole overall volume of
             distribution

Examples of plots for these studies in accordance with Equation
(22) are given in Figure 2, where the ratio of cumulative amounts
of the N^4-acetyl metabolite in the urine at a time (t) to the area
under the plasma concentration-time curve of sulfisoxazole up to
that time:

$$U_M/AUC_t = U_{N^4}/AUC_S$$

is plotted against the ratio of the N^4-acetylsulfisoxazole concentration to the sulfisoxazole plasma concentration-time curve area
up to that time:

$$C_m/AUC_t = [N_4]/AUC_S$$

The values at earlier times deviate from linearity, a probable
consequence of the fact that the metabolite is not instantaneously
equilibrated in the overall volume of distribution, and that there
is a time-dependent distribution of the metabolite in the body
which initially yields a higher concentration in the central compartment.   The linearities of the plots at later times indicates
when the one-compartment body model can be assigned for the
metabolite.

The solid lines through the experimental N^4-acetylsulfi-
soxazole plasma concentrations in Figure 3 were calculated from the
parameters $V_d^{N_4}$ and $CL_{S \to N^4}^{met}$ obtained in accordance with Equation
(23) and, as anticipated, underestimated the experimental values at
the earlier times.   The parameters of a two-compartment body
model for N^4-acetylsulfisoxazole could be obtained by deconvolution

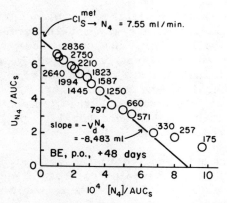

Figure 2. Plot in accordance with Equation (22) for the determination of the metabolic clearance, $CL_{S \to N4}^{met}$ for sulfisoxazole to the N^4-acetylsulfisoxazole metabolite and the
overall volume of distribution V_d^{N4}, of this metabolite
when the metabolite plasma concentrations, $[N_4]$, and
cumulative amounts excreted in urine, U_{N^4}, were
monitored with time. The AUC_S is the area under the
sulfisoxazole plasma concentration-time curve at that
time. Reprinted from (12) by permission of John Wiley
and Sons, Ltd.

$$S \xrightarrow{CL_{met_1}} M_1 \xrightarrow{CL_{met_2}} M_2 \xrightarrow{CL_{R_2}} U_{M_2}$$

$$M_1 \xrightarrow{CL_{R_1}} U_{M_1}$$

of the data in these plots. The dashed lines in Figure 3 were
calculated with the assumption of a first-order introduction of N^4-
acetylsulfisoxazole into a two-compartment body model. Such a
model can be characterized by the sum of two exponentials on
intravenous bolus administration of the N^4-acetylsulfisoxazole
(12). That the dashed lines are coincident with the experimentally
determined metabolite plasma concentrations shows the validity of
the conceptual basis for their calculation.

Sequential Formation of Metabolites That Are Renally Excreted

The elimination and metabolic sequence can be constructed as:

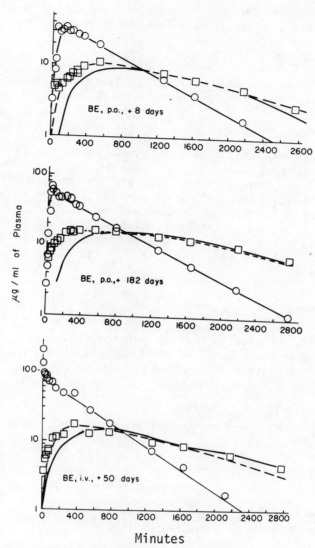

Figure 3. Plots of experimental sulfisoxazole (circles) and N⁴-acetylsulfisoxazole (squares) plasma concentrations with time in humans upon i.v. and p.o. administration of 1 g sulfisoxazole. The solid lines through the metabolite values were calculated from Equation (23). The dashed lines were calculated on the premise of a first-order introduction of the metabolite in a two-compartment model where the plasma profile could be characterized by the sum of two exponentials on i.v. bolus administration of the metabolite. Reprinted from (12) by permission of John Wiley and Sons, Ltd.

The stoichiometry for the cumulative amount of metabolite (M_1) formed from the drug at any time can be formulated as:

$$M_1 = CL_{met_1} AUC_S = U_{M_1} + V_{m_1} C_{m_1} + M_2 \tag{24}$$

where M_2 is the cumulative amount of the second metabolite formed from M_1 at that time and can be calculated from:

$$M_2 = CL_{met_2} AUC_{M_1} \tag{25}$$

where the AUCs are the respective areas under the plasma concetration-time curves at that time for the drug (S) and the metabolite (M_1). The CL_{met_2} value can be obtained by the method given in the previous case with the additional restrictions that the metabolite M_1 must have a concentration-independent metabolic clearance and that M_2 is relatively rapidly equilibrated in an apparent overall volume of distribution, V_{m2}. The pertinent equation equivalent to Equation (21) for the estimation of V_{m2} and CL_{met_2} from the appropriate plots is:

$$U_{M_2}/C_{m_2} = -V_{m_2} + CL_{met_2} \ (AUC_{M_1}/C_{m_2}) \tag{26}$$

The cumulative amounts of urinary metabolites, (U_{M1} and U_{M2}), and the plasma concentrations of drug (C_S) and of metabolites (C_{m_1} and C_{m2}) are monitored with time. Equation (24) can be rearranged to:

$$\frac{U_{M_1} + M_2}{AUC_S} = \frac{U_{M_1} + CL_{met_2} AUC_{M_1}}{AUC_S} = -V_{m_1} \frac{C_{m_1}}{AUC_S} + CL_{met_1} \tag{27}$$

or to:

$$\frac{U_{M_1} + M_2}{C_{m_1}} = U_{M_1} + \frac{CL_{met_2} AUC_{M_1}}{C_{m_1}} = -V_{m_1} + CL_{met_1} \frac{AUC_S}{C_{m_1}} \tag{28}$$

and, as from similar plots, CL_{met_1} and V_{m_1} can be estimated.

Metabolite Is Excreted Into Both Urine and Bile

The stoichiometry for the cumulative amount of metabolite formed is:

$$M = CL_{met} AUC = U_M + B_M + V_m C_m \tag{29}$$

When biliary (B_M) and urinary (U_M) amounts excreted are monitored with respect to time and there is no enterohepatic circulation:

$$(U_M + B_M)/C_m = -V_m + CL_{met} \ (AUC/C_m) \tag{30}$$

or:

$$(U_M + B_M)/AUC = -V_m \ (C_m/AUC) + CL_{met} \tag{31}$$

Typical plots in accordance with Equations (30) and (31) are given in Figure 4 for the pharmacokinetics of morphine in the bile-cannulated dog with complete bile collection where:

biliary amounts: $\quad B_M = \Sigma \ B_{MG}$

urinary amounts: $\quad U_M = \Sigma \ U_{MG}; \ U = \Sigma \ U_M$

plasma concentrations: $\quad C_p = [M], \ C_m = [MG]$

of morphine (M) and its glucuronide metabolite (MG) were monitored with respect to time (1).

The values of $[MG]_{calc}$ were obtained from an equation similar to Equation (23):

$$[MG]_{calc} = \frac{CL_{met}AUC - \Sigma \ U_{MG} - \Sigma \ B_{MG}}{V_{MG}} \tag{32}$$

and are plotted as the solid line through the experimental glucuronide plasma concentrations ($[MG]_{exp}$) shown in Figure 5, for the high intravenous bolus dose of 7.68 mg/kg of morphine. These calculated values underestimated the initial experimental values for up to 70 minutes after morphine administration (initial dashed line, Figure 5), probably for the same reason discussed previously; a period of time may be necessary for the conjugate to equilibrate in its overall distribution volume. The only underlying assumptions for this case are a constant metabolic clearance for morphine and an instantaneous equilibration of the systemically available conjugate in its overall volume of distribution. It should be noted in Figure 5 that there is no additional slow phase evident for glucuronide (MG) elimination from the plasma which indicates that there is not a deep compartment.

An interesting lag in the renal excretion of morphine ($\Sigma \ U_M$) and its glucuronide ($\Sigma \ U_{MG}$) can be observed. This is due to the temporary renal shutdown encountered at these high morphine doses. The lines drawn through these experimental values of cumulative amounts in the urine were calculated from the integral expressions for renal clearance (Eq. (4)) modified for no operative renal function before a time (t) in accordance with:

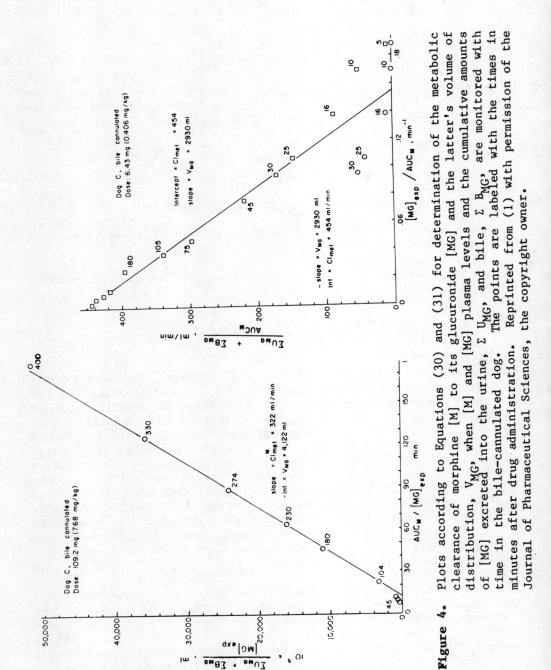

Figure 4. Plots according to Equations (30) and (31) for determination of the metabolic clearance of morphine [M] to its glucuronide [MG] and the latter's volume of distribution, V_{MG}, when [M] and [MG] plasma levels and the cumulative amounts of [MG] excreted into the urine, ΣU_{MG}, and bile, ΣB_{MG}, are monitored with time in the bile-cannulated dog. The points are labeled with the times in minutes after drug administration. Reprinted from (1) with permission of the Journal of Pharmaceutical Sciences, the copyright owner.

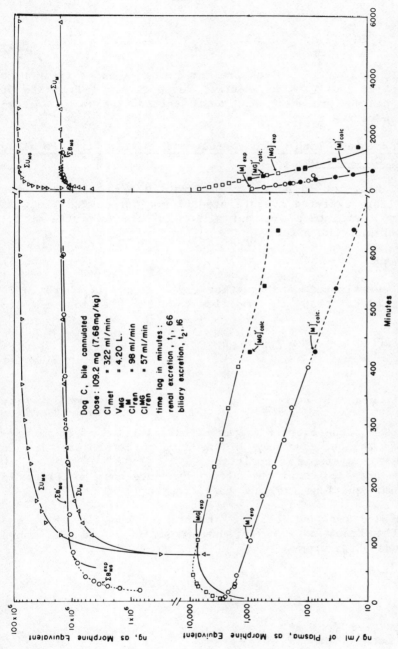

Figure 5. Example of plot of experimental plasma levels of morphine (M) and morphine glucuronide (MG), of cumulative amounts of (M) and (MG) excreted into the urine, and of cumulative amounts excreted into the bile of a biliary cannulated dog. The solid line through the (MG) plasma concentrations was calculated from Equation (32). The solid lines through the cumulative urinary amounts, Σ U, were calculated from Equations (33) and (34) where the areas were diminished by the area up to 66 minutes. Reprinted from (1) with permission of the Journal of Pharmaceutical Sciences, the copyright owner.

$$\Sigma \ U_M = CL_R^M (AUC_t^M - AUC_{t_1}^M) \tag{33}$$

and:

$$\Sigma \ U_{MG} = CL_R^{MG} \ (AUC_t^{MG} - AUC_{t_1}^{MG}) \tag{34}$$

where the AUC_t and AUC_{t_1} values are for the area under the curves up to a time (t) and t_1 = 66 minutes, respectively. Prior to 66 minutes, it can be presumed that renal elimination of both compounds is inoperative.

Metabolite Excreted Both Into Urine and Bile, With Possible Enterohepatic Circulation

The stoichiometry is as given in Equation (29). In the case where the biliary excreted amounts are not monitored with time, it is possible to postulate a constant biliary clearance of the metabolite secreted into the bile:

$$B_M = CL_B AUC \tag{35}$$

which can be substituted into Equation (29). Thus, if there is no enterohepatic circulation, the modified Equation (29) can be rearranged to:

$$U_M/C_m = -V_m + (CL_{met} - CL_B) \ (AUC/C_m) \tag{36}$$

or:

$$U_M/AUC = -V_m C_m/AUC + CL_{met} - CL_B \tag{37}$$

The parameters for the overall volume of distribution of the metabolite (V_m) and the net clearance of the drug to metabolite that is available to the systemic circulation $[(CL_{met})_{systemic} = CL_{met} - CL_B]$, can be obtained from the slope and intercept of plots in accordance with Equations (36) and (37), respectively.

The presumed constant biliary clearance (CL_B) can be calculated from the known total clearance (Dose/AUC_∞) and the known renal clearance (CL_R) from:

$$CL_{met} = CL_B + (CL_{met})_{systemic} = CL_{tot} - CL_R \tag{38}$$

Thus:

$$CL_B = CL_{met} - (CL_{met} - CL_B) \tag{39}$$

where the latter parenthetical expression is determined from the application of Equations (36) or (37).

Morphine was administered intravenously into the normal, non-bile-cannulated dog and the urinary amounts of drug ($U = \Sigma\ U_M$) and metabolite ($U_M = \Sigma\ U_{MG}$) and plasma concentrations ($C_p = [M]$, $C_m = [MG]$) of morphine (M) and its glucuronide conjugate (MG) were monitored with time (1). A typical plot in accordance with Equation (37) is shown in Figure 6 to obtain the $CL_{met} - CL_B$ and V_{MG} values from the intercept and slope, respectively.

The values of $[MG]_{calc}$ were obtained from an equation similar to Equation (23):

$$[MG]_{calc} = \frac{(CL_{met} - CL_B)\ AUC - \Sigma\ U_{MG}}{V_{MG}} \tag{40}$$

These values are plotted as the solid lines through the experimentally determined glucuronide plasma concentrations in Figures 7 and 8. Bolus doses of morphine of 7.60 (Fig. 7) and 0.070 (Fig. 8) mg/kg were administered intravenously to normal, non-bile-cannulated dogs. The calculated and experimental values for [MG] agree well up to 200–350 minutes; the subsequent calculated values underestimate the experimental values (terminal dashed lines). This can readily be explained by the postulation of enterohepatic circulation of the glucuronide excreted in the bile to the systemic volume; in effect this is an additional infusion of glucuronide after the time lag necessary for transit through the bile to the site of reabsorption. This fact also explains the deviation of the data from the expected linearity (Fig. 6) at later time points when plotted in accordance with Equation (37).

Such analyses also permit the calculation of the amount ($\Sigma\ MG_{ent}$) of metabolite enterohepatically circulated. The cumulative amount secreted into the bile is:

$$\Sigma\ B_{MG}^{tot} = CL_B AUC_{MG} \tag{41}$$

where CL_B can be estimated from Equation (39). The actual amount of glucuronide in the biliary system at any time, $\Sigma\ B_{MG}^{calc}$, can be calculated on stoichiometric grounds; the total glucuronide formed ($\Sigma\ MG_{tot}$) must equal the sum of the amounts in the bile ($\Sigma\ B_{MG}^{calc}$), urine ($\Sigma\ U_{MG}^{exp}$), and body ($\Sigma\ MG_{body}$), so that the calculated amount in the bile would be:

$$\Sigma\ B_{MG}^{calc} = \Sigma\ MG_{tot} - \Sigma\ U_{MG}^{exp} - \Sigma\ MG_{body}$$

$$= CL_{met} AUC_M - \Sigma\ U_{MG}^{exp} - V_{MG}[MG]_{exp} \tag{42}$$

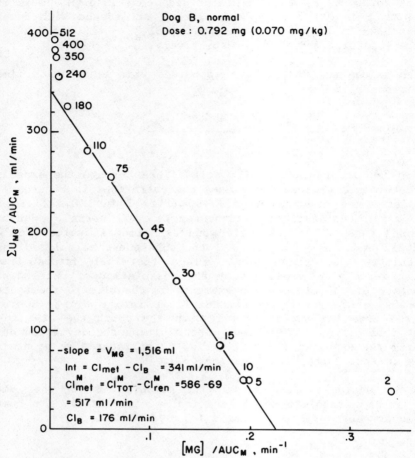

Figure 6. Plot in accordance with Equation (37) for the determination of the net metabolic clearances of morphine to systemically introduced glucuronide ($CL_{met} - CL_B$) and the
latter's volume of distribution, V_{MG}, when morphine [M]
(and the corresponding AUC_M) and glucuronide [MG] plasma
concentrations as well as the cumulative amounts of
glucuronide excreted into the urine, $\Sigma\ U_{MG}$, are monitored with time in the normal dog. The points are
labeled with time in minutes after drug administration.
Reprinted from (1) with permission of the Journal of
Pharmaceutical Sciences, the copyright owner.

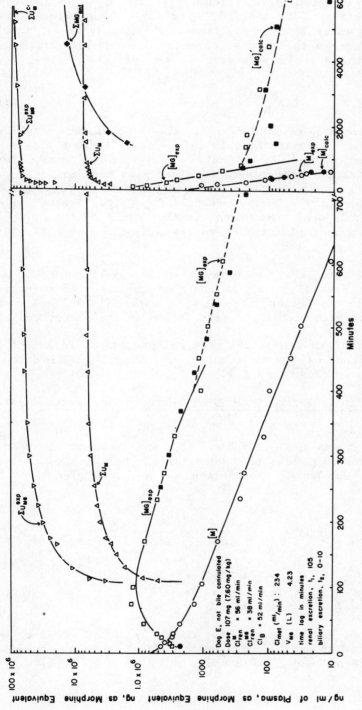

Figure 7. Example of plot of experimental plasma concentrations of morphine (M) and morphine glucuronide (MG), and of cumulative amounts of (M) and (MG) excreted into the urine of a normal dog for a 7.60 mg/kg i.v. bolus dose of (M). The solid line through the (MG) plasma concentrations was calculated from Equation (40). The line for the amount of enterohepatically circulated (MG), Σ MG$_{ent}$, was calculated from Equation (43). Reprinted from (1) with permission of the Journal of Pharmaceutical Sciences, the copyright owner.

where CL_{met} was estimated from Equation (38) and V_{MG} from the application of Equations (36) and (37) (Fig. 6). Thus, the amount enterohepatically circulated at any time ($\Sigma\ MG_{ent}$) can be estimated from the difference in the cumulative amount secreted in the bile (Eq. (41)) and the calculated amount in the biliary system (Eq. (42)):

$$\Sigma\ MG_{ent} = \Sigma\ B_{MG}^{tot} - \Sigma\ B_{MG}^{calc} \tag{43}$$

Plots of amounts of enterohepatically circulated morphine glucuronides ($\Sigma\ MG_{ent}$), calculated in this manner, against time are shown in Figures 7 and 8. The slow additional phase for glucuronide elimination from plasma is clearly evident in Figure 7 and indicates the presence of a deep compartment that was not present in the case of the bile-cannulated dog (Fig. 5) whose bile was collected. This deep compartment is the result of the delayed enterohepatic return of glucuronide to the systemic circulation in the normal dog.

It should be noted that there is no apparent renal shutdown at the low morphine dose (Fig. 8) in contrast to the high morphine dose (Fig. 7). In the former case, AUC_t^{MG} and AUC_t^{M} in Equations (33) and (34) were zero, but had finite values in the latter case.

The power of these simple analyses and procedures in defining and quantifying complex pharmacokinetic processes is well demonstrated in this particular case (1).

A Common Metabolite is Formed From Two Precursors and Excreted into Urine and Bile

Heroin (H) forms both morphine (M) and monoacetylmorphine (AcM) and both compounds can form morphine glucuronide (MG). The simplified scheme for heroin disposition can be constructed as:

$$
\begin{array}{ccccccc}
 & & \Sigma\ U_{AcM} & & & & \\
 & & \uparrow & & & & \\
[H] & \rightarrow & [AcM] & \rightarrow & [MG] & \rightarrow & \Sigma\ U_{MG} \\
\downarrow & \searrow & \downarrow & \nearrow & & & \\
\Sigma\ U_H & & [M] & \rightarrow & \Sigma\ U_M & & \Sigma\ B_{MG}
\end{array}
$$

The stoichiometric expression for the total amount of glucuronide (MG_{tot}) formed at any time can be formulated as being produced from both morphine and monoacetylmorphine:

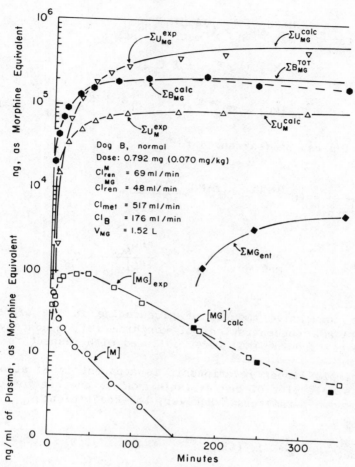

Figure 8. Example of plot of experimentally determined plasma concentrations of morphine (M) and morphine glucuronide (MG), and of cumulative urinary amounts of morphine and its glucuronide in a normal dog for a 0.070 mg/kg i.v. bolus dose of morphine. The solid line through the glucuronide plasma concentrations was calculated from Equation (40) The solid line, $\Sigma\, B_{MG}^{tot}$, through the calculated amount of glucuronide in the biliary system ($\Sigma\, B_{MG}^{calc}$, Eq. (42)), was calculated on the premise of a constant biliary clearance with no enterohepatic circulation (Eq. (41)). The line for the amount of enterohepatically circulated morphine glucuronide, $\Sigma\, MG_{ent}$, was calculated from Equation (43). Reprinted from (I) with permission of the Journal of Pharmaceutical Sciences, the copyright owner.

$$\Sigma \; MG_{tot} = CL_{met}^{M\rightarrow MG} AUC_M + CL_{met}^{AcM\rightarrow MG} AUC_{AcM}$$

$$= V_{MG}[MG] + \Sigma \; B_{MG} + \Sigma \; U_{MG}$$

$$= V_{MG}[MG] + CL_B^{M\rightarrow MG} AUC_M + CL_B^{AcM\rightarrow MG} AUC_{AcM} + \Sigma \; U_{MG} \quad (44)$$

This equation can be rearranged to:

$$\frac{U_{MG}}{[MG]_{exp}} = (CL_{met}^{M\rightarrow MG} - CL_B^{M\rightarrow MG})\frac{AUC_M}{[MG]_{exp}}$$

$$+ (CL_{met}^{AcM\rightarrow MG} - CL_B^{AcM\rightarrow MG})\frac{AUC_{AcM}}{[MG]_{exp}} - V_{MG} \quad (45)$$

where the cumulative amounts of glucuronide in the urine ($\Sigma \; U_{MG}$) and the plasma concentrations of morphine [M], monoacetylmorphine [AcM] and glucuronide [MG] were monitored with respect to time (2).

No simple linear relationship is apparent in Equation (45) to permit a simple plot of one variable against another for estimation of the unknown parameters. However, the coefficients:

$$(CL_{met}^{M\rightarrow MG} - CL_B^{M\rightarrow MG}), \; (CL_{met}^{AcM\rightarrow MG} - CL_B^{AcM\rightarrow MG}), \; V_{MG}$$

are determinable by multiple linear regression (2,13). The plasma concentrations of glucuronide ($[MG]_{calc}$) could thus be estimated at any given time from:

$$[MG]_{calc} = \frac{(CL_{met}^{M\rightarrow MG} - CL_B^{M\rightarrow MG})AUC_M + (CL_{met}^{AcM\rightarrow MG} - CL_B^{AcM\rightarrow MG})AUC_{AcM}}{V_{MG}} \quad (46)$$

When the plasma concentrations of glucuronide were calculated on these premises from Equation (46), the fit to the experimentally determined glucuronide data was excellent (Fig. 9) up to the time of enterophepatic return of glucuronide secreted into the bile. The fit based on the premise that glucuronide was formed solely from morphine was not as satisfactory (2).

CRITIQUES AND LIMITATIONS

Calculation and Prediction of Time Courses of Drug and Metabolite
in Plasma, Urine and Bile from Pharmacokinetic Parameters Derived
from Integral Expressions

The plasma concentration-time curve of a drug that has dose-independent pharmacokinetics can be described by a mathematical expression, generally a linear sum of exponentials. The area under this plasma concentration-time curve (AUC_t) can be measured or calculated at any time (t). The total amounts of any metabolites concentration-independently formed or eliminated at any time can be determined from the product of a constant clearance (CL) and the area: $CL(AUC_t)$, (Eqs. (2) – (5) and Fig. 1).

The plasma concentrations of any rapidly equilibrating, systemically circulating metabolite can be calculated (Eq. (23)) at any time from the known metabolic clearance (CL_{met}) of the drug or precursor to the metabolite, the calculated plasma concentration-time area of the drug or precursor, the apparent volume of

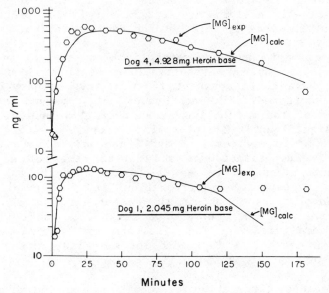

Figure 9. Fitting of experimental glucuronide plasma concentrations $[MG]_{exp}$ by application of Equation (44) (solid line, $[MG]_{calc}$) on the premise that glucuronide is formed both from morphine and monoacetylmorphine in the dog after i.v. administration of heroin. Reprinted from (2) with permission of the Journal of Pharmaceutical Sciences, the copyright owner.

distribution of the metabolite and the known amounts of metabolite eliminated or transformed. Practical examples were given in Figures 2, and 4-7.

If the metabolite is only renally eliminated, the plasma concentration of metabolite at any time can be calculated from the experimentally determined renally excreted amounts. If the metabolite (M_I) is both renally eliminated and transformed to another metabolite (M_{II}), the plasma concentrations of the precursor metabolite (M_I) can be calculated when the sum of the amounts renally excreted and further transformed are known.

Determination of Parameters from Integral Expressions

The metabolic clearance of a drug or any precursor to a metabolite, and the equilibrated overall volume of distribution of this metabolite used in the calculation and prediction of the time course can be obtained for multiple metabolites by the methods described in this chapter. The methods require the concomitant monitoring of plasma concentrations and urinary amounts of drug and metabolite(s) with time, but not necessarily to infinity. No explicit knowledge of the compartmental model of the drug, or the fraction of drug transformed to metabolite, or the bioavailability of the systemically acting drug is necessary. The procedures are independent of the mode or rate of drug administration.

Concentration-independent metabolic clearances of the drug and metabolite(s), if any, are required, but renal or biliary clearances do not have to be constant if cumulative urinary or biliary amounts are monitored. The achievement of a pseudo-steady-state equilibration of the metabolite in an overall volume of distribution for a significant time interval is a prerequisite. Linearity of plots such as in Figures 2, 4 and 6 can only occur over such an interval. The non-coincidence at initial times of experimental plasma concentrations and values calculated with the assumption of instantaneous metabolite equilibration in the overall volume permits deconvolutions to obtain the sum of exponentials necessary to characterize the time course of a metabolite if it were intravenously administered. The fraction of administered drug transformed to metabolite is needed for exact determination of the coefficients of the exponentials.

Enterohepatic circulation of drug can be indicated by the deviation from linearity at later times of plots such as Figures 2, 4 and 6. This enterohepatic circulation of a metabolite can be quantified from the differences between experimental plasma concentrations of metabolite at later times, and those concentrations calculated on the premise of no enterohepatic return (Eq. (43)).

Clearing organ inhibition or shutdown can be deduced from the failure of expressions such as Equations (4) and (5) to predict amounts of metabolite formed or drug excreted. Such equations can be modified (Eqs. (33) and (34)) to permit determination of the duration of such organ shutdown.

Methods have been developed to determine the metabolic clearances of two precursors to the same metabolite as well as the latter's overall volume of distribution. The procedure can be applied to the determination of the apparent overall volume of distribution, and the first-order absorption and elimination rate constants of a drug, when the fractions of drug absorbed and renally excreted are known. These procedures provide an alternative method to "feathering" for the determination of the sequential and parallel rate constants for first-order degradations in solution, even in the absence of highly discrepant rate constants which are needed for "feathering" processes.

The primary restriction in all of the above cases is that metabolic or transformation clearances must be constant. Such transformations must be first-order and the apparent first-order rate constants must be concentration-independent.

Caveats with Statistical Ramifications

Plots, such as in Figures 2, 4 and 6, that are based on the derived paired equations (Eqs. (21), (22); (30), (31); and (36), (37)) are functions of multiple variables: quotients, quotients of sums, and so forth. Each of these variables would have its own error and contribute to the greater error of the complex variable. For example, the variance (σ^2) of a quotient (x/y) of two variables x and y with their individual variances (σ_x^2, σ_y^2), can be approximated by:

$$\sigma^2 = \frac{x^2}{y^2} \left(\frac{\sigma_x^2}{x^2} + \frac{\sigma_y^2}{y^2} \right) \tag{47}$$

In fact, the weighting of values for individual times would be widely different for the linear regressions of each of the above cited paired equations, even though they were obtained by rearrangements of the same expression. Thus, slightly different sets of pharmacokinetic parameters would result from the linear regression analyses of plots of differently transformed but presumably equivalent equations. Notwithstanding this valid statistically-based criticism of the linearization procedure used to obtain the estimates of pharmacokinetic parameters by regression of such complex functions, the methodology does give estimates of these parameters (see Figs. 2, 4 and 6) that lead to a close fit between the experimentally obtained values and the calculated values (see

Figs. 3, 5, 7-9). Deviations from expected linearity provide evidence for clearing organ shutdown (see Figs. 5-7; Equations (33) and (34)) and data for the evaluation of the sum of exponentials to describe metabolite disposition (see Fig. 3).

If the weightings introduced by the complex variables and the chosen equation are unacceptable for any reason, nonlinear regression analyses can be used if the simple variables are given the appropriate weightings. Examples would be to fit the data by nonlinear regression to Equation (12) instead of by linear regression in accordance with Equations (13) or (14); to Equation (17) instead of Equations (18) or (19); to Equation (20) instead of Equations (21) or (22); to Equation (24) instead of Equations (27) or (28); to Equation (29) instead of Equations (30) or (31); and to Equation (29) with the incorporation of Equation (35) instead of Equation (36) or Equation (37). However, it is recommended that the data first be plotted in accordance with the anticipated linear relationships of the transformed equations in order to determine and restrict the interval within which the theoretical premises underlying the nonlinear regressions are valid. An alternative statistical approach is the use of multiple linear regression of the non-transformed equations within the chosen interval for the best estimate of the pharmacokinetic parameter, as in the example (Eq. (45)) where a common metabolite is formed from two precursors and excreted into both bile and urine (2, 13).

Acknowledgment. The experimental aspects of this work were supported in part by Grant 2-R01-DA-00743 from the National Institute of Drug Abuse, Rockville, MD.

REFERENCES

1. E.R. Garrett and A. Jackson, Pharmacokinetics of morphine and its surrogates III: Morphine and morphine 3-monoglucuronide in the dog as a function of dose, J. Pharm. Sci. 68:753-771 (1979).
2. E.R. Garrett and T. Gürkan, Pharmacokinetics of morphine and its surrogates IV: Pharmacokinetics of heroin and its derived metabolites in the dog, J. Pharm. Sci. 69:1116-1134 (1980).
3. M. Rowland, L.Z. Benet and G.G. Graham, Clearance concepts in pharmacokinetics, J. Pharmacokin. Biopharm. 1:123-136 (1973).
4. G.R. Wilkinson and D.G. Shand, A physiological approach to hepatic drug clearance, Clin. Pharmacol. Ther. 18:377-390 (1975).
5. E.R. Garrett, Pharmacokinetics and clearances related to renal processes, Int. J. Clin. Pharmacol. 16:155-172 (1978).
6. E.R. Garrett, Classical pharmacokinetics to the frontier, J. Pharmacokin. Biopharm. 1:341-361 (1973).

7. E.R. Garrett, Theoretische Pharmakokinetik, in "Klinische Pharmacologie and Pharmakotherapie," (Vol. 3), H. Kuemmerle, E.R. Garrett and K.H. Spitzy, eds., Urban and Schwarzenberg, München (1976).

8. E.R. Garrett and H.J. Lambert, Pharmacokinetics of trichloroethanol and metabolites and the interconversions among variously referenced pharmacokinetic parameters, J. Pharm. Sci 62:550-572 (1973).

9. E.R. Garrett, J. Bres and K. Schnelle, Pharmacokinetics of saturably metabolized amobarbital, J. Pharmacokin. Biopharm. 2:43-103 (1974).

10. L.Z. Benet and R.L. Galeazzi, Noncompartmental determination of the steady-state volume of distribution, J. Pharm. Sci. 68:1071-1074 (1979).

11. E.R. Garrett, Evidence for general base catalysis in an ester hydrolysis II. Hydrolysis of an aminoalkyl acetylsalicylate, J. Amer. Chem. Soc. 80:4049-4056 (1958).

12. E.R. Garrett, R.S. Süverkrüp, K. Eberst, R.L. Yost and J.P. O'Leary, Surgically affected sulfisoxazole pharmacokinetics in the morbidly obese, Biopharm. Drug Disp. 2:329-365 (1981).

13. Program stat-1-27A Multiple Linear Regression in HP-65, stat Pac 1, Hewlett-Packard Co., Palo Alto, California (1974): Based on A.M. Mood and F.A. Grayhill, "Introduction to the Theory of Statistics", McGraw-Hill, New York, NY (1963).

Chapter 21

PHARMACOKINETICS AT THE INTERFACE BETWEEN PHARMACOLOGY AND PHYSIOLOGY

Gerhard Levy

Department of Pharmaceutics, School of Pharmacy
State University of New York at Buffalo
Amherst, New York

It is customary to consider the activity of enzyme or transport systems or the perfusion rate of organs as rate determining or limiting in the elimination of drugs from the body. However, some drug conjugation processes are limited by the availability of an endogenous cosubstrate. A comprehensive characterization of the pharmacokinetics of drugs that are affected by limited cosubstrate availability requires models that include representation of all processes affecting the concentration-time profile of the cosubstrate. The latter may be subject to a number of physiologic controls that facilitate homeostasis, including feedback control of formation rate and concentration-dependent renal clearance. These processes can be affected by pathophysiologic variables, and their effects on drug disposition can be both dose- and time-dependent. Additional complexity of the system may arise from drug and endogenous cosubstrate concentration-dependent changes in apparent V_{max} and K_m of drug biotransformation processes that are bisubstrate reactions. The pharmacokinetics of these complex nonlinear systems have important pharmacologic implications and exemplify the interrelationship between metabolic processes involving both exogenous and endogenous substrates. Thus, drug biotransformation processes that are associated with and affected by depletion of an endogenous cosubstrate illustrate the interdigitation of pharmacology and physiology and emphasize the need for appreciating the role of both pharmacologic and physiologic factors in pharmacokinetic research.

It has been established that several endogenous cosubstrates (or precursors of cosubstrates) of drug biotransformation processes can become depleted so that the rate of biotransformation (and therefore the rate of cosubstrate utilization) can exceed the rate of formation or mobilization of the endogenous cosubstrate. Examples of such cosubstrates are glutathione (1), (activated) glucuronic acid (2), glycine (3) and (activated) sulfate (4). Cosubstrate depletion as a cause of nonlinear or time-dependent drug biotransformation kinetics can be distinguished from other potential causes, i.e., limited capacity of enzyme systems responsible for drug or cosubstrate activation or for transfer of cosubstrate to the drug, by the increased drug biotransformation rate following direct administration of the cosubstrate. For example, the formation rate of hippuric acid from benzoic acid can be increased by administration of glycine (3). On the other hand, glycine administration has no effect on the formation of salicylurate from salicylate; that process is rate-limited by the activation of salicylate (3,5). Some endogenous cosubstrates cannot be replenished by exogenous administration because they do not penetrate to the site of biotransformation. Examples are activated sulfate (3'-phosphoadenosine 5'-phosphosulfate) and glutathione. It is possible, however, to replenish some of these substances by administration of precursors.

An excellent example of the interrelationship between the pharmacokinetics of a drug and an endogenous cosubstrate of the biotransformation of that drug is the conversion of acetaminophen to acetaminophen sulfate. Acetaminophen (also known as paracetamol) is a widely used nonprescription analgesic and antipyretic. It is eliminated almost entirely by biotransformation, largely to the glucuronide and sulfate conjugates. There are also several minor metabolites, including one that is highly reactive and capable of causing serious damage to vital tissues, particularly the liver but including the kidneys and the heart (6). Such damage, which can be produced by overdoses of acetaminophen, arises from several concomitant occurrences: the absolute amount of the reactive metabolite formed increases with increasing dose; that increase is more than proportional to the increase of the dose of acetaminophen due to relatively decreased formation of the major metabolites (the glucuronide and sulfate conjugates) of acetaminophen with increasing dose (7); the inactivation of the reactive metabolite is relatively decreased with increasing dose due to the limited availability of the cosubstrate glutathione (1).

Our first attempts to characterize the pharmacokinetics of acetaminophen disposition in humans over a wide dose range, including doses large enough to be lethal eventually, were based on results of earlier studies which revealed that both the glucuronidation and sulfation of acetaminophen are processes of relatively limited capacity (8). We therefore developed a pharmacokinetic model of acetaminophen disposition in humans that consisted of two Michaelis-Menten type processes for formation of the two major conjugates, and two apparent first-order processes for renal excretion of unmetabolized drug and for formation of the reactive metabolite, respectively. All four processes operate in parallel and are therefore competing. The dose-dependence of the composition of urinary acetaminophen excretion products predicted by this model is in excellent agreement with clinical data over a wide dose range (7), but there is one notable discrepancy between the model and clinical observations. The pharmacokinetic model predicts that a semilogarithmic plot of post-absorption and post-distribution plasma concentrations versus time after ingestion of a large amount of acetaminophen ($\geq$ 10 g in adults) curves downward and becomes apparently exponential only when the amount of drug in the body has decreased to 1 or 2 g in adults (7). Actual clinical studies have shown no such downward curvature; acetaminophen concentrations appear to decline exponentially over a wide range, irrespective of dose, but with a half-life that increases with increasing dose (9). It was tempting to ascribe this phenomenon to dose-dependent hepatic damage which becomes increasingly apparent with time after drug ingestion, thereby exerting a gradually increasing adverse effect on acetaminophen biotransformation which in turn causes an increasing difference between actual and model-predicted drug concentrations. However, we did not find this argument sufficiently persuasive and elected to search for a more plausible explanation.

The rat was found to be a useful model for investigation of the unusual dose-dependence of acetaminophen pharmacokinetics. As do humans, rats eliminate acetaminophen mainly by formation of the glucuronide and sulfate conjugates (10). Moreover, rats exhibit the same apparently exponential decline of plasma or serum acet-aminophen concentrations with a half-life that increases with increasing dose* (Fig. 1). The increasing half-life was accompa-nied by a pronounced decrease in the fraction of the dose converted to the sulfate conjugate. Serum concentrations of endogenous inorganic sulfate, ordinarily approximately 1 mM in the rat, decreased appreciably after administration of as little as 15 mg/kg acetaminophen and became close to zero after administration of 150 or 300 mg/kg (Fig. 2). In subsequent clinical studies we found that a single 1.5 g dose of acetaminophen caused a definite decrease of endogenous inorganic sulfate in serum of normal volunteers (11).

The depletion of endogenous inorganic sulfate produced by large doses of acetaminophen and the consequent relatively decreased formation of acetaminophen sulfate are responsible for the apparently exponential dose-dependent elimination of the drug

---

*Significantly, the rat is very resistant to acetaminophen-induced hepatotoxicity. Even the largest single dose used in our studies, 300 mg/kg, is not toxic to rats.

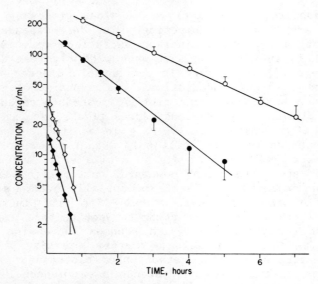

Figure 1. Acetaminophen concentrations in plasma of rats after i.v. injection of 15 (filled diamonds), 30 (open diamonds), 150 (filled circles) and 300 (open circles) mg/kg. Mean of five animals. Bars represent ± one SD. Open and closed symbols represent two cross-over studies with different groups of animals. Reprinted from Galinsky and Levy (10), with permission.

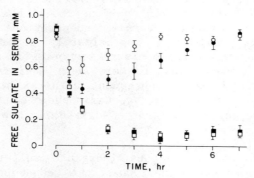

Figure 2. Effect of acetaminophen administration on concentrations of free sulfate in serum of rats. The drug was injected i.v. at zero time as a single dose of either 15 (open circles), 30 (filled circles), 150 (open squares) or 300 (filled squares) mg/kg body weight. Data are mean values; n = 5-7. Vertical bars represent ± one SEM Reprinted from (17), with permission from Pergamon Press, Ltd.

over a wide dose range.   If depletion of inorganic sulfate is
prevented by continuous i.v. infusion of sodium sulfate, the plasma
acetaminophen concentration profiles become typically Michaelis-
Menten (Fig. 3).

As long as the rate of formation of acetaminophen sulfate
exceeds the rate of formation or mobilization of inorganic sulfate,
the latter will eventually become depleted if acetaminophen is
administered long enough.   This depletion can occur, therefore,
even at acetaminophen concentrations well below the K_m for the
conjugation process.   The injection of a small (30 mg/kg) dose of
acetaminophen and the subsequent prolonged infusion of the drug, at
a rate designed to produce acetaminophen concentrations comparable
to those obtained initially after the injected dose, yield information that proves this contention (Fig. 4).   Contrary to pharmacokinetic predictions for apparent first-order processes, plasma
acetaminophen concentrations during the infusion did not level off
at approximately 1 hour after the start of the infusion but continued to increase at a substantial rate.   This drug accumulation was
associated with a pronounced quantitative change in the formation
of acetaminophen conjugates;   the initially predominant sulfation

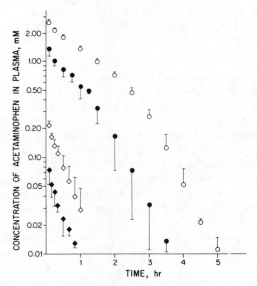

Figure 3. Acetaminophen concentrations in plasma of rats after
i.v. injection of 15 (filled diamonds), 30 (open
diamonds), 150 (filled circles) and 300 (open circles)
mg/kg.   These animals also received sodium sulfate, 71
mg/kg by i.v. injection at −1 hr, followed immediately
by an infusion of 76.7 mg/kg/hr from −1 to 5 hr.   Mean ±
SD, n = 4 or 5.   From Lin and Levy (to be published).

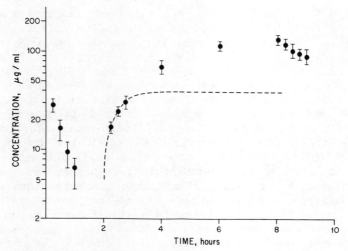

Figure 4. Acetaminophen concentrations in plasma of rats after i.v. injection of 30 mg/kg at 0 hr and intra-arterial infusion of about 60 mg/kg/hr from 2 to 8 hr. Mean ± SD, n = 6. The dashed line is the calculated concentration-time profile based on the pharmacokinetics of acetaminophen after i.v. injection of 30 mg/kg and assuming first-order elimination kinetics. Reprinted from Galinsky and Levy (10), with permission.

diminished with time and relatively more of the drug was metabolized to the glucuronide (Fig. 5). Of interest is the eventual acetaminophen sulfate concentration plateau after 4 hours of infusion (that is, after 6 hours on the time scale in Figure 5). It reflects formation of the metabolite at a basal rate dictated by the rate at which endogenous inorganic sulfate becomes available for activation and conjugate formation. If depletion of inorganic sulfate is prevented by concomitant infusion of sodium sulfate, the kinetics of acetaminophen accumulation are apparent first-order, with plasma concentrations in excellent agreement with theoretical predictions (i.e., the stippled line in Figure 4). This experiment illustrates an important feature of cosubstrate depletion, namely its time-dependent effect on drug elimination kinetics. This is of obvious importance in the design and interpretation of chronic toxicity studies and should also be taken into consideration when one attempts to predict drug concentration profiles after repeated dosings, from kinetic data obtained after administration of single doses.

When drug biotransformation and endogenous cosubstrate kinetics are interrelated, changes in physiologic status that modify the formation or disposition of the cosubstrate can have pronounced

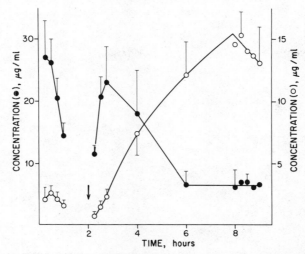

Figure 5. Concentrations of acetaminophen sulfate (filled circles) and acetaminophen glucuronide (open circles) in plasma obtained in the experiment described in Figure 4. All concentrations are expressed in terms of acetaminophen. The arrow indicates the start of the acetaminophen infusion. Reprinted from Galinsky and Levy (10), with permission.

effects on the pharmacokinetics of the drug. For example, endogenous inorganic sulfate levels are greatly elevated in renal failure (12), thereby preventing or delaying the depletion of inorganic sulfate during acetaminophen infusion. Consequently, there are pronounced differences in the acetaminophen concentration profiles during infusion of the drug in normal rats and in rats with experimental renal failure, respectively (Figs. 6 and 7). Of additional interest is the fact that elevated levels of endogenous inorganic sulfate had no effect on the pharmacokinetics of the initial small (15 mg/kg) bolus dose of acetaminophen. One cannot increase acetaminophen sulfate formation rate by increasing the concentration of inorganic sulfate to above the normal physiologic level; one can only prevent the decrease in acetaminophen sulfate formation rate arising from hyposulfatemia. The reasons for this became apparent from the results of more detailed enzyme kinetic studies.

Use of isolated rat hepatocytes incubated in a medium of essentially constant known concentrations of acetaminophen and inorganic sulfate permitted the determination of enzyme kinetic constants for formation of acetaminophen sulfate (13). It was found that the apparent K_m and V_{max} values for this process change as a function of inorganic sulfate concentration when the latter is

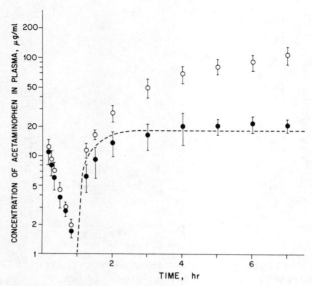

Figure 6. Acetaminophen concentrations in plasma of control rats (open circles) and rats with ligated ureters (filled circles) after injection of 15 mg/kg followed one hour later by infusion of about 36 mg acetaminophen/kg/hr for 6 hours. Mean ± SD, n = 5. The stippled line is the calculated concentration-time profile based on the pharmacokinetics of the 15 mg/kg dose, assuming first-order kinetics. Reprinted from Lin and Levy (12), with permission.

less that 1 mM (Fig. 8). Above that concentration, K_m and V_{max} values are independent of inorganic sulfate concentration. It so happens that the normal physiologic concentration of inorganic sulfate in the plasma of rats is about 1 mM. Since this anion is not significantly plasma protein bound, it is likely that its concentrations in plasma and in interstitial water are similar. Thus, the failure of hypersulfatemia to increase acetaminophen sulfate formation rate in vivo is readily explained by the in vitro data. Moreover, the in vitro experiments revealed an additional interesting facet of sulfate conjugate formation. This bisubstrate reaction proceeds by two parallel pathways: formation of a drug-enzyme complex which then reacts with activated sulfate to form acetaminophen sulfate, or formation of an activated sulfate-enzyme complex which then reacts with acetaminophen to form the same metabolite. Depletion of inorganic sulfate (and, therefore, of activated sulfate) favors the formation of the drug-enzyme complex and vice versa. Since the enzyme kinetic constants for the two reaction pathways differ, the observed apparent K_m and V_{max} values

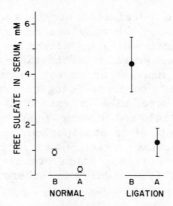

Figure 7. Concentrations of free sulfate in serum of rats immediately before injection (B) and at the end of the infusion (A) of acetaminophen in the experiments described in Figure 6. Mean ± SD. Based on data from Lin and Levy (12).

depend on the relative contribution of each pathway to the formation of the metabolite. This accounts for the inorganic sulfate concentration-dependence of the apparent K_m and V_{max} for acetaminophen sulfate formation.

From a different perspective, the decrease of the apparent K_m and V_{max} for acetaminophen sulfate formation with decreasing inorganic sulfate concentrations represents a mechanism by which the

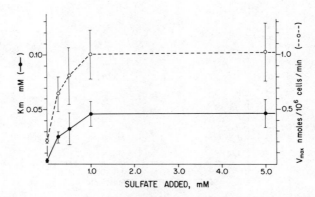

Figure 8. Effect of sodium sulfate concentration added to incubation medium on the apparent values of enzyme kinetic constants for the formation of acetaminophen sulfate from acetaminophen by isolated rat hepatocytes. Mean ± SD, n = 5. From Lin and Levy (13).

body can counteract the depletion of the endogenous cosubstrate.
But the body seldom depends on only one mechanism for homeostasis.
In the case of inorganic sulfate, direct homeostatic control is
provided by a pronounced serum concentration-dependence of sulfate
renal clearance (14).   Many other investigators have explored this
in the physiologic and superphysiologic concentration range of
inorganic sulfate; we were able to extend this to the subphysio-
logic range in rats (14) and humans (11) by making use of the
sulfate-depleting effect of acetaminophen.   The renal clearance
profile of inorganic sulfate (Fig. 9) reflects largely the effect
of a specialized tubular reabsorption process of low capacity but
there is also evidence, from studies by others, of a minor specialized renal tubular secretion mechanism.

    Endogenous inorganic sulfate is derived mainly from the catab-
olism of sulfur-containing amino acids.   Some of that sulfate is
utilized anabolically but most is excreted as such by the kidneys.
The question arises whether depletion of endogenous sulfate caused
by formation of a drug sulfate conjugate initiates a feedback
process leading to increased formation rate of inorganic sulfate as
yet another means of homeostatic control.   This is of considerable
interest because increased catabolism of sulfur-containing amino
acids could have appreciable physiologic implications.   We investigated this problem by determining the urinary excretion rate of
total (free and conjugated) sulfate during control periods and
during prolonged acetaminophen infusion (15).   The control studies
showed essentially constant excretion rate of total sulfate by rats
over 14 to 16 hours;   most of the excreted sulfate was in inorganic

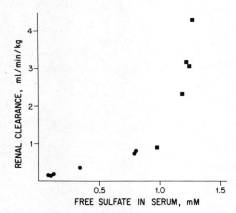

Figure 9. Relationship between renal clearance and serum concen-
          tration of inorganic sulfate in two rats.   One animal
          received   acetaminophen   (circles)   while   the   other
          received sodium sulfate (squares).   From Lin and Levy
          (14), reproduced with permission of the copyright owner.

form.   Prolonged acetaminophen infusion eventually depleted endogenous inorganic sulfate and caused acetaminophen sulfate excretion
to decrease to a constant, relatively low rate (Fig. 10).   Since
most of an injected dose of acetaminophen sulfate can be recovered
in the urine (10) and since the urinary excretion products of
acetaminophen under appropriate conditions account for essentially
all of the administered drug (10), the constant excretion rate of
acetaminophen   sulfate   by   sulfate   depleted   animals   should
approximate their rate of formation of endogenous sulfate.   We
found that rate to be consistently higher than the rate of total
sulfate excretion under control conditions (Fig. 10), suggesting

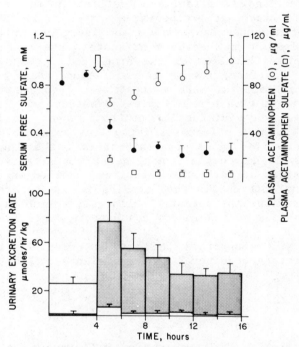

Figure 10. Availability of endogenous inorganic sulfate for formation of acetaminophen sulfate during acetaminophen-
induced sulfate depletion in rats. Upper panel: serum
concentrations of inorganic sulfate before and during
acetaminophen administration (30 mg/kg at 4 hr and 10
mg/hr/rat thereafter) and plasma concentrations of acetaminophen and acetaminophen sulfate.   Lower panel:
urinary excretion of free (open bars) and conjugated
(shaded bars) sulfate. Mean ± SD, n = 8. The ratio of
the total sulfate excretion rate, 14 to 16 hr period/
control period, is 1.36 ± 0.26 (p < 0.01). From Lin,
Galinsky and Levy (15).

that inorganic sulfate formation rate is under feedback control. However, the magnitude of this increase (approximately 40%) is modest and considerably less than what we would expect of a feedback mechanism. We therefore favor the view that the observed increase represents a change in the utilization of sulfate whereby the fraction of this anion that is normally used for anabolic purposes (such as cartilage formation) is diverted to, and utilized for drug sulfate conjugate formation.

The composite picture of acetaminophen sulfate formation and its interrelationship with the availability of endogenous inorganic sulfate provides a fascinating example of the pharmacokinetic implications of endogenous cosubstrate depletion. It appears that the information now available is sufficient to account for all quantitatively important processes; a comprehensive pharmacokinetic model of acetaminophen disposition and inorganic sulfate formation and elimination which describes adequately the concentration- and time-dependent elimination of the drug and the associated changes of inorganic sulfate plasma concentrations has been developed (16). The experimental studies that were required to develop the model provided us with a remarkable and esthetically inspiring view of the body's many interacting control mechanisms that serve to minimize the adverse effects of intrusions by xenobiotics or other perturbations. To the pharmacokineticist, the investigation of processes involving complex, nonlinear, concentration- and time-dependent systems is both stimulating and challenging. I expect to see increasing interest in such studies in the future as pharmacokineticists realize the potential clinical, toxicologic and physiologic implications of endogenous cosubstrate depletion.

Acknowledgement. Supported in part by grant GM 19568 from the National Institute of General Medical Sciences, National Institutes of Health.

REFERENCES

1. J.R. Mitchell, S. Thorgeirsson, W.Z. Potter, D.J. Jollow and H. Keiser, Acetaminophen-induced hepatic injury: Protective role of glutathione in man and rationale for therapy, Clin. Pharmacol. Ther. 16:676-684 (1974).
2. L.A. Reinke, S.A. Belinsky, R.K. Evans, F.C. Kauffman and R.G. Thurman, Conjugation of p-nitrophenol in the perfused rat liver: The effect of substrate concentration and carbohydrate reserves, J. Pharmacol. Exp. Ther. 217:863-870 (1981).
3. L.P. Amsel and G. Levy, Drug biotransformation interactions in man II. A pharmacokinetic study of the simultaneous conjugation of benzoic and salicylic acids with glycine, J. Pharm. Sci. 58:321-326 (1969).

4. G. Levy and T. Matsuzawa, Pharmacokinetics of salicylamide elimination in man, J. Pharmacol. Exp. Ther. 156:285-293 (1967).

5. E. Nelson, M. Hanano and G. Levy, Comparative pharmacokinetics of salicylate elimination in man and rats, J. Pharmacol. Exp. Ther. 153:159-166 (1966).

6. H.J. Zimmerman, Effects of aspirin and acetaminophen on the liver, Arch. Intern. Med. 141:333-342 (1981).

7. J.T. Slattery and G. Levy, Acetaminophen kinetics in acutely poisoned patients, Clin. Pharmacol. Ther. 25:185-195 (1979).

8. G. Levy and H. Yamada, Drug biotransformation interactions in man. III. Acetaminophen and salicylamide, J. Pharm. Sci. 60:215-221 (1971).

9. L.F. Prescott, Kinetics and metabolism of paracetamol and phenacetin, Br. J. Clin. Pharmacol. 10:291S-298S (1980).

10. R.E. Galinsky and G. Levy, Dose- and time-dependent elimination of acetaminophen in rats: Pharmacokinetic implications of cosubstrate depletion, J. Pharmacol. Exp. Ther. 219:14-20 (1981).

11. M.E. Morris and G. Levy, Serum concentrations and renal excretion by normal adults of inorganic sulfate after acetaminophen, ascorbic acid or sodium sulfate, Clin. Pharmacol. Ther. 33:529-536 (1983).

12. J.H. Lin and G. Levy, Effect of experimental renal failure on sulfate retention and acetaminophen pharmacokinetics in rats, J. Pharmacol. Exp. Ther. 221:80-84 (1982).

13. J.H. Lin and G. Levy, Effect of inorganic sulfate concentration on kinetics of conjugation of acetaminophen with sulfate by isolated rat hepatocytes, to be published.

14. J.H. Lin and G. Levy, Renal clearance of inorganic sulfate in rats: Effect of acetaminophen-induced depletion of endogenous sulfate, J. Pharm. Sci. 72:213-217 (1983).

15. J.H. Lin, R.E. Galinsky and G. Levy, Availability of endogenous inorganic sulfate for conjugation during acetaminophen-induced sulfate depletion in rats, to be published.

16. J.H. Lin and G. Levy, manuscript in preparation.

17. J.H. Lin and G. Levy, Sulfate depletion after acetaminophen administration and replenishment by infusion of sodium sulfate or N-acetylcysteine in rats, Biochem. Pharmacol. 30:2723-2725 (1981).

Chapter 22

METHODS FOR DRUG DOSAGE INDIVIDUALIZATION: PAST, PRESENT AND FUTURE

Lewis B. Sheiner

Department of Laboratory Medicine and
Division of Clinical Pharmacology
Department of Medicine
University of California
San Francisco, California

There is considerable interest in the measurement and interpretation of concentrations of drugs in plasma (Cp). Much of this interest stems from the hope that such measurements will provide a means, at least in some instances, of controlling drug therapy so as to achieve desired pharmacologic effects (and avoid undesired ones) with more precision than heretofore. The methodologic issues in doing so concern how to use population information and the information in Cp measurements from the individual of concern. It is the purpose of this chapter to discuss and review these issues.

A DOSAGE OPTIMIZATION PROBLEM

In this chapter, only the simplest possible dosage optimization problem will be considered: choosing a steady-state drug input rate, R, so as to achieve a target average plasma steady-state concentration for a linear pharmacokinetic system (the target is C_T). Further, assuming that dosage is parenteral, or bioavailability is unity, the model governing the outcome of interest, the steady-state plasma drug concentration, Cpss, is:

$$Cpss = \frac{R}{CL} \tag{1}$$

when CL is set to the drug clearance of the individual to be treated.

The Loss Function

The desire for Cpss to equal C_T can be formalized by defining a quadratic loss function, $\ell(CL,R)$:

$$\ell(CL,R) = (Cpss - C_T)^2 \tag{2}$$

where Cpss is given by Equation (1). The optimal R, R_{opt}, is the one which minimizes the loss function (Eq.(2)) for $CL = CL^*$, the true clearance for the individual:

$$\ell(CL^*, R_{opt}) = \frac{Min}{R} \; \ell(CL^*, R) \tag{3}$$

Given Equation (1), it is evident that:

$$R_{opt} = CL^* \cdot C_T \tag{4}$$

Posterior Expected Loss

Thus, computation of the optimal dosage represents no problem when CL* is known. Difficulties arise, however, because CL* is not, in general, known. In that case, there will always be some uncertainty about the Cpss that will result from any choice of R. Consequently, a single dosage that is best for all (realistically) possible values of CL* cannot be chosen, and one must be content to choose a dosage that is expected to yield the best average outcome, or, according to Bayesian decision theory, the action associated with least "posterior expected loss" (1). This is defined as:

$$L(R) = \int \ell(CL,R) \; p(CL) \; dCL \tag{5}$$

where the integral is over the real positive line (the range of values for CL*) and p(CL) is the (posterior) probability density function for CL*; p(CL) is denoted the posterior density because it reflects not only the (prior) probability of CL*, based on population parameters and the individuals' values of physiologic factors (such as renal function) that may influence clearance, but also on all information available from past observations of drug concentrations. This will be discussed further below. Equation (5) simply says that the "expected loss" for dose rate R is a weighted average of the losses associated with R under all the different possible values of CL*. The weights are numbers proportional to the probabilities of the possible values of CL*, given by p(CL).

Although the loss function (Equation (2)) depends on CL, the expected loss (L) does not. The integration removes the effect of CL by averaging over all of its possible values. The optimal

(Bayesian) decision rule now is to choose R_{opt} so as to minimize posterior expected loss. That is:

$$L(R_{opt}) = \frac{Min}{R} L(R) \tag{6}$$

A Simplified Version of Expected Loss

It is traditional, although not universally favored (see reference 2), to try to avoid the computational complexity of the integration implied by Equation (5). To do so, an estimate of CL*, CL, is used to define L(R). That is:

$$L(R) = \ell(\hat{CL}, R) \tag{7}$$

is used instead of Equation (5). In this case, it is once more evident that the solution, R_{opt}, to Equation (6) is given by:

$$R_{opt} = \hat{CL} \cdot C_T \tag{8}$$

Note that Equation (7) says that the loss associated with dosage R is no longer the average loss with respect to the possible values of CL*, but rather is the single loss associated with some particular value of CL, CL. In light of the resemblance of Equation (4) and Equation (8), it seems intuitive that CL should be chosen so as to be "close to" CL*; all the suggestions to be discussed herein share this objective.

INFORMATION SOURCES

By adopting Equation (7), the problem of choosing R_{opt} has been reduced to that of choosing CL, an estimate of CL*. To do so, there are two sources of information available: prior knowledge and feedback knowledge. The distinction between the two is that the former does not depend on the patient at hand having taken the drug of concern, while the latter does. Prior knowledge consists of knowledge gained from the study of other patients taking the drug (such as, the proportionality constant linking renal clearance of drug and creatinine clearance), and patient data unrelated to drug experience (such as, the patient's creatinine clearance). Feedback knowledge consists of measured drug concentrations from the patient at hand, plus the dosing history prior to those measurements.

Prior knowledge of clearance can be summarized by a prior probability distribution $\pi(CL)$, adjusted for the patient at hand. The prior distribution characterizes the probability of all possible clearance values for the patient before any feedback knowledge is available. The first two moments of the distribution are frequently of interest. They are the mean, $\overline{CL}$, and the variance ω^2_{CL}. Note that $\overline{CL}$ may be different for different patients as it may depend on patient size, age, renal function, and so forth. ω^2_{CL} is usually assumed to be the same for all patients. Similarly a prior distribution for some other parameter(s), such as volume of distribution, V, may be defined as $\pi(V)$, with mean $\overline{V}$ and variance ω^2_V. (For simplicity, it is assumed that CL* and V are statistically independent.)

Feedback (Cp) data must be related to CL. This is done via a pharmacokinetic/statistical model:

$$Cp_j = \hat{Cp}(D,V,CL,t_j) + \varepsilon_j; \quad j=1,N \qquad (9)$$

Cp_j is the jth of N observed concentrations, observed at time t_j; while $\hat{Cp}(.)$ is the pharmacokinetic model. For the purposes of this chapter, the model is assumed to predict Cp_j using only the parameters volume of distribution (V), clearance (CL), past dosage (D) and the time of the observation (t_j). The prediction, Cp_j, will not, of course, exactly equal the observation, and the random variable, ε_j, represents this discrepancy. The ε_j are assumed to be independent and identically distributed, with variance equal to σ^2, a quantity that is part of prior knowledge.

For the purposes of this discussion, all items of prior knowledge are assumed known; ways of estimating them from routine patient data are described and discussed elsewhere (3-6). Note that Cp_j is not an estimate of Cpss (see Eq. (1)). It is assumed that although the target concentration is expressed in terms of an average steady-state value, observations may have been made at any time, under any (reasonable) circumstances. All such observations are to be used so that $\hat{Cp}(.)$ must model them.

The general idea behind using prior information and feedback information together is to use the latter to modify the prior distribution of CL ($\pi(CL)$) so as to reflect its information content (Bayes theorem is one way to do so). After the modification, the probability of various CL values is given by the modified distribution, the one called the posterior distribution above, and denoted either p(CL), or more completely, p(CL; Cp), meaning the probability of CL given (the observed) Cp values. When choosing CL, if some distribution of CL is to be used as a basis for the choice, p(CL) should obviously be used rather than $\pi(CL)$.

APPROACHES TO ESTIMATING CLEARANCE

A number of approaches to estimating clearance (in general, for estimating individual pharmacokinetic parameters) have been proposed and used. The theoretical basis of these will be discussed beginning with those that use the least information and progressing to those that use the most. This order correlates with both the sophistication and performance of the methods. For the moment, no general restriction on the type or number of feedback observations of Cp that are available is assumed. The next section will discuss a hierarchy of these, and briefly review and categorize, according to the hierarchies defined herein, many of the suggestions for dosage optimization appearing in the pharmaco-kinetic literature.

Use Prior Mean Only. The first (traditional) method uses no feedback information. It chooses $CL = \overline{CL}$, the prior mean, and thus uses only a limited amount of prior information. Nonetheless, when no feedback information is available, all workers agree that this approach is near optimal, and no alternative method has been seriously considered.

Use Only Feedback Information. It is traditional that when some feedback information becomes available, this is used. The usual approach at this point is to use only the feedback informa-tion and ignore the prior information. To do so requires that N be greater than or equal to the number of model parameters (2 in the example herein; generally, M). The method used is Ordinary Least Squares (OLS).

The Ordinary Least Squares estimate of CL, $\hat{CL}_{OLS}$, minimizes the OLS objective function:

$$O_{OLS}(CL,V) = \sum_{j=1}^{N} (Cp_j - \hat{Cp}_j)^2 \tag{10}$$

Note that although an estimate of V is of no direct interest, it must be obtained along with CL_{OLS} in order to obtain the latter. The estimate, CL_{OLS}, minimizes the sum of squared differences of predictions of Cp_j from observed values of Cp_j; that is, it minimizes the sum of the squared estimates of the ε_j.

When (as assumed) the ε_j are independent and identically distributed, statistical theory states that the OLS procedure yields an estimate with a number of useful properties. First, the estimate will yield CL* when N approaches infinity. Second, when Cp(.) is a linear function, CL_{OLS} is most precise among a rather large class of estimators (perhaps this feature carries over to some extent when Cp(.) is nonlinear in CL, as is usually the case in pharmacokinetics). Finally, when N is large, CL_{OLS} is itself distributed about CL* according to the normal distribution law. Although of little concern here, this last property is helpful when estimating confidence intervals for CL*.

The OLS estimate depends only on the data, Cp_j, and takes no notice of any features of the prior distribution, $\pi(CL)$. Thus CL_{OLS} cannot be seen as any particular point on $p(CL)$, since this is never computed. It is true, however, that when N is large and the distribution of ε is as stated, CL_{OLS} will correspond to the mean of $p(CL)$, when the latter is computed according to Bayes theorem. However, when N is small, CL_{OLS} has no such property. This at least partly explains why CL_{OLS} behaves rather poorly when N is near zero. Indeed, at this limit (when N = 0) the method says nothing whatever about how to choose estimates. Nor could it; it ignores the prior and has no observations on which to base an estimate. Because of poor behavior at the limit, poor behavior in the neighborhood of the limit is expected, and this is what is found: when N = M (the number of parameters of the model), there will be no minimization; each squared deviation is simply set equal to its minimum value, zero, and M equations in M unknowns are solved. When N is less than M, some ad hoc solution must be proposed since there will be fewer constraints (squares) than parameters to be estimated.

Use Feedback and Prior Mean(s). The usual solution to the problem of N < M is to begin to use some prior information: M − N parameters are arbitrarily chosen to be set equal to their prior mean values, and then the other N parameters are estimated, using OLS, as for the N = M case. For example, if N were 1, one would set $V = \bar{V}$ and choose CL to minimize $(Cp(D,\bar{V},CL,t)-Cp)^2$; that is, such that $(Cp(D,\bar{V},CL,t) = Cp$.

There is no sound theoretical basis for proceeding as just outlined, and it must be regarded as simply an ad hoc solution to the problem posed by attempting to apply OLS when N < M.

Use Feedback, Prior Means, Variances and σ^2. As just discussed, OLS needs improvement when data are sparse. A theoretically sound means to do so has largely been advocated by the present author and his co-workers (3,4,7-12). The essential idea is simply to recognize that there continues to be information about CL in the prior, $\pi(CL)$, even after observations become available. To take advantage of this information, one can regard the prior mean values of CL and V as additional observations of the system (of a different kind, to be sure, but in the same spirit as Cp). Thus:

$$CL = \overline{CL} + \eta \tag{11}$$

which is analogous to Equation (9). Equation (11) says that the "observation" of CL is the population mean value, $\overline{CL}$, and the "error," an individual shift, η, is the random part of CL and thus has variance ω^2_{CL}; the η's for two different individuals are, of course, independent. By analogy, the estimates of CL and V should minimize the sum of squared "errors" of this type, as well as of the other type. This is where the variance of the prior distribution (of CL or η), ω^2_{CL}, becomes relevant. Using it and a similar quantity for V, a weighted least squares (WLS) estimator of CL, CL_{WLS}, can be defined. CL_{WLS} minimizes the sum of both types of squared errors by minimizing the objective function (for example):

$$O_{WLS}(CL,V) = \sum_{j=1}^{N} \frac{(\hat{Cp}_j - Cp_j)^2}{\sigma^2} + \frac{(CL-\overline{CL})^2}{\omega^2_{CL}} + \frac{(V-\overline{V})^2}{\omega^2_V} \tag{12}$$

where, in the general case there would be M terms on the right after the first summation, one for each parameter of the model.

There are two sets of "squares" in Equation (12), one for the estimated errors in observations of Cp_j, and one for the estimated errors in "observations" of the model parameters. Each squared error is weighted by the reciprocal of its variance. Thus, the differing scales of the drug concentrations and the various parameters are normalized to a common scale as each is weighted by a quantity, in its own units, that expresses the typical value of a squared error of that type. (Recall that the average squared deviation of a random variable from its mean is its variance.)

Although Equation (12) can be used simply because of its intuitive appeal, there are two stronger justifications. First, under the distributional assumptions stated for CL (and V) and ε, statistical theory asserts that the WLS procedure has the same properties as OLS. Now that two types of observations with different variances are recognized as relevant, the OLS estimate per se is no longer the most precise in its class; the WLS estimator is. It is more precise because it incorporates more information (the information present in the prior distributions of the parameters). Second, and perhaps as compelling, if the further assumption is made that the form of the distribution of both the parameters and ε's is Normal, then Equation (12) defines a Bayes estimate. That is, CL_{WLS} is the mode (highest point) of $p(CL)$ when the latter is computed from $\pi(CL)$ and the Cp according to Bayes theorem. Thus CL_{WLS} is the "most probable" value of CL*.

Examination of Equation (12) reveals that it does accomplish its original purpose. Its behavior at the limit (N = 0) is just what it ought to be; each parameter is estimated to be equal to its (population) mean. When N is small compared to M, there is no necessity for an ad hoc procedure; there are always at least as many constraints (squares) as there are parameters to be estimated.

It is instructive to compare OLS and Bayesian approaches. The estimates of the latter will coincide with the OLS estimates in two circumstances: first, when there is "overwhelming evidence." This occurs when N so far exceeds M that the first sum of squares in Equation (12) overwhelms the second in magnitude. The coincidence of the estimates in this case is as it should be; there is so much evidence on which to base estimates that prior beliefs are appropriately abandoned. The second case in which the OLS and Bayesian estimates will coincide is in the condition of "prior ignorance." In this condition all the ω^2 are very large relative to σ^2, and $N \geq$ M. Then, relatively small deviations of the Cp_j from the Cp_j will count a great deal, while even large deviations of any parameter from its prior mean will be relatively inconsequential. In this circumstance, the Bayes estimates and those of OLS will properly coincide. There is so little reason to favor prior belief, that estimates should (and will) depend virtually entirely on the data, no matter how sparse they are (so long as $N \geq M$).

Finally, consider the ad hoc procedure using OLS for the case when N is small. To fix certain parameters to their mean values, and to use the observed outcomes to estimate the others according to OLS is equivalent to using the Bayes approach, but the assumption is made that the variances of the fixed parameters are all infinitesimal relative to those of the parameters that are not fixed. When the prior variance of a parameter is infinitesimal, the Bayes procedure accords any deviations of that parameter from its prior mean a very large weight. Consequently that parameter estimate will not deviate from its prior mean. This corresponds exactly to the ad hoc procedure. Thus, when $N \leq M$ and the ad hoc adaptation of OLS is used, the Bayes procedure is actually being used, but with the wrong weights. Hence, the ad hoc OLS estimates cannot be (on average) as precise as the Bayes ones. The same argument holds, of course, even when N exceeds M. These theoretical expectations are borne out by empirical study.

Use Feedback and $\pi(CL)$. As noted above, $\hat{CL}$ in the Bayes method is chosen as the mode of p(CL), whereas certain theoretical considerations may lead one to prefer to choose CL as its mean. A final sophistication is to do just this. The method uses Bayes theorem to define p(CL) and performs numerical integration (over the range of both CL and V) to find its mean (12,13).

OBSERVATION STRATEGIES AND LITERATURE SUGGESTIONS

Just as for the estimation of CL, so a number of suggestions have been made for how many and which observations of Cp are to be used with proposed dosage optimization methods. Again, these can be ordered (from most restrictive to least restrictive) to correspond to increasing sophistication and practical applicability. If a primary ordering of suggestions for dosage optimization made in the clinical pharmacokinetic literature is carried out according to the method of the previous section, and within this primary ordering, a secondary ordering according to the observation hierarchy just alluded to is also made, then an overall hierarchy of literature suggestions will result. It will run from least to most sophisticated, and least to most general. Such an ordering is presented in Table I, where overall performance of the various methods is also indicated.

To understand the table, the hierarchy of observation strategies must be explained, as must the measure of performance used. To dispense with the latter, the magnitude of the ε_j, the differences between the predictions, $Cp_{j,\lambda}$ and the observations, Cp_j, when the former are made using the CL of the method, is a natural performance measure. Their coefficients of variation (standard deviation of ε_j/Cp_j) is the measure used in Table I, called "typical percent error," to express method performance. While it might have been preferable to use the error, $C_T - Cpss$, or $CL - CL^*$, these are not always (or even ever) available in studies of dosage optimization methods, whereas the measure used herein is almost always available, or can be estimated from the data presented.

The items that may be fixed for an observation strategy are N, D and t. The most restrictive strategies fix all of these.

No Feedback. The first strategy of this type fixes N = 0 (D and t become irrelevant), and corresponds to the "no feedback" method of the previous section. This method has been common practice for years, although Jelliffe (see references 14 and 15) must be given credit for bringing to the attention of the American medical community the importance of adjusting drug dosage (of digitalis glycosides) in accordance with (prior) patient characteristics (notably renal function).

The seminal work on adjusting dosage of aminoglycosides for differences in renal function was that of Orme and Cutler for kanamycin (16). Gentamycin has become a more important drug, and the dependence of its clearance on renal function has been clearly documented, among others, by Chen et al. (17) and McHenry et al. (18), who each proposed nomograms for maintenance dosage based on prior knowledge of renal function and size. Subsequently, investigators (see reference 19, for example), feeling that dosage adjustment based on such nomograms was insufficiently precise, attempted to produce better nomograms using adjustments for prior knowledge of age and sex, in addition to the others. Despite this, their data show a percent error on the order of 30-40%. Jelliffe's original digoxin method is also based entirely on prior knowledge (14); data from a subsequent evaluation suggests a percent error in excess of 50% (15), a value confirmed by others (20-22). The same error magnitude seems to hold for the "no feedback" approach to theophylline predictions (23), and to other drugs. The value of

50% for percent error in Table I reflects this experience. The
message appears to be that predictions of individual drug kinetics
from such items as age, size, renal function, and so forth, simply
do not capture interindividual kinetic variation very well. This
is not to say that renal function does not affect the kinetics of
gentamicin or digoxin or many other drugs. Rather it says that
there are many other factors that modify individual kinetics, and
that most of these factors are unknown and/or unpredictable from
prior knowledge alone.

Fixed N, Dosage and Time. The next most restrictive observation strategies demand that N be some fixed number, and that both
dosage and sampling time be fixed. Such a strategy leaves little
flexibility, and, to the extent that the fixed dosage strategy is
not identical with clinically optimum initial therapy, will delay
efficacy. The usual reason for the restriction is the desire to
use the Cp observation in a simple (proportional) formula to arrive
at CL. Since the simple formula cannot model the general Cp to
dosage relationship, a fixed relationship must be built into the
observation strategy.

Because the "fixed" N is usually 1, no such methods are proposed that use only feedback, and these methods first appear at the
3rd level of the outer (methodologic) hierarchy in Table I, where
feedback plus prior means are to be used (although the use of the
latter may be implicit rather than explicit). The first suggestion
along these lines was that of Cooper et al. (24) who found that a
lithium concentration drawn 24 hours after an initial dose
correlated well with the ultimate steady-state concentration. They
then advocated use of this test-dose-single-sample method for
choosing steady-state dosage.

This success led to similar applications in psychiatry. Both
Brunswick et al. (25) and Potter et al. (26) advocate the use of a
single 24-hour sample after a test dose of desmethylimipramine or
imipramine to optimize dosage.

Chiou et al. (27) propose a "fixed N" method for theophylline.
Although the dosage route (an infusion) is fixed, the rate itself
is not fixed and some latitude as to sampling time is allowed.
Thus, this method is not as rigid as the other single sample
methods just discussed. Chiou et al. wish to deal with the common
clinical situation of a patient who has taken an unknown prior dose
(perhaps before entry into the hospital). They propose to determine a drug concentration before beginning a long-term infusion;
then to begin it, having chosen the rate from prior knowledge
alone. They then suggest sampling another drug concentration some-
time later, and computing drug clearance from this and the first
concentration. Although this approach appears to depend on two
concentrations, the first concentration actually serves to replace

Table I. Examples of observation strategies.

Method Uses	Allowable Observations[a]	First Author (ref.)	Drug(s)	Typical Percent Error[b]
1. Population means	none	Jeliffe (15) Orme (16) Chen (17)	digoxin kanamycin gentamycin	∿50
2. Observed C_p	Min N ($\geq$M); Usual D,t	Monjanel (37) Pancorbo (38) Cipolle (39) Jelliffe (40) Ludden (41)	methotrexate theophylline tobramycin many phenytoin	10 – 20 (N $\leq$ 4)[c]
3. Population means + Observed C_p	Fixed N,D,T	Cooper (24) Brunswick (25) Chiou (27) Richens (28)	lithium desmethylimipramine theophylline phenytoin	20 – 30
	Fixed N,D,T; t "optimal"	Koup (36)	chloramphenicol theophylline	20 – 30
4. Population means + Population variances + Observed Cp	any	Vozeh (9) Sheiner (7) Peck (8)	phenytoin digoxin theophylline	10 – 20 (N $\leq$ 2)[c]

[a] N is the number of Cp observations; M is the number of model parameters; D is the dosage; t is the sampling time.

[b] Percent error of estimate is mean ((obs-est)/est) x 100, where the est are the estimates of Cp made by the method and the obs are the observed Cp's. When steady state is considered, this percent error applies equally to the estimated (predicted) drug clearance.

[c] For monoexponential model.

knowledge of prior doses. Only the difference in the two concentrations is used to compute clearance. Hence the method is, mathematically, a "single sample" method. Chiou et al. explicitly retain the population estimate of volume of distribution in their computation of a clearance estimate, which is based on an approximation to the area under the curve joining the two concentrations.

In a series of papers since 1975, Richens and co-workers have proposed (28,29), corrected (30) and revised (31) a nomogram for phenytoin dosage based on the observation of a single steady-state dosage-Cpss pair. Since phenytoin exhibits nonlinear kinetics, two parameters, Km and Vm (see below), govern clearance. Further, since only one observation is available, the authors fix Km to the prior mean and use the single dosage–Cpss pair to solve for an individual estimate of Vm. They then offer a nomogram to compute the steady–state dosage designed to achieve a target Cpss for these parameter estimates. This is, as previously noted, equivalent to using the Bayes approach with the variance of both Km and the ε error set to an infinitesimal value while the variance of Vm remains finite.

Chiba et al. (32) use the same basic strategy to compute dosage, but in their version of the ad hoc approach they elect to fix Vm to the prior mean and compute a new estimate of Km for each individual. Their study in a group of pediatric patients suggests somewhat poorer performance than the method of Richens et al. (31).

A representative performance range, culled from all of these studies, is indicated in Table I. Percent errors of 20–30% appear typical, with most drugs (methods) represented at the upper limit. Nonetheless, the great value of even limited feedback information, suboptimally used, is clear.

<u>Arbitrary N and Dosage: "Optimal" Time</u>. Although this approach still removes any choice from all three items, it can be considered more sophisticated than the previous method in that an attempt is made to take some advantage of the rigid specifications. This is done by attempting to choose the sampling time so that the resulting drug concentration yields a more precise estimate of CL* than would a concentration at any other time. That, at least, is the idea, although in the methods of this type recently suggested, the goal is not quite reached. Before discussing these, the theory behind what must be regarded as the currently accepted approach to this problem is outlined.

Assume a fixed dosage design, D, and a fixed interval of time (t_1 to t_2) within which, for simplicity, only one observation is to be obtained. The problem is to choose the sampling time for the observation so as to maximize some measure of the precision of the subsequent estimate of CL*. For additional simplicity, assume the method for estimating CL will be the third method previously discussed: OLS with V fixed to $\bar{V}$.

Precision of an estimate of CL* can be measured by the magnitude of the average squared deviation of the estimate from its mean. This is the variance of the estimate. Given an unbiased estimator (that is, one that estimates CL*, on the average), minimizing the variance of the estimate is equivalent to minimizing the squared distance of the estimate from the true value. (Thus, the loss function here is identical in form to that used to optimize dosage. If the Bayes estimate, rather than OLS were to be used, one would seek an observation strategy minimizing the variance of p(CL).)

Under the previous assumptions about the distribution of the ε error, the variance of the OLS estimate of CL, $\text{var}(\hat{CL}_{OLS})$ can be estimated as:

$$\text{var}(\hat{CL}_{OLS}) = s^2 \left(\frac{\partial \hat{Cp}_j}{\partial CL}\right)^{-2} \tag{13}$$

where s is a proportionality constant fixed by the data and the OLS procedure, and $\partial Cp_j/\partial CL$ is the first derivative of the model $(Cp_j(.,t_j))$ taken with respect to CL, and evaluated at the estimate, $\hat{CL}_{OLS}$ and $\bar{V}$. Since the estimate $\hat{CL}_{OLS}$ is not available when choosing sampling times, some preliminary estimate of it must be used when evaluating Cp_j: a logical choice is the prior mean, $\bar{CL}$. Equation (13), is then minimized with respect to sampling time, t, on the interval t_1 to t_2 to obtain t^*, the optimal sampling time.

An intuitive justification for this procedure arises from recalling that sampling time should be chosen so that the then present drug concentration contains as much information about the parameter of interest as possible. To make the idea of information more precise, consider a drug concentration at time t_j, Cp_j. Assuming constant error magnitude, it is intuitive that for a unit difference in the value of CL, the more Cp_j would change, the more information about CL it would contain. But Cp_j is approximately $\hat{Cp}_j$ (if $\hat{CL}$ is near CL*) and the first derivative of Cp_j with respect to CL directly measures the change in Cp_j caused by a unit change in CL. If (positive) information is measured as the square of the partial derivative (so as to remove its sign), then to maximize information, its reciprocal can be minimized, and this is precisely what minimizing Equation (13) implies.

To illustrate the procedure, and to provide some insight for later discussion, consider the following problem: a single sample can be taken at any time, $t^* \geq 0$ from a monoexponential model after a single bolus dose, D:

$$\hat{Cp} = \hat{Cp}(D,V,CL,t) = \frac{D}{V} \exp\left(-\frac{CL}{V}t\right) \tag{14}$$

The squared partial derivative of Equation (14) with respect to CL is:

$$z = \left(\frac{\partial \hat{Cp}}{\partial CL}\right)^2 = \frac{D^2 t^2}{V^4} \exp\left(-2\frac{CL}{V}t\right) \tag{15}$$

To find the value of t that maximizes Equation (15) (i.e., that minimizes its reciprocal), its partial derivative with respect to t is set to zero and solved for t^*; the expression is then evaluated at $V = \bar{V}$, $CL = \overline{CL}$. An observation at this value of t has maximum information about CL and is therefore the optimal sampling time. The following equations detail this procedure:

$$\frac{\partial z}{\partial t} = \frac{2tD^2}{V^4} \exp(-2\frac{CL}{V} t) - \frac{D^2 t^2}{V^4} \exp(-2\frac{CL}{V} t) (\frac{2CL}{V}) = 0;$$

$$\frac{t*CL}{V} = 1; \quad t* = V/CL; \quad t* = \overline{V}/\overline{CL} \tag{16}$$

The optimal sampling time for estimating clearance under the conditions and model defined above thus occurs at the mean transit time of a drug molecule though the system, equal to the reciprocal of the rate constant of the monoexponential decline.

The method above is easily extended to several parameters, non-constant error and $N > 1$. It was first put forth by Box and Lucas (33), and a recent review is given by St. John and Draper (34); in its general form it is called D-optimality.

Inspired, no doubt, by the work of Cooper et al. (24), Koup et al. (36) describe a single sample, optimal sampling time method for chloramphenicol and theophylline. Slattery et al. (35) justify the sampling time of Koup et al. (36), 6 hours, by considering the ratio of the steady-state drug concentration to a drug concentration, Cp*, obtained at a fixed time, t*, after a single dose (assuming a monoexponential model). They argue that since CL will be estimated as proportional to Cp*, the particular sampling time, t*, that renders the ratio, Cpss/Cp*, closest to a constant despite variation in clearance and volume of distribution is the best value. After some consideration, it becomes clear that the authors have, in this case, rather ingeniously rediscovered D-optimality. However, their criterion of "least change in the proportionality constant" is related only to convenience and not to any intuitive notion of optimality, as D-optimality is. It is simply fortunate (and in this particular case, inevitable) that the two should coincide. Because 24 hours, the sampling time arbitrarily chosen for the psychiatric drugs previously discussed, is fortuitously very near the time corresponding to the reciprocal of the terminal rate constant for those drugs, one may expect the performance of those methods and the one of Koup et al. (36) to be similar. This is indicated in Table I.

Minimum N, Flexible Dosage and Time. The next approach to be discussed demands a certain minimum number of Cp observations, but allows them to be taken during usual therapeutic dosage schedules, without excessive sampling time restrictions. Since this approach may be less sophisticated than the optimal sampling time one and it is not clear whether a minimum N or a fixed t is harder to attain in practice, it should perhaps be regarded as on a par with, rather than preferable to, the latter.

The strategy is to ignore prior information and use the OLS approach. Therefore suggestions of this type are found in Table I under the second primary (method) heading. Many authors, (2,38-41) have advocated taking general Cp observations and fitting a model (involving CL) to them by OLS. In this case, N > M. As indicated in Table I, one usually finds a marked reduction in percent error from the no feedback case, with final percent error between 10 and 20%. This is probably as well as one can do since, at least for a number of drugs, irreducible day-to-day kinetic variability in actual patients may be of this order of magnitude (4,9,23). It appears that when using the simple (monoexponential) model, OLS-based approaches that ignore prior information can achieve percent errors on the order of 10-20% after use of only 4 Cp observations (40). This is indicated in Table I.

When N = M, the simple OLS approach does not fare quite so well. Phenytoin provides an example. As previously noted, the model usually used to describe the relationship between phenytoin dosage rate and steady-state drug concentration involves two parameters: Km, the phenytoin concentration at half-maximal elimination rate, and Vm, the maximal elimination rate itself. The model equation can be rearranged so that it is a linear function of (transformed) dosage and (transformed) concentration. Ludden et al. (41) advocate using a linear form and two measured concentrations at different steady-state dosages to solve for the two parameters of the model. In a retrospective study, Vozeh et al. (9) found that in 13 patients the Ludden method yielded a percent error of 26%, a value typical of the "arbitrary N" case, above. Moreover, another study (5) points out that the method can yield patently absurd parameter estimates; in a group of 32 patients each having at least two dosage-concentration pairs, one patient's parameters were estimated to be Vm = 30 mg/kg, Km = 102 µg/ml (typical actual values might be Vm = 5 mg/kg, Km = 7 µg/ml). This highlights the problem with OLS estimates when N is near M.

Any N, Dosage and Time. Ultimate flexibility is provided by an approach that can use any observed Cp (within reason), without arbitrary restriction as to number, prior dosage or sampling time. Only the Bayesian method previously discussed can deal with this case, and so it alone appears under the fourth primary (method) heading of Table I.

In the previously cited study of Vozeh et al. (9), the arbitrary N method for phenytoin of Richens and Dunlop (reference 28, and see above) was compared to the Bayesian method. Data from 32 patients, each with at least two dosage-Cpss pairs were used. When the first of two dosage-Cpss pairs was used by each method to predict the dosage required to achieve the second observed Cpss, the percent error of the Richens and Dunlop method was 12%, and of the Bayesian method, 8.7%. These remarkably low values are undoubtedly due, at least in part, to each method having been optimized for the data at hand. One cannot, of course, expect this performance prospectively. Nonetheless the purpose of the comparison is served. The relative percent error of the non-Bayesian method is seen to be 35% larger than that of the Bayesian method.

The Bayes method has also been applied to other drugs, notably digoxin (7,8) and theophylline (42). A typical finding is that predictions of minimum possible percent error (10-20%; see above) can often be obtained with as few as two Cp observations. This is to be contrasted with the four required for this performance by the OLS method (see above).

CONCLUDING REMARKS

The Past. Space does not permit mention of the many other dosage optimization suggestions made in the clinical pharmacokinetic literature. Yet, without detracting from the originiality of those works, this paper does outline the basic approaches that have been taken to the problem. These approaches can be seen to lie along two independent gradients. First, a gradient of increasing sophistication of data analysis methodology (and hence exploitation of all available information) and second, a gradient of increasing latitude with respect to the type and amount of feedback information (observed drug concentrations) that can be used.

The least sophisticated and most restrictive methods require that one adhere to a rigid schedule of number of Cp observations, dosage and sampling time, and fail optimally to exploit prior (population) information. That such methods remain popular may be due to their (deceptive) simplicity. At the other extreme, the most sophisticated and least restrictive method, the Bayes method, allows use of virtually any (number and type of) drug concentration observation, and attempts fully to exploit both this and prior information.

The Present. Indeed, the Bayes method is never worse than the other methods, is often better, and must be considered the current "state of the art." First of all, it is entirely general. It can be defined for virtually any drug for which a reasonable pharmacokinetic model can be written. There is no restriction on the form of this model or on the form of the relationships between patient variables (such as age or weight) and prior means. It can, as noted, deal with any dosage, sampling pattern and number of observations: Second, it is quite practical, and can be implemented on a desk-top microcomputer (see reference 42). Finally, it is likely to perform better than the alternatives precisely in those circumstances in which they perform worst; when observed drug concentrations actually provide little information about underlying parameters.

The Future. When considering what improvements the future may bring, it seems likely that the minimum 10-20% error discussed previously (but now regarded as the percent error in achieving the target concentration) will not be reduced further, as it appears to represent unavoidable intraindividual, random kinetic variation plus Cp measurement error. Rather, one may look for improvement in the number of Cp observations required to achieve it. Perhaps, using a (hitherto untried) combination of optimum sampling time methods (34) and Bayesian estimation (8), a single Cp observation may suffice.

Another fruitful avenue for exploration is to attempt to use loss functions other than the quadratic. The latter undoubtedly penalizes Cp deviations from the midpoint of the therapeutic range too severely when the attained Cpss is within the therapeutic range, and penalizes deviations insufficiently when the Cpss is outside this range. Moreover, asymmetric loss functions, with greater penalties for exceeding the target than for being too low, are probably clinically appropriate. In the same spirit, robust estimation methods, that is, those that respond less to "outlier" observations than do least squares type methods (to which latter class both OLS and the Bayesian method belong), may also prove useful in increasing the stability of optimization procedures. It should be recognized, however, that to use either a nonquadratic loss function or robust methods will entail additional computational effort (although not to an insurmountable degree), as the simplification of Equation (8) may now be inappropriate.

Finally, one may also hope for the exploration and use of more complete pharmacokinetic/dynamic models in dosage optimization systems so that even greater flexibility in use of feedback information is achieved. Perhaps the day is not far off when drug concentration measurements in saliva, urine or other sites can easily be used, as can observations of clinical effects of drugs.

Acknowledgement. This work was supported in part by USDHHS Grant GM 26676.

REFERENCES

1. J.O. Berger, "Statistical Decision Theory," Springer Verlag, New York (1980).

2. A. Schumitzky, Adaptive control in drug therapy, in: "Computer Aid to Drug Therapy and to Drug Monitoring," H. Ducrit, ed., Amsterdam, North Holland (1974), pp. 357-364.

3. L.B. Sheiner, B. Rosenberg and K.L. Melmon, Modelling of individual pharmacokinetics for computer-aided drug dosage, Comp. Biomed. Res. 5:441-459 (1972).

4. L.B. Sheiner, B. Rosenberg and V.V. Marathe, Estimation of population characteristics of pharmacokinetic parameters from routine clinical data, J. Pharmacokin. Biopharm. 5:445-479 (1977).

5. L.B. Sheiner and S.L. Beal, Evaluation of methods for estimating population pharmacokinetic parameters. I. Michaelis-Menten Model: routine clinical pharmacokinetic data, J. Pharmacokin. Biopharm. 8:553-571 (1981).

6. L.B. Sheiner and S.L. Beal, Analysis of nonexperimental pharmacokinetic data, in: "Drug Absorption and Disposition," K.S. Albert, ed., Amer. Pharm. Assoc., Washington, D.C. (1981), pp. 31-49.

7. L.B. Sheiner, H. Halkin, C. Peck, B. Rosenberg and K. Melmon, Improved computer-assisted digoxin therapy, Ann. Intern. Med. 82:619-627 (1975).

8. L.B. Sheiner, S.L. Beal and B. Rosenberg, Forecasting individual pharmacokinetics, Clin. Pharmacol. Ther. 26:294-305 (1979).

9. S. Vozeh, K.T. Muir, L.B. Sheiner and F. Follath, Predicting individual phenytoin dosage, J. Pharmacokin. Biopharm. 9:131-146 (1981).

10. E. Martin, T.N. Tozer, L.B. Sheiner and S. Riegelman, The clinical pharmacokinetics of phenytoin, J. Pharmacokin. Biopharm. 5:579-596 (1977).

11. L.B. Sheiner and S.L. Beal, Bayesian individualization of pharmacokinetics: a simple implementation and comparison with non-Bayesian methods, J. Pharm. Sci. 71:1344-1348 (1982).

12. D. Katz, A. Schumitzky, S. Azen and D. D'Argenio, Bayesian analysis of pharmacokinetic models with applications to dosing regimen determination, Proc. 4th Ann. Symp. on Comp. Appl. Med. Care, November (1980).

13. D. Katz, S.P. Azen and A. Schumitzky, Bayesian approach to the analysis of nonlinear models: implementation and evaluation, Biometrics 37:137-143 (1981).

14. R.W. Jelliffe, An improved method of digoxin therapy, Ann. Intern. Med. 69:703-717 (1968).

15. R.W. Jelliffe, J. Buell and R. Kalaba, Reduction of digitalis toxicity by computer-assisted glycoside dosage regimens, Ann. Intern. Med. 77:891-906 (1972).

16. B.M. Orme and R.E. Cutler, The relationship between kanamycin pharmacokinetics: distribution and renal function, Clin. Pharmacol. Ther. 10:543-550 (1969).

17. R.A. Chen, E.J. Benner and P.D. Hoeprich, Gentamicin therapy in renal failure: a nomogram for dosage, Ann. Intern. Med.

76:773-778 (1972).

18. M.C. McHenry, T.L. Gavan, R.W. Gifford, N.A. Geurkink, R.A.
     Van Ommen, M.A. Town and J.G. Wagner, Gentamicin dosages for
     renal insufficiency: adjustments based on endogenous creati-
     nine clearance and serum creatinine concentration, Ann.
     Intern. Med. 74:192-197 (1971).

19. J.H. Hull and F.A. Sarubbi Jr., Gentamicin serum concentra-
     tions: pharmacokinetic predictions, Ann. Intern. Med. 85:183-
     189 (1976).

20. C.C. Peck, L.B. Sheiner, C.M. Martin, D.T. Coombs and K.L.
     Melmon, Computer-assisted digoxin therapy, N. Engl. J. Med.
     289:441-446 (1973).

21. S.M. Dobbs, G.E. Mawer, E.M. Rodgers, B.G. Woodcock and S.B.
     Lucas, Can digoxin dose requirements be predicted?, Br. J.
     Clin. Pharmacol. 3:231-237 (1976).

22. J.K. Aronson, Monitoring digoxin therapy. III. How useful
     are the nomograms?, Br. J. Clin. Pharmacol. 5:55-64 (1978).

23. J.R. Powell, S. Vozeh, P. Hopewell, J. Costello, L.B. Sheiner
     and S. Riegelman, Theophylline disposition in acutely ill
     hospitalized patients, Amer. Rev. Resp. Dis. 118:1123-1127
     (1978).

24. T.B. Cooper, P-E. Berner and G.M. Simpson, The 24-hour serum
     lithium level as a prognosticator of dosage requirements,
     Amer. J. Psychiat. 130:601-603 (1973).

25. D.J. Brunswick, J.D. Amsterdam, J. Mendels and S.L. Stern,
     Prediction of steady-state imipramine and desmethylimipramine
     plasma concentrations from single-dose data, Clin. Pharmacol.
     Ther. 25:605-610 (1975).

26. W.Z. Potter, A.P. Savadil, I.J. Kopin and F.K. Goodwin,
     Single-dose kinetics predict steady-state concentrations of
     imipramine and desipramine, Arch. Gen. Psychiat. 37:314-320
     (1980).

27. W.L. Chiou, M.A.D. Gadalla and G.W. Peng, Method for the rapid
     estimation of the total body drug clearance and adjustment of
     dosage regimens in patients during a constant-rate intravenous
     infusion, J. Pharmacokin. Biopharm. 6:135-151 (1978).

28. A. Richens and A. Dunlop, Serum phenytoin levels in management
     of epilepsy, Lancet II:247-248 (1975).

29. A. Richens, A study of the pharmacokinetics of phenytoin
     (diphenylhydantoin) in epileptic patients, and the development
     of a nomogram for making dose increments, Epilepsia 16:627-646
     (1975).

30. A. Richens and A. Dunlop, Phenytoin dosage nomogram, Lancet
     II:1305-1306 (1976).

31. B. Rambeck, H.E. Boenigk, A. Dunlop, P.W. Mullen, J. Wadsworth
     and A. Richens, Predicting phenytoin dose - a revised nomo-
     gram, Ther. Drug Monitor. 1:325-333 (1979).

32. K. Chiba, T. Ishizaki, H. Miura and K. Minagawa, Michaelis-
     Menten pharmacokinetics of diphenylhydantoin and application
     in the pediatric age patient, Pediatrics 96:479-484 (1980).

33. G.E.P. Box and H.L. Lucas, Design of experiments in nonlinear situations, Biometrika 46:77–90 (1959).

34. R.C. St. John and N.R. Draper, D-optimally for regression designs: a review, Technometrics 17:15–23 (1975).

35. J.T. Slattery, M. Gibaldi and J.R. Koup, Prediction of maintenance dose required to attain a desired drug concentration at steady-state from a single determination of concentration after an inital dose, Clin. Pharmacokin. 5:377–385 (1980).

36. J.R. Koup, C.M. Sack, A.L. Smith and M. Gibaldi, Hypothesis for the individualization of drug dosage, Clin. Pharmacokin. 4:460–469 (1979).

37. S. Monjanel, J.P. Rigault, J.P. Cano, Y. Carcassone and R. Favre, High-dose methotrexate: Preliminary evaluation of a pharmacokinetic approach, Cancer Chemother. Pharmacol. 3:189–196 (1979).

38. S. Pancorbo, R.J. Sawchuk, C.H. Dashe and M. Schallock, Use of a pharmacokinetic model for individualizing intravenous doses of aminophylline, Eur. J. Clin. Pharmacol. 16:251–254 (1979).

39. R.J. Cipolle, R.D. Seifert, D.E. Saske and R.G. Strate, Systematically individualizing tobramycin dosage regimens, J. Clin. Pharmacol. 20:570–580 (1980).

40. R.W. Jelliffe, A. Schumitzky, J. Rodman, D.Z. D'Argenio, T. Forest, T. Gilman and E. Kolb, Computer programs for adaptive control (AC) of drug dosage regimens, Abstract #0564, World Conference on Clinical Pharmacology and Therapeutics, London (1980).

41. T.M. Ludden, J.P. Allen, W.A. Valutsky, A.V. Vicuna, J.M. Nappi, S.F. Joffman, J.E. Wallace, D. Lalka and J.L. McNay, Individualization of phenytoin dosage regimens, Clin. Pharmacol. Ther. 21:187–293 (1977).

42. C.C. Peck, W.D. Brown, L.B. Sheiner and B.G. Schuster, A microcomputer drug (theophylline) dosing program which assists and teaches physicians, Proc. 4th Ann. Symp. on Comp. Appl. Med. Care, November (1980), pp. 988–994.

Chapter 23

TREATMENT OF DEPRESSION – PHARMACOKINETIC AND PHARMACOGENETIC CONSIDERATIONS

Gunnar Alván and Folke Sjöqvist

Department of Clinical Pharmacology
Karolinska Institute
Huddinge University Hospital
Huddinge, Sweden

In spite of rapid progress in neurobiology, the brain remains the least explored organ in clinical pharmacology and its responses to drugs are notoriously difficult to assess in a reproducible way. In the mid-'60s, we began to study the mechanisms behind interindividual differences in response to tricyclic antidepressant drugs (TCA) using a pharmacokinetic research strategy. This paper summarizes some of the results obtained and the methodological problems encountered in this work.

A crucial decision in this research was to establish long-term collaboration with academic psychiatrists trained in assessing the quality and quantity of depressive symptoms with reproducible methods (1). A major reason for the different opinions regarding drug efficacy in depression has been the failure of many clinical trials to recognize the existence of subtypes of depressive illnesses, such as endogenous (vital) and neurotic depression. In the former condition many symptoms are suggestive of disturbed monoaminergic functions; for example, psychomotor retardation, disturbance of the sleep pattern, suicidal thoughts, and the diurnal and seasonal variation in symptomatology. While the therapeutic effects of TCA's are unequivocal in patients with endogenous depression, their efficacy in other depressive states is less impressive. Thus, studies attempting to relate plasma concentrations of TCA's to clinical effects ought to be carried out in endogenously depressed patients (see reference 2). In general, clinical pharmacokinetic studies in psychiatry are likely to go wrong unless the research protocol adheres to the principles summarized in Table I.

315

Another problem in earlier years was to find analytical methods which were sensitive enough to pick up nanogram quantities of the drugs in plasma. Our early finding of a 36-fold inter-individual difference in steady-state plasma concentrations of desmethylimipramine in patients on a fixed-dosage regimen (3,4) received a rather cool reception because the sceptics believed that our method yielded erroneous results. The method was based on in vitro acetylation of secondary amines with tritiated acetic anhydride. Fortunately, subsequent applications of mass fragmentography some years later confirmed the major findings obtained with the relatively primitive techniques of the early '60s (5). Nortriptyline appears to be one of the first drugs whose kinetics

Table I. Clinical prerequisites for correlating steady-state plasma concentration of a psychotropic drug and clinical outcome.

1. The drug works in the psychiatric condition and patient group being studied; e.g., low numbers of placebo-responders and drug nonresponders.

2. The selection criteria and clinical characteristics of the patients are given.

3. The patient group is defined in terms of age, sex, drug history, previous response to drugs, and, most important, intensity and duration of disease.

4. The patient group is sufficiently large.

5. Appropriate rating scales are used for assessing the effect of the drug; inter-rater reliability should be established.

6. The clinical raters are kept blind to drug plasma concentrations.

7. No other drugs likely to affect drug-receptor interaction are used.

8. Time course of clinical effects as well as final outcome are assessed.

9. Adequate statistical analysis and unbiased interpretation of the data; raw data should be presented.

and metabolism were explored with mass fragmentography which makes
it well suited as a pharmacogenetic reference compound (6).

The pharmacokinetic features of the TCA's are summarized in
Table II. A major research interest has been to evaluate the
clinical importance of these marked interindividual differences in
pharmacokinetics.

Table II. Unequivocal pharmacokinetic features of tricyclic antidepressants.

Feature	Comments	Original Reference
Marked interindividual variability in steady-state plasma concentration on fixed doses (5-10-fold, occasional high outliers)	Confirmed for all drugs in the group	(3, 4 and 7)
Genetic control of C_{ss}, k_{el}, V_d and plasma protein binding	Shown for NT but indirectly also for DMI	(8, 9 and 10)
Substantial first-pass metabolism after oral administration	Shown initially for NT and subsequently for IP and AT	(11, 12, 13, 14, 15)
C_{ss} predictable from single oral dose studies	Confirmed for NT, DMI and IP	(16, 10)
Comparatively small interindividual variability in plasma protein binding	Confirmed for several TCA's	(17, 18)
Importance of α_1-acid glycoprotein for binding	True for several basic drugs (21)	(19, 20)

Abbreviations: TCA = tricyclic antidepressants
                AT = amitriptyline
                NT = nortriptyline
                IP = imipramine
                DMI = desmethylimipramine

Our initial attempt to correlate plasma concentrations of nortriptyline to clinical outcome gave a rather surprising result, with an indication of a curvilinear relationship between steady-state plasma concentrations and antidepressant effects (1). At the time this was a controversial result but it has now been confirmed by colleagues in Denmark (22), England (23) and the U.S. (24). Thus, a therapeutic window of plasma concentrations (50-150 ng/ml) seems to exist for nortriptyline, possibly because the drug at high concentrations becomes phenothiazine-like in its actions on mono-aminergic neurons. On the basis of this finding it has been possible to design a rational dosage schedule of nortriptyline for patients in Sweden since the kinetic variability in this population has been characterized (Fig. 1).

Table III summarizes the main indications for monitoring TCA concentrations during therapy as they have emerged from a number of clinical studies performed in different countries. A major indication is to identify slow hydroxylators of these drugs. In pharmacogenetic studies Alexanderson (26) showed that the phenotype at risk to develop excessive plasma concentrations of a TCA is the poor hydroxylator. Recent studies in pharmacogenetics using debrisoquine as a drug probe (27) refocused our interest on slow hydroxylators of TCA's. The research on debrisoquine has provided strong support for the existence of polymorphism in drug hydroxyla-tion. Mellström et al. (28) found that the metabolic clearance of NT by E-10 (but not Z-10) hydroxylation correlated well with the debrisoquine hydroxylation index (the ratio between parent compound and the 4-OH-metabolite in urine) (Fig. 2). Slow debrisoquine hydroxylators are also slow in hydroxylating NT, and an association between this phenotype and increased side effects of the anti-depressant has been demonstrated (29).

These _in vivo_ observations agree well with recent _in vitro_ observations made by von Bahr and co-workers (30). They studied 4-hydroxylation of debrisoquine and 10-hydroxylation of NT in human liver microsomes obtained from different individuals and found a strong intraindividual correlation between these two reactions (Fig. 3). This suggests that similar if not identical enzymes in the cytochrome P-450 family may be involved in the metabolism of these two drugs.

The debrisoquine hydroxylation index is bimodally distributed in Caucasians (27). However, in the case of NT it has been impos-sible so far to get a clear separation of the two phenotypes using metabolite data or clearance values. The clearance of nortripty-line is nevertheless largely determined by its 10-hydroxylation. A tentative explanation for this discrepancy may be that a second hydroxylase, other than the monogenically controlled debrisoquine hydroxylase, is involved in this process.

Table III. Clinical indications for measuring TCA's in plasma.

Indications	Drug	Comments
To check compliance with the drug regimen	Any TCA	Urinary main metabolites may be measured also
To explore mechanisms of exaggerated drug response	Any TCA	Look for slow hydroxylators
In patients with coexisting cardiac disease and in the elderly to avoid toxic drug levels	AT,IP,NT[a]	As a rule of thumb, more than 200 ng/ml should be avoided
When effects of standard doses are inadequate after at least two weeks treatment	NT	Responders generally improve at concentrations between 50–150 ng/ml. The drug is less effective at lower and higher concentrations. Studies were performed mainly in hospitalized patients with endogenous depression
	IP	Responders generally improve at concentrations between 150–200 ng/ml (imipramine + desmethylimipramine). Relationship established only in endogenous depression and does not occur in unipolar delusional depressives (25)

[a]See Table II for abbreviations.

     During the course of our studies it became apparent that poor
clinical response was not always associated with low or high plasma
concentrations of NT, but could also occur within the "therapeutic
window." We therefore began to explore the hypothesis that a
biochemical difference in monoaminergic brain function may exist
between responders and nonresponders. Focusing on the function of
central serotonin and noradrenaline neurons, mass fragmentographic
methods were developed for measuring monoamine metabolites in

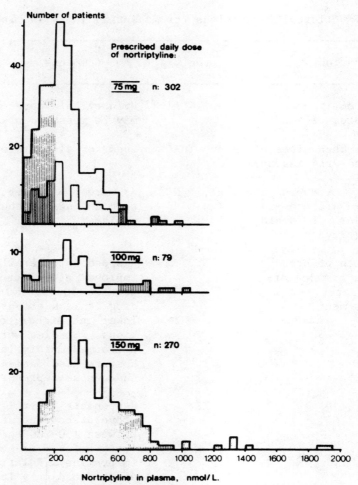

Figure 1. Distributions of plasma concentrations of nortriptyline
at three dose levels in clinical treatment. The
shadowed area in the upper distribution represents
patients older than 65. The "therapeutic window" is
indicated. Reprinted with permission from M. Åsberg and
F. Sjöqvist, Communications in Psychopharmacology 2:381-
391, (1978), Pergamon Press, Ltd.

cerebrospinal fluid (CSF) (31). Moreover, the clinical conditions
under which the lumbar punctures were performed were standardized
to permit reproducible measurements (32). It was then possible to
demonstrate that endogenously depressed patients had lower
concentrations of 5-hydroxyindoleacetic acid (5-HIAA) and homo-
vanillic acid (HVA) in CSF than controls (33). An apparent bimodal

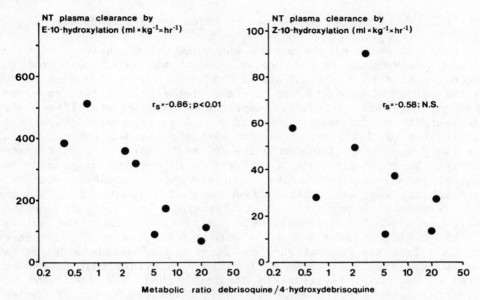

Figure 2. Correlation between nortriptyline plasma clearance by E-
10- and Z-10-hydroxylation and debrisoquine metabolic
ratio.   From Mellström et al. (28), with permission of
Clinical Pharmacology and Therapeutics.

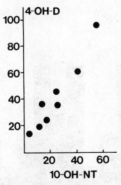

Figure 3. Relationship between rates of formation (pmol/mg · min)
of 10-hydroxy-nortriptyline (10-OH-NT) and 4-hydroxyde-
brisoquine (4-OH-D) in eight human livers.   The liver
with the lowest hydroxylation capacity originated from a
poor debrisoquine hydroxylator assessed <u>in vivo</u>.   Reprinted from von Bahr et al. (30), with permission.

distribution of 5-HIAA in CSF was reported in 1973 by Åsberg et al. (34) (Fig. 4).

The existence of a separate subpopulation of patients with 5-HIAA concentrations in CSF below 15 ng/ml was later confirmed in extensive studies (33). A higher incidence of suicidal behaviour in this group of subjects has also been reported. It thus appeared that patients with endogenous depression might be stratified into biochemical subgroups. This turned our interest toward the utilization of different types of monoamine uptake inhibitors in the two groups of patients with low and high 5-HIAA in CSF, respectively. We found differential effects of NT and chlorimipramine on central noradrenaline and serotonin neurons. Moreover, clinical observations suggested that patients with low levels of 5-HIAA in CSF responded better to chlorimipramine, a serotonin uptake inhibitor than to nortriptyline, a typical noradrenaline uptake inhibitor (18). These and other attempts to predict the response to TCA's from biochemical subclassifications of depressed patients suffer from the small amounts of patient materials that have been examined so far. Nevertheless, better methods must be found to guide clinicians in the selection of the antidepressant of choice for a particular patient. It is possible that receptor binding techniques may be useful in the future.

A rational approach to the treatment of depression must be based on clinical, biochemical and pharmacokinetic considerations. The former two are important for drug selection while individualization of drug dosage largely depends on knowledge of the concentration-effect curve of the antidepressant used. Differences

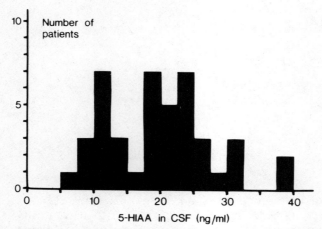

Figure 4. Distribution of 5-HIAA in CSF of depressed patients. From Åsberg et al. (34), with permission of Clinical Pharmacology and Therapeutics.

between patients in the number of drug receptors may also contribute to interindividual differences in drug response. Pharmacokinetically controlled investigations are needed to explore this possibility.

REFERENCES

1. M. Åsberg, B. Cronholm, F. Sjöqvist and D. Tuck, Relationship between plasma level of nortriptyline and therapeutic effect, Br. Med. J. 3:331-334 (1971).
2. W.Z. Potter, L. Bertilsson and F. Sjöqvist, Clinical pharmacokinetics of psychotropic drugs - Fundamentals and practical aspects, in: "Handbook of Biological Psychiatry," H.M. van Praag, M.H. Lader, O.J. Rafaelsen and E.J. Sachar, eds., Marcel Dekker Inc., New York (1980).
3. W. Hammer, C.M. Idestrom and F. Sjöqvist, Chemical control of antidepressant drug therapy, in: "Proceedings of the First International Symposium on Antidepressant Drugs," S. Garattini and M.N.G. Dukes, eds., Excerpta Med. Congr. Ser., Vol. 122, Milan (1967), pp. 301-310.
4. W. Hammer and F. Sjöqvist, Plasma levels of monomethylated tricyclic antidepressants during treatment with imipramine-like compounds, Life Sci. 6:1895-1903 (1967).
5. O. Borgå L. Palmér, A. Linnarsson and B. Holmstedt, Quantitative determination of nortriptyline and desmethylnortriptyline in human plasma by combined gas chromatography-mass spectrometry, Anal. Letters 4:837-849 (1971).
6. B. Alexanderson and F. Sjöqvist, Pharmacokinetic and genetic studies of nortriptyline and desmethylimipramine in man: The predictability of therapeutic plasma levels from single dose plasma concentration data, in: "Pharmacology and the Future of Man," Proc. 5th Int. Congr. Pharmacology (Vol. 3), Karger, Basel (1973), pp. 150-162.
7. J.P. Moody, A.C. Tait and A. Todrick, Plasma levels of imipramine and desmethylimipramine during therapy, Br. J. Psychiatry 113:183-193 (1967).
8. B. Alexanderson, D.A. Price Evans and F. Sjöqvist, Steady-state plasma levels of nortriptyline in twins: Influence of genetic factors and drug therapy, Br. Med. J. 2:764-768 (1969).
9. M. Åsberg, D. Price Evans and F. Sjöqvist, Genetic control of nortriptylline kinetics in man - A study of the relatives of propositi with high plasma concentrations, Br. J. Med. Genet. 8:129-135 (1971).
10. B. Alexanderson, Prediction of steady-state plasma levels of nortriptyline from single oral dose kinetics: A study in twins, Eur. J. Clin. Pharmacol. 6:44-53 (1973).
11. B. Alexanderson, O. Borgå and G. Alván, The availability of orally administered nortriptyline, Eur. J. Clin. Pharmacol.

5:181-185 (1973).

12. C. von Bahr, O. Borgå, E. Fellenius and M. Rowland, Kinetics of nortriptyline (NT) in rats in vivo and in the isolated perfused liver: Demonstration of a "first-pass disappearance" of NT in the liver, Pharmacology 9:177-186 (1973).

13. L.F. Gram and K. Fredrickson-Overø, First-pass metabolism of nortriptyline in man, Clin. Pharmacol. Ther. 18:305-314 (1975).

14. L.F. Gram and J. Christiansen, First-pass metabolism of imipramine in man, Clin. Pharmacol. Ther. 17:555-563 (1975).

15. G. Alván, O. Borgå, M. Lind, L. Palmér and B. Siwers, First-pass hydroxylation of nortriptyline: Concentrations of parent drug and major metabolites in plasma, Eur. J. Clin. Pharmacol. 11:219-224 (1977).

16. B. Alexanderson and F. Sjöqvist, Individual differences in the pharmacokinetics of monomethylated tricyclic antidepressants: Role of genetic and environmental factors and clinical importance, Ann. N.Y. Acad. Sci. 179:739-751 (1971).

17. O. Borgå, D.L. Azarnoff, G. Plym-Forshell and F. Sjöqvist, Plasma protein binding of tricyclic antidepressants in man, Biochem. Pharmacol. 18:2135-2143 (1969).

18. F. Sjöqvist, L. Bertilsson and M. Åsberg, Frontiers in therapeutic drug monitoring - tricyclic antidepressants, in: "Frontiers in Therapeutic Drug Monitoring," G. Tognoni and W. Jusko, eds., Raven Press, (1980). Also published in Therapeutic Drug Monitoring, (1980).

19. K. Piafsky and O. Borgå, Plasma protein binding of basic drugs. II. Importance of α_1-acid glycoprotein for inter-individual variation, Clin. Pharmacol. Ther. 22:545-549 (1977).

20. K. Piafsky, O. Borgå, I. Odar-Cederlöf, C. Johansson and F. Sjöqvist, Increased plasma protein binding of propranolol and chlorpromazine mediated by disease-induced elevations of plasma α_1-acid glycoprotein, N. Engl. J. Med. 229:1435-1439 (1978).

21. D. Fremstad, K. Bergerud and J.F.W. Haffner, Increased plasma binding of quinidine after surgery: A preliminary report, Eur. J. Clin. Pharmacol. 10:441-444 (1976).

22. P. Kragh-Sørensen, C. Eggert-Hansen, P.C. Baastrup and E.F. Hvidberg, Self-inhibiting action of nortriptyline's effect at high plasma levels, Psychopharmacology 45:305-312 (1976).

23. R. Braithwaite, S. Montgomery and S. Dawling, Nortriptyline in depressed patients with high plasma levels, Clin. Pharmacol. Ther. 23:303-314 (1978).

24. V.E. Ziegler, P.J. Clayton, J.R. Taylor, B.T. Co and J.T. Biggs, Nortriptyline plasma levels and therapeutic response, Clin. Pharmacol. Ther. 20:458-463 (1976).

25. A.H. Glassman, J.M. Perel, M. Shostak, S.J. Kantor and J.L. Fleiss, Clinical implications of imipramine levels for depressive illness, Arch. Gen. Psychiatry 34:197-204 (1977).

26. B. Alexanderson, On interindividual variability in plasma levels of nortriptyline and desmethylimipramine in man: A pharmacokinetic and genetic study, MD thesis, Linkoping, (1972).

27. A. Mahgoub, J.R. Idle, L.G. Dring, R. Lancaster and R.L. Smith, Polymorphic hydroxylation of debrisoquine in man, Lancet, II:584-586 (1977).

28. B. Mellström, L. Bertilsson, J. Sawe, H.-U-. Schulz and F. Sjöqvist, E- and Z-10-hydroxylation of nortriptyline in man - relationship to polymorphic hydroxylation of debrisoquine, Clin. Pharmacol. Ther. 30:190-193 (1981).

29. L. Bertilsson, B. Mellström, F. Sjöqvist, B. Mårtensson and M. Åsberg, Slow hydroxylation of nortriptyline and concomitant poor debrisoquine hydroxylation: Clinical implications, Lancet, I:560-561 (1981).

30. C. von Bahr, H. Glaumann, B. Mellström and F. Sjöqvist, In vitro assessment of hepatic drug metabolism in man - a clinical pharmacological perspective, Trends in Pharmacological Sciences 3:487-490 (1982).

31. L. Bertilsson, Quantitative mass fragmentography - A valuable tool in clinical psychopharmacology, in: "Clinical Pharmacology in Psychiatry," J. Davies and E. Usdin, eds., Elsevier, North Holland, New York (1980).

32. L. Bertilsson, M. Åsberg, O. Lantto, G.-P. Scalia-Tomba, L. Traskman and G. Tybring, Gradients of monoamine metabolites and cortisol in cerebrospinal fluid of psychiatric patients and healthy controls, Psych. Res. 6:77-83 (1982).

33. M. Åsberg, L. Bertilsson, E. Ryding, D. Schalling, P. Thoren and T. Traskman-Bendz, Monoamine metabolites in cerebrospinal fluid in relation to depressive illness, suicidal behaviour and personality, Proc. 12th CINP Congress, in: "Recent Advances in Neuropsycho-Pharmacology, Advances in the Bio-Sciences" (Vol. 31), B. Angrist, G.D. Burrows, M. Lader, O. Lingjaerde, G. Sedvall and D. Wheatley, eds., Pergamon Press, Oxford and New York (1981).

34. M. Åsberg, L. Bertilsson, D. Tuck, B. Cronholm and F. Sjöqvist, Indoleamine metabolites in the cerebrospinal fluid of depressed patients before and during treatment with nortriptyline, Clin. Pharmacol. Ther. 14:277-286 (1973).

Chapter 24

KINETICS OF DRUG ACTION

Lennart K. Paalzow,[1] Gudrun H.M. Paalzow[2] and
Peer Tfelt-Hansen[3]

[1] Department of Biopharmaceutics and Pharmacokinetics
Faculty of Pharmacy
University of Uppsala
Uppsala, Sweden

[2] Department of Pharmacology
Central Research and Control Laboratory
National Corporation of Swedish Pharmacies
Solna, Sweden

[3] Department of Neurology,
Rigshospitalet
Copenhagen, Denmark

We all probably agree that the rapid progess in pharmacokinetics observed over the past decade has not been matched by a rapid
development in our knowledge of the kinetics of drug action. The
main reasons for this can probably be found in our limited ability
to obtain precise pharmacodynamic data, especially in humans, and
in the emphasis pharmacologists place upon the determination of
qualitative and quantitative measures of effect rather than the
kinetic aspects of the effects. However, with a combined knowledge
of the pharmacodynamic events at the receptor sites and the
pharmacokinetic properties of a specific drug we can learn quite a
lot about drug action.

In this chapter, I give examples from our current work dealing
with different aspects of drug action in relation to pharmacokinetics. I will first discuss some dynamic aspects of interindividual
variability in drug response and then present some data emphasizing
the importance of a careful characterization of dose (concentration)-response relationships.

INTERINDIVIDUAL VARIABILITY IN DRUG RESPONSE

Many of us would like to consider variability in pharmacokinetics to be the main source of variable drug responses. This, in fact, may be true in many cases and, therefore, less attention has been paid to the ability of an individual patient to produce a certain degree of drug response at a given receptor (biophase) concentration of the drug. Recently, we have examined such variability in the pharmacodynamics of ergotamine and apomorphine.

Ergotamine

Ergotamine has been and remains the mainstay in the treatment of migraine attacks (1). The proper and safe use of this drug, however, is limited by the poor knowledge of its clinical pharmacology. Due to the lack of sensitive and specific analytical techniques for the determination of ergotamine in tissues, the pharmacokinetics of this drug are poorly defined.

Recently, a sensitive and specific high performance liquid chromatographic method using a fluorescence detector has been developed in our laboratory (2). The limit of detection of the assay is 50-100 picogram/ml of plasma. This technique has now been used to evaluate the pharmacokinetic characteristics of ergotamine after different modes of administration and with different dosage forms.

One of our first findings was the very low bioavailability of ergotamine after oral administration (3). No ergotamine was detected in plasma after the intake of the recommended oral dose of 2 mg to patients. As we have also evaluated the kinetics of ergotamine after intravenous administration (4), we know that the limit of detection of the analytical assay (100 pg/ml) will yield a biological availability of about 2%. These results raised the question of whether ergotamine given orally really is an active drug in the treatment of migraine attacks. Since migraine attacks are difficult to measure clinically in quantitative terms, we used a strain gauge technique to investigate the effects of ergotamine on peripheral arteries. The effect was expressed as the systolic blood pressure gradient between the toe and the arm (as has been extensively described, see reference 5). To standardize the experiments from a kinetic point of view, ten patients were given ergotamine by the intramuscular route of administration. The pharmacokinetic characteristics of ergotamine after intramuscular injection are listed in Table I and the time course of plasma concentrations after a dose of 0.5 mg is shown in Figure 1.

Ergotamine is a drug with a high plasma clearance (717 ml/min for a 70 kg man) which is close to the normal hepatic plasma flow. Absorption is rapid with a mean half-life of about 10 minutes. The biological half-life is short, averaging about 2 hours (Table I); 8

Table I. Pharmacokinetic parameters of ergotamine after intramuscular administration of 0.5 mg of ergotamine tartrate to 10 patients.

	V (L/kg)	k_a (hr^{-1})	Total plasma clearance (L/hr/kg)	Elimination half-life (hr)
Mean[a]	0.418 ± 0.009	3.96 ± 0.14	0.615 ± 0.026	2.02 ± 0.04
Range	0.235 – 0.644	1.16 – 9.10	0.324 – 2.340	0.70 – 3.01

[a]Values represent mean ± SD.

hours after administration, plasma concentrations have declined below 100 pg/ml. The effects on peripheral arteries were measured simultaneously at each blood sampling time. The activity developed slowly, reached a maximum at about four to six hours following injection, and declined slowly as seen in Figure 1.

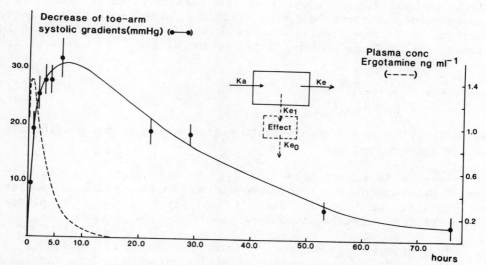

Figure 1. Plasma concentration and effect relationship versus time for 10 patients receiving 0.5 mg of ergotamine tartrate i.m. The solid line represents the best fit of the proposed model (inserted in the figure) to the data. The data points represent the mean ± SE from 10 patients.

Obviously, there is a pronounced dissociation between the time course of the pharmacodynamic effects and the concentration of ergotamine in plasma. To resolve this discrepancy we adopted the effect model described by Sheiner et al. (6). In their model, drug pharmacokinetics are described by a mammillary compartment model to which a hypothetical effect compartment is linked by a first-order rate constant (k_{el}, see Fig. 1). The effect compartment actually receives a negligible mass of drug and its exponential, therefore, does not enter into the pharmacokinetic solution for the mass of drug in the body. Drug dissipation from the effect compartment occurs by means of another first-order rate constant, k_{e0}. The rate constant k_{el} is assumed to be very small in magnitude compared to the other rate constants of the pharmacokinetic model. The rate constant k_{e0} will characterize the temporal aspects of equilibration between plasma concentrations and effects.

The pharmacokinetic characteristics of ergotamine could be described by a one-compartment open model after intramuscular administration:

$$C_P = \frac{F \cdot Dose \cdot k_a}{(k_a - k_e) \cdot V_d} (e^{-k_e t} - e^{-k_a t}) \tag{1}$$

The equations describing the effect site concentrations have been derived for different compartment models (7,8). These equations include the parameters of the pharmacokinetic model for plasma concentrations and, additionally, the equilibrium rate constant k_{e0}. As suggested by Sheiner et al. (6), the experimental time-effect data can then be fitted to the Hill equation (Eq. (2)):

$$E = \frac{E_{max} \cdot C_{pss}^s}{C_{pss}^s + C_{pss}(50)^s} \tag{2}$$

where $C_{pss}(50)$ is the steady-state plasma concentration causing 50% of the maximum response.

As seen in Figure 1, a good fit of this model to the experimental data was obtained. The resulting pharmacodynamic parameter estimates can be found in Table II, and Figure 2 shows the plasma concentration-effect relationships predicted from these values.

The average $C_{pss}(50)$ was 260 pg/ml and the equilibration (k_{e0}) half-life was 10.8 hours. This relatively long half-life for loss of drug from the effector sites can probably be explained by a slow dissociation from the receptors since it has recently been reported that ergotamine induced contraction of human arteries in vitro is resistant to repeated washings (9). An interesting finding was the 40-fold interindividual variability in the steady-state plasma

Table II. Pharmacodynamic parameter estimates for ergotamine after intramuscular administration of 0.5 mg of ergotamine tartrate to 10 patients. Equilibration half-life is $0.693/k_{e_0}$.

	Equilibration half-life (hr)	s	$C_{pss}(50)$ (ng/ml)
Mean[a]	10.76 ± 0.73	0.787 ± 0.113	0.260 ± 0.028
Range	$4.12 - 27.8$	$0.272 - 1.384$	$0.033 - 1.381$

[a]Values represent mean $\pm$ SD.

concentration for 50% of maximal effect. A range from 33 pg/ml to 1381 pg/ml was found in the ten patients studied (Table II). This should be compared to the largest range for the individual kinetic parameters, where the rate of absorption showed the highest range with an 8-fold variability. The implications of these findings are that even if ergotamine plasma concentrations are less than 100 pg/ml and we are unable to measure it in plasma, ergotamine can nevertheless be an active drug. It may therefore be necessary to carefully titrate the optimum dose in the individual patient. This is required also because ergotamine has many serious side effects.

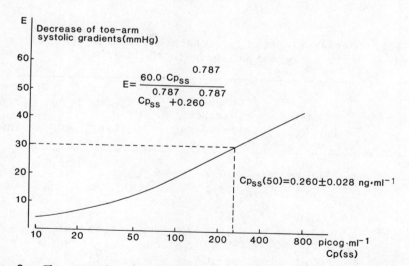

$$E = \frac{60.0 \cdot C_{pss}^{0.787}}{C_{pss}^{0.787} + 0.260^{0.787}}$$

$C_{pss}(50) = 0.260 \pm 0.028 \ ng \cdot ml^{-1}$

Figure 2. The steady-state plasma concentration-response data for the effect of ergotamine on peripheral arteries obtained from the data given in Figure 1.

Apomorphine

Emesis is a characteristic sign of postsynaptic dopaminergic activity. In a collaborative study we investigated the emetic potency of a number of newly synthesized central dopaminergic stimulating compounds. We used an intravenous infusion technique in dogs to find the minimum dose required for emesis.

The rate of infusion was adjusted to give emesis after about 5-10 minutes, at which point the infusion was stopped. After a few days rest, the animals were then used again for a new test. Apomorphine was used as a reference drug for postsynaptic dopaminergic agonism and the individual dogs were repeatedly tested for sensitivity to this drug during a one-year experimental period. During these experiments, we noted an interindividual difference in sensitivity to apomorphine and a remarkable stability of the emetic dose of apomorphine in the dogs, and we therefore decided to investigate the kinetic properties of apomorphine in relation to the emetic properties.

Apomorphine was injected i.v. into three dogs at two dose levels (30 µg/kg and 60 µg/kg) and blood samples were drawn for three hours and analyzed for unchanged drug by an HPLC procedure using fluorescence detection (10). Plasma clearances and volumes of distribution showed small interindividual variabilities among the animals (Table III). The model-predicted plasma concentrations in the different dogs during the intravenous infusion fitted well to the measured plasma concentrations (Fig. 3).

Table III. Pharmacokinetic parameters of apomorphine after i.v. bolus doses of 30 µg/kg and 60 µg/kg in the dog.

	Dose (µg/kg)	Total plasma clearance (ml/min/kg)	V (L/kg)	$t_{1/2z}$ (min)
Dog 1	30.0	70.7	2.73	26.8
	60.0	64.1	3.56	38.5
Dog 2	30.0	69.7	3.11	31.0
	60.0	56.6	2.99	36.7
Dog 3	60.0	67.6	3.13	32.1
Mean ± SD		65.7 ± 5.7	3.10 ± 0.30	33.0 ± 4.7

Since the rate of infusion was kept constant, these time-concentration curves were then used to calculate the plasma concentration for emesis in the individual dogs tested at different times over a whole year. As seen in Table IV, the concentration for emesis was stable over the year of study. An interesting observation was the individual sensitivity toward apomorphine induced emesis in the different dogs; for example, dog 3 required a concentration about 7 times higher for emesis than dog 1 (Table IV). Emesis is elicited from the trigger zone of the area postrema which is located outside the blood-brain barrier, thus the individual plasma concentrations for emesis should reflect the drug concentration at the site of action.

These two studies with ergotamine and apomorphine show that we should not only focus our interest on pharmacokinetic reasons for

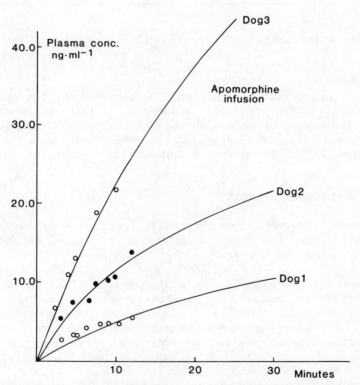

Figure 3. Plasma concentration of apomorphine in three dogs during i.v. infusion. The solid line represents the predicted levels from pharmacokinetic data in Table III and the data points are experimentally determined values. The dogs received their infusions at a constant, individually determined rate.

Table IV. Plasma concentrations of apomorphine calculated at the time of emesis during intravenous infusion.

	Plasma concentration at emesis (ng/ml)[a]	Range of plasma concentrations for emesis during 1 year (ng/ml)
Dog 1	3.0 ± 0.1 (N = 8)[b]	2.8 - 3.1 (N = 8)
Dog 2	8.8 ± 0.5 (N = 8)	7.3 - 10.5 (N = 8)
Dog 3	20.6 ± 1.4 (N = 6)	17.9 - 24.2 (N = 6)

[a]Mean ± SE.
[b]N represents the number of experiments.

interindividual variability in drug response, but also on the possibility of varying receptor responses. This interest in the relation between biophase concentrations and pharmacodynamic effects leads into a discussion of the importance of careful characterization of the dose- or concentration-response curves.

MULTIPLE RECEPTOR RESPONSES

In discussing a pharmacological effect, we must be aware that one specific drug can bind to different receptors depending upon the concentration or the dose.

Clonidine, for example, is a drug which at low concentrations has been found to activate α_2-receptors, which leads to an inhibition of the neuronal activity of the noradrenergic neurons. Higher concentrations have been shown to activate α_1-receptors leading to a functional response similar to increased noradrenergic activity. In a small area of neuronal tissue, we can thus activate two different types of receptors which can produce opposite functional responses. When we elicit a pharmacological effect we can thus observe a response from a single receptor interaction or a sum of responses from several types of interactions (11). If we know the kinetics of the drug concentration at the site of action, we can express the observed effect E as the sum of the individual receptor responses, such that $E = E_1 + E_2 \ldots E_n$. Expressed in accordance with the Hill equation we obtain the following relationship:

$$E = \frac{E_{1max} \cdot C_1^{s1}}{C_1^{s1} + C_1(50)^{s1}} + \frac{E_{2max} \cdot C_2^{s2}}{C_2^{s2} + C_2(50)^{s2}} \tag{3}$$

where C_1 and C_2 are the concentrations of the drug at the two receptor sites, assuming only two effects are involved. $C(50)$ is the concentration that produces 50% of the maximal effect and s is a number influencing the slope of the concentration-effect curve.

Studies With Clonidine

Investigation of the effects of clonidine on the arterial blood pressure in conscious rats yielded the results shown in Figure 4 (12). Plasma concentrations of clonidine were maintained at different steady-state levels by intravenous infusions, and

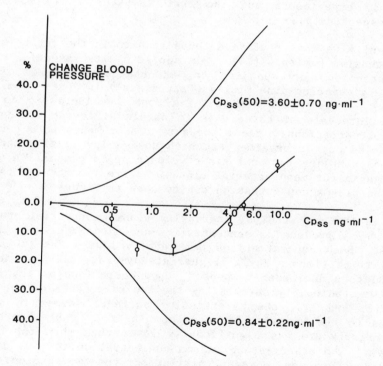

Figure 4. Effects of clonidine on blood pressure at different steady-state plasma concentrations in the normotensive rat. Each point represents the mean ± SE from 3-5 animals. The observed effect was separated into two components by the best fit of Equation (3) to the experimental data.

arterial blood pressure was measured. Steady-state concentrations
less than 1 ng/ml produced a decrease in blood pressure (Fig. 4).
With increasing drug concentration, the effect decreased and concentrations above 5 ng/ml increased the pressure. If we assume
that the fall in blood pressure is a consequence of an interaction
at α_2-receptors and the rise is due to the α_1-receptors, we should
be able to describe the observed concentration-effect relationship
according to Equation (3). Since we have experimental results from
pharmacokinetic investigations of clonidine (13) which indicate
that the two types of receptors are located kinetically in the same
tissues, C_1 equals C_2 in Equation (3). From the observed effect
values (E), the two components (E_1 and E_2) of the effect were calculated using the nonlinear least squares regression program NONLIN
and the results are depicted in Figure 4. The steady-state plasma
concentration for 50% of maximal response ($C_{pss}(50)$) for the effector site producing a decrease in blood pressure was 0.84 ± 0.22
ng/ml, and for the site increasing pressure, 3.60 ± 0.70 ng/ml.
The values of E_{1max} and E_{2max} were obtained (11) from other i.v.
bolus dose experiments and the best computer fits (-55.0% and
90.0%, respectively).

Recently we have confirmed these results in the rat by studies
in hypertensive patients (14). Six subjects with essential arterial hypertension corresponding to WHO stages I-II participated.
They were given clonidine orally (Catapresan®) in doses from 150 µg
to 600 µg, three times a day. The dose was increased in three
steps at intervals of three days to obtain different steady-state
plasma concentrations. Blood pressure measurements were performed
on the third day of treatment at each dosage level, simultaneously
with blood sampling for analysis of clonidine in plasma. A plot of
the change in the mean arterial blood pressure for the six patients
versus the plasma concentration can be seen in Figure 5.

As in the rat studies, increasing plasma concentrations up to
about 1 ng/ml produced a concentration-dependent decrease in blood
pressure. Such concentrations were achieved with the lowest dose
(150 µg, three times a day). Higher steady-state plasma concentrations led to a decreased response. Upon comparison of the results
of the two studies, by calculating the two components of the effect
in man (E_1 and E_2), the hypertensive patients seemed to be more
sensitive to the pressor effects since their $C_{pss}(50)$ for the increase in pressure was significantly lower than that for the rat
(Table V). The steady-state plasma concentration for 50% decrease
in blood pressure was, however, similar for the two species.

An interesting consequence of the concentration-effect relationship seen for clonidine (Figs. 4,5) is the influence of the
mode of administration on the time course of effects on blood pressure. After an i.v. bolus dose we essentially proceed along the
concentration-effect curve from the right to the left since the

Table V. Pharmacodynamic parameter estimates for clonidine under steady-state conditions in humans and rats. The observed effects on blood pressure were separated into two components by the best fit of Equation (3) to the experimental data.

	Decrease in blood pressure		Increase in blood pressure	
	$C_{pss}(50)$ (ng/ml)	s1	$C_{pss}(50)$ (ng/ml)	s2
Rat[a]	0.84 ± 0.22	1.64 ± 0.66	3.60 ± 0.70	1.18 ± 0.11
Man[a]	0.65 ± 0.07	1.86 ± 0.08	1.28 ± 0.16	2.36 ± 0.54

[a]Mean ± SD.

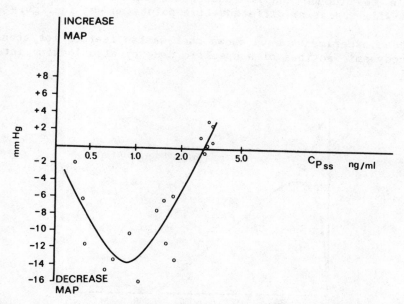

Figure 5. Effects on blood pressure at different steady-state plasma concentrations in six hypertensive patients. Clonidine was given orally in different doses to produce different steady-state concentrations.

concentrations are continuously declining. The initial increase in pressure will be followed by a decrease and then a return to the preinjection value. Other modes of administration yielding a rising concentration due to an absorption phase can be exemplified by a 100 µg/kg dose of clonidine given subcutaneously to rats. The plasma concentration curve obtained is shown in Figure 6. If the dose is sufficiently high we will proceed left to right in Figure 4 through the minimum of the concentration-effect curve (E_{min}) during the absorption phase and further to the right on that curve. During the elimination phase when the concentrations are declining, we retrace the concentration-effect curve proceeding from right to left. The predicted changes in blood pressure with time after subcutaneous injection of 100 µg/kg clonidine were found. As seen in Figure 7, a short decrease in pressure is predicted during the absorption phase, which is then followed by a pronounced increase in blood pressure. During the clonidine elimination phase, the effect decreases, with the maximum decrease at about 170 minutes following administration, a point in time at which the concentration passes through the minimum of the curve in Figure 4 (E_{min}).

Simulations of the effects after 50 µg/kg and 25 µg/kg subcutaneous doses can also be seen in Figure 7. As a consequence of the two opposite blood pressure effects, these two doses should cause the same maximal decrease in pressure as 100 µg/kg if they are able to produce the concentrations needed for E_{min}, but the maximum will appear at different time points as see in Figure 7.

These experiments have shown that we can learn a lot about the pharmacodynamic actions of a specific drug by also looking into the

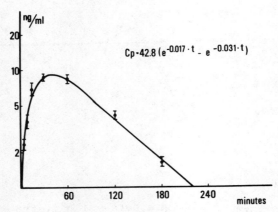

Figure 6. Plasma concentrations of clonidine in the rat after subcutaneous administration of 100 µg/kg. Each point represents the mean ± SE from 5-8 rats.

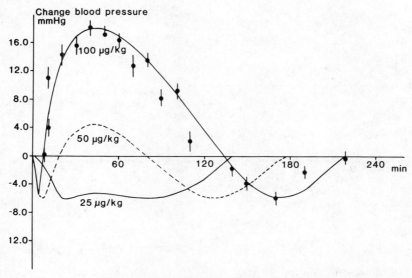

Figure 7. The effect of clonidine on arterial blood pressure in the rat after subcutaneous injection of 100 µg/kg. Each point represents the mean ± SE from 5 rats and the solid line represents the best fit of Equation (3) to the data points. The effects after 50 µg/kg and 25 µg/kg were calculated from the data obtained at 100 µg/kg.

time course of activity after different doses. To point out the importance of the multiple receptor concept (11) another example will be given from our studies on central mechanisms for analgesia and hyperalgesia.

Studies With Yohimbine

Yohimbine in low doses is considered to be a rather specific α_2-noradrenergic antagonist. In a recent study (15) we found that this drug produced an increased pain sensitivity at low subcutaneous doses, whereas higher doses induce analgesia in the rat. The effects on the pain threshold were determined by following the threshold for a vocalization response (graded response), using Caroll and Lim's technique for registering pain (16). The experimental dose-response curve for yohimbine can be seen in Figure 8.

As previously described, the two components (E_1 and E_2) of the observed effect were calculated and the ED50 values are shown in Figure 8. Evidently, about 0.5 mg/kg was needed to produce a 50% decrease in the pain threshold (E_2) whereas a dose about ten times higher was necessary for the opposite effect (E_1) in the absence of

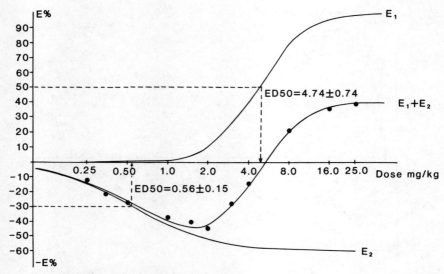

Figure 8. The dose-response relationship for the effects of yohimbine HCl on the threshold for vocalization in the rat.
The effect is expressed as the percentage change of the
predrug threshold (graded response).   The observed
effects were separated into two components by the best
fit of Equation (3) to the experimental data and the ED
50 values of the components are given in the figure.
Each data point represents the mean of 9-10 animals. C_1
and C_2 in Equation (3) are replaced by the dose.

E_2.   These results give a measurement of the specificity of yohimbine for activation of these two types of responses (receptors).

The time course of the pharmacodynamic effect after subcutaneous administration of 8 mg/kg yielded the experimental data shown
in Figure 9.   Obviously one single dose yields different effects on
pain transmission.   During the absorption phase when the concentration is rising, the α_2-receptor antagonism is detectable and five
minutes following injection the pain threshold is decreased briefly
by about 50%.   Forty-five minutes after administration the observed
effect is dominated by the analgesic response (E_1) (Fig. 9); the
effect then slowly declines.

The fact that a decrease in the pain threshold does not
reappear during the elimination phase (as observed in clonidine's
effect on blood pressure) could be explained by a slow elimination
of yohimbine.   Since we did not know the kinetics of yohimbine but
we did know the parameters of the dose-response curve of yohimbine
(s1, s2, $ED50_1$, $ED50_2$)   and the time course of the pharmacodynamic

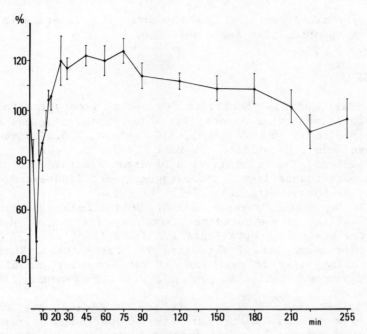

Figure 9. The effect of yohimbine HCl on the threshold for vocalization after subcutaneous administration of 8 mg/kg.
Each point represents the mean ± SE from 9–10 rats.

effects (as given in Fig. 9) we could calculate the rates of absorption and elimination of yohimbine into and out of the site of
action. The half-life for the absorption phase was found to be
13.9 ± 2.2 min (SD) and for the elimination phase, 2.9 ± 0.2 hr.

Considering this elimination half-life, it is understandable
that during an experimental period of about 4 hours, no terminal
maximal decrease in the effect was observed (Fig. 9).

Although pharmacological experiments many times produce smooth
and sigmoid dose-response curves, especially when isolated organs
are used, in vivo dose-response relationships are probably more
complex than anticipated. We believe that future studies require
increased efforts to characterize the dose-response curves or preferably the concentration-response curves. This should be done in
vivo over a dose range large enough to make it possible to detect
multiple receptor interactions. Furthermore, a careful evaluation
of the time course of the pharmacodynamic activity will allow us to
learn more about the mechanisms of action at the receptor level and
may, hopefully, also explain findings which initially only can be
interpreted as irregularities in the time course of effects.

Combined pharmacodynamic and pharmacokinetic experiments create interesting opportunities for the future.

REFERENCES

1. T.W. Rall and L.S. Schleifer, Oxytocin, prostaglandins, ergot alkaloids and other agents, in: "The Pharmacological Basis of Therapeutics," (6th Edition), A.G. Gilman, L.S. Goodman and A. Gilman, eds., Macmillan, New York (1980), p. 946.

2. P.O. Edlund, The determination of ergot alkaloids in plasma by high performance liquid chromatography and fluorescence detection, J. Chromatogr. 226:107-115 (1981).

3. K. Ekbom, L.K. Paalzow and E. Waldenlind, Low biological availability of ergotamine tartrate after oral dosing in cluster headache, Cephalalgia 1:203-207 (1981).

4. J.J. Ibraheem, L.K. Paalzow and P. Tfelt-Hansen, Kinetics of ergotamine after intravenous and intramuscular administration in migrainous patients, Eur. J. Clin. Pharmacol. 23:235-240 (1982).

5. P. Tfelt-Hansen, J.H. Eickhoff and J. Olesen, The effect of single dose ergotamine tartrate on peripheral arteries in migraine patients: Methodological aspects and time effect curve, Acta Pharmacol. Toxicol. 47:151-156 (1980).

6. L.B. Sheiner, D.R. Stanski, S. Vozeh, R.D. Miller and J. Ham, Simultaneous modeling of pharmacokinetics and pharmacodynamics: Application to d-turbocurarine, Clin. Pharmacol. Ther. 25:358-371 (1979).

7. W.A. Colburn, Simultaneous pharmacokinetic and pharmacodynamic modeling, J. Pharmacokin. Biopharm. 9:367-388 (1981).

8. N.H.G. Holford and L.B. Sheiner, Understanding the dose-effect relationship: Clinical application of pharmacokinetic-pharmacodynamic models, Clin. Pharmacokin. 6:429-453 (1981).

9. E. Mikkelsen, O. Ledeballe Pedersen, J.R. Østergaard and S. Ellebaek Pedersen, Effects of ergotamine on isolated human vessels, Arch. Int. Pharmacodyn. 252:241-252 (1981).

10. P.O. Edlund, Determination of apomorphine in plasma. A comparison between capillary gas chromatography with electron capture detection and HPLC with fluorescence detection, in preparation.

11. L.K. Paalzow and P.O. Edlund, Multiple receptor responses: A new concept to describe the relationship between pharmacological effects and pharmacokinetics of a drug: Studies on clonidine in the rat and cat, J. Pharmacokin. Biopharm. 7:495-510 (1979).

12. S. Christersson, M. Frisk-Holmberg and L.K. Paalzow, Steady-state plasma concentration of clonidine and its relation to the effects on blood pressure in normotensive rats, J. Pharm. Pharmacol. 31:418-419 (1979).

13. L.K. Paalzow and P.O. Edlund, Pharmacokinetics of clonidine in the rat and cat, J. Pharmacokin. Biopharm. 7:481-494 (1979).

14. M. Frisk-Holmberg and L.K. Paalzow, to be published.

15. G.H.M. Paalzow and L.K. Paalzow, Yohimbine both increases and decreases nociceptive thresholds in rats: Evaluation of the dose-response relationship, Naunyn-Schmiedeberg's Arch. Pharmacol. 322:193-197 (1983).

16. M.N. Caroll and R.K.S. Lim, Observations on the neuropharmacology of morphine and morphine-like analgesia, Arch. Int. Pharmacodyn. 125:383-403 (1960).

Chapter 25

CANCER DRUG DELIVERY SYSTEMS: MACROMOLECULAR PRODRUGS OF MITOMYCIN C

Hitoshi Sezaki and Mitsuru Hashida

Department of Basic Pharmaceutics
Faculty of Pharmaceutical Sciences
Kyoto University
Kyoto, Japan

With the development of new cancer drugs based on advanced knowledge of the mechanism of drug action and with the introduction of effective dosage regimens, cancer chemotherapy has now become an essential part of oncology therapy (1). However, due to the heterogeneity of tumors and the wide variety of complex roles played by the host, various therapeutic measures and rational drug delivery are urgently needed to overcome such problems as toxicity and the lack of drug specificity. Hence, elucidation of the pharmacokinetics of each class of cancer drugs will play an important role, not only in understanding the mechanism of action of the drugs and in designing clinical trials, but also in developing the means of drug delivery to the tumor.

Due to the development of analytical methods to measure cancer drugs in biological fluids and the advances in pharmaceutical technology, a great deal of research effort has been expended to follow and to attempt to control the pharmacokinetic profile of cancer drugs. For the design of successful cancer drug delivery systems, it will ultimately be necessary to convert these fragmental but sophisticated research efforts, as well as such basic information as the physico-chemical characteristics of drugs and drug products, conditions of tumors and the condition of the host, into a concrete therapeutic regimen (2).

For the past decade we have studied cancer drug delivery systems from the viewpoints of utilization of physical devices (3-8) and chemical transformation of the drug molecule (9,10). Some of these delivery systems have been clinically investigated and

positive results have been achieved (2,11). In this chapter, we
have selected mitomycin C (MMC) and its macromolecular prodrugs as
model compounds, and an attempt is made to demonstrate the implications of the biopharmaceutical approach for the optimization of
cancer drug delivery.

PHYSICO—CHEMICAL AND BIOLOGICAL CHARACTERISTICS OF MITOMYCIN C PRODRUGS

MMC is an antitumor antibiotic isolated from Streptomyces
caespitosus by Wakaki and his associates in 1958 (12). It contains
a urethane and a quinone group in its structure, as well as an
aziridine ring, which is essential for antineoplastic activity
(13). Although therapeutic responses to MMC have been reported for
a variety of human neoplasms, treatment with MMC has been only
palliative because it is often necessary to halt therapy short of a
cancer-destroying dose because of the drug's high toxicity. However, the drug is experiencing a renaissance of interest, both in
clinical studies and in the preparation of newer analogs and dosage
forms, which may result in greater efficacy and safety (14).

We have synthesized soluble macromolecular derivatives of MMC
(15), mitomycin C-dextran conjugates (MMCD) (Fig. 1). Three types
of dextran having average molecular weights of 10,000 (T-10),
70,000 (T-70) and 500,000 (T-500), purchased from Pharmacia Fine
Chemicals, were activated with cyanogen bromide; ε-aminocaproic
acid was introduced as a spacer. MMC was then conjugated through a
carbodiimide catalyzed reaction. These conjugates were estimated
to contain MMC to an almost equal extent of about 10% (w/w) and the
degree of substitution by MMC of dextran was estimated to be one

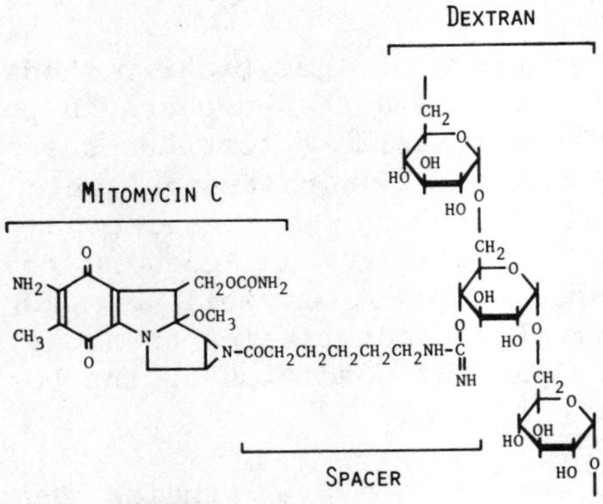

Figure 1. Representative structure of a mitomycin C-dextran conjugate.

molecule of MMC per approximately 12-14 glucose units (16). These prodrugs appear to be more stable to acidic degradation and metabolic transformation than the parent drug. In a basic environment between pH 7-10, MMC is released from MMCD by a general base catalyzed reaction; the regenerated MMC was found to possess antimicrobial activity equal to that of the original MMC. At pH 7.4 and 37°C, free MMC is released from MMCD with a rate constant and a half-life of about 0.029 hr^{-1} and 24 hr, respectively, regardless of the conjugate molecular weight. No increase in the conversion rate was seen upon addition of tissue homogenates.

Although various conjugates of cytotoxic agents with high molecular weight materials such as proteins, polysaccharides, synthetic polymers or immune carriers have been synthesized and evaluated as candidates for tumor specific devices (17-19), surprisingly little is known about the relationship between the antitumor activities and the physico-chemical characteristics of the conjugates. The latter properties are among the most important factors governing the in vivo fate and activity of the conjugates. Furthermore, the crucial role that the carrier moiety may play in the overall kinetic behavior of delivery systems is almost completely unexplored. We have developed several techniques, including spectrophotometric, bioassay, radiometric and anthrone colorimetric methods (20), to follow the fate of MMCD, and to characterize the various in vitro and in vivo properties of the prodrugs. Previous in vitro biological activity tests (one hour contact time) of MMCD demonstrated that antimicrobial activity against E. coli B was about one-fiftieth that of the parent compound; against L1210 murine leukemia cells, activity was about one-tenth of that for the parent. However, in vivo antitumor activity of these conjugates in mice bearing various murine tumors was higher than that of MMC (Table I).

Although the antitumor activity of these prodrugs is due mainly to the MMC released from MMCD, it seems probable that some prodrugs themselves have some sort of activity as intact forms. Animal tests were carried out employing tumor systems having various kinds of inherent physiological characteristics including growth behavior, tumor lethality, metastases and chemotherapeutic response (21). MMCD yielded an increase in life span (ILS) value about three times as large as that of MMC with B16 melanoma, which is considered to be an adequate model for solid tumors since B16 melanoma has a relatively long volume doubling time and a rather small growth fraction. The improved localization of MMCD and prolonged supply of potential parent drug in the peritoneal cavity are thought to increase effectiveness against B16 melanoma implanted there. This hypothesis is consistent with the findings of Barlogie and Drewinko (22) that the cytotoxicity of MMC is governed by a given exposure time, regardless of the drug concentration. In Ehrlich ascites carcinoma and P388 leukemia,

Table I. Comparison of antitumor activities of mitomycin C (MMC) and mitomycin C-dextran conjugate (MMCD, T-70) against various murine tumors in mice[a].

Tumor		ILS_{30}[b] (mg/kg)	ILS_{max}[c] (mg/kg)	TI[d]	Maximum ILS %	Survivors at 60 days
L1210 leukemia	MMCD	2.12	10.0	4.7	55.3	0/6
	MMC	1.43	5.0	3.5	70.3	0/6
P388 leukemia	MMCD	1.94	10.0	5.2	113.9	0/6
	MMC	1.28	5.0	3.9	90.0	0/6
Ehrlich ascites carcinoma	MMCD	1.49	15.0	10.1	>141.5	2/6
	MMC	1.09	5.0	4.6	123.7	0/6
B16 melanoma	MMCD	3.72	8.0	2.2	>183.9	3/8
	MMC	2.29	5.0	2.2	68.6	0/6

[a]Single intraperitoneal dose given 24 hours after intraperitoneal tumor inoculation.
[b]Dose producing a 30% increase in life span (ILS) over the control group calculated from the regression line between the dose and the obtained ILS value by the least squares method.
[c]Dose producing maximal antitumor effect.
[d]Therapeutic index (ILS_{max}/ILS_{30}).

MMCD also showed higher maximal ILS values than MMC, whereas MMCD appears to have lower efficacy in the treatment of L1210 leukemia. Failure of MMCD in the L1210 leukemia system may in some instances be associated with early entry of leukemia cells into the brain (23) and their continued multiplication at this site in spite of intraperitoneal administration of sufficient MMCD to partially suppress the advancement of the disease at the inoculation site. Intravenous injection of MMCD afforded only a modest prolongation of life span for mice bearing leukemia, suggesting poor permeation of MMCD through the blood-brain barrier.

These differences between the activities of MMCD and MMC in various experimental tumor systems are considered to reflect the improved biopharmaceutical properties of MMCD resulting from the modification of MMC into polymeric prodrugs. The effects of carrier moiety molecular weight are illustrated in Figure 2 which

shows the antitumor activities of MMC and three different types of
MMCD in P388 leukemia bearing mice. Single intraperitoneal injections of MMCD (T-70) and MMCD (T-500) showed maximum ILS values of
124.9% at doses of 10 mg/kg and 5 mg/kg, respectively. MMCD (T-10)
showed a maximum ILS value of 83.2% at a dose of 15 mg/kg.
Although there is no difference in the release rates or amounts of
MMC among the three conjugates, the shift of the dose-response
curves toward higher doses with decreased carrier molecular size
indicates that the prodrugs may exhibit different pharmacokinetic
properties after intraperitoneal injection which results in
modified bioavailability of free MMC depending on prodrug molecular
weight.

SYSTEMIC APPLICATION OF MITOMYCIN C PRODRUGS

To obtain more knowledge of the _in vivo_ fate of MMCD, plasma
concentration-time curves were plotted based on the concentrations

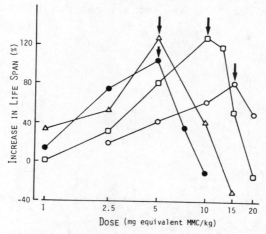

Figure 2. Effect of mitomycin C and mitomycin C-dextran conjugates
on the survival time of mice bearing P388 leukemia.
Filled circles, MMC; open circles, MMCD (T-10); squares,
MMCD (T-70); triangles, MMCD (T-500).   P388 leukemia
cells were given to BDF$_1$ mice by intraperitoneal injection; chemotherapy was given intraperitoneally 24 hours
later. Antitumor activity was evaluated by comparing the
mean survival times of the treated animals (T) and the
control group (C); that is, by calculating the percentage increase in life span (ILS): (T/C-1)x100(%).   The
mean survival period for the control group was 10.1
days.   Each point represents the mean value for six
mice; arrows indicate the peak effect for each compound.

of free MMC and MMCD after intravenous injection in rats (Fig. 3); a pharmacokinetic model for MMCD, illustrated in Figure 4, was obtained.   Plasma concentrations were determined by bioassay directly (MMC) or after hydrolysis (MMCD).   In this scheme, it is assumed that the MMC concentration data can be described by the one-compartment open model of volume V_F and that hydrolytic conversion of MMCD to MMC can also take place in the peripheral compartment for the conjugate, C2.   Curve fitting and parameter estimation were done using the nonlinear least squares program MULTI (24).   Concentrations of free and conjugated MMC were fitted simultaneously.   The conversion rate constants (k_4) calculated using the least squares method, are almost identical to the ones obtained in the in vitro MMC release experiment (about 0.029 hr^{-1}) (16), regardless of the size of the carrier portion of the prodrugs.   The excellent agreement between the experimental and theoretical mean plasma concentrations, as shown in Figure 3, substantiates the unique in vivo kinetic behavior of different molecular weight forms of MMCD, with all processes following apparent first-order kinetics.   Extension of the concentration and effects of drugs by employing rate-limiting conversion has generally been thought to be impractical due to the loss of the

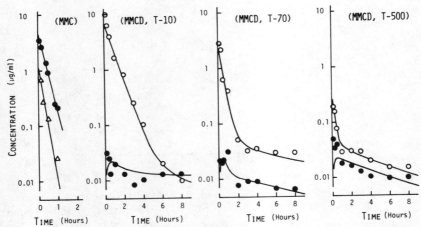

Figure 3. The observed and simultaneously fitted (solid line) plasma concentration-time data for MMC after i.v. injection of MMC or MMCD conjugates to rats.   Filled circles, free MMC after injection of MMC (5 mg/kg) or MMCD (5 mg equivalent MMC/kg);   triangles, free MMC after injection of MMC (1 mg/kg); open circles, dextran-conjugated MMC after injection of MMCD (5 mg equivalent MMC/kg).   Each point represents the mean value of at least three rats.   The curves are computer generated fits to the model depicted in Figure 4.

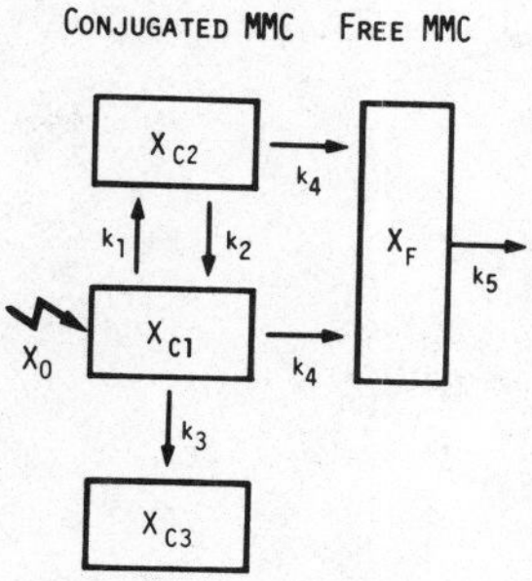

Parameter	Free MMC		MMC-D (5 mg/kg)		
	(5 mg/kg)	(1 mg/kg)	T-10	T-70	T-500
k_1 (hr^{-1})			0.575	0.872	2.906
k_2 (hr^{-1})			0.004	0.122	0.497
k_3 (hr^{-1})			0.536	1.579	1.036
k_4 (hr^{-1})			0.026	0.030	0.027
k_5 (hr^{-1})	3.31	4.81	4.81	4.81	4.81
V_{C1} (ml)			150.4	369.9	2359.2
V_F (ml)	214.2	186.1	186.1	186.1	186.1

Figure 4. Pharmacokinetic model and estimated parameters for the disposition behavior of MMC and MMCD conjugates. The curve fittings and parameter estimations were done using the nonlinear least squares program MULTI (24). Values for k_5 and V_F were assumed to be identical whether MMC or MMCD was administered. Concentrations of free and conjugated drug were fitted simultaneously.

intact prodrug through competing elimination mechanisms (25). However, we could prolong plasma drug concentrations by means of macromolecular prodrugs with rate-limiting conversion.

To obtain further information concerning the biopharmaceutical behavior of MMCD, tissue distribution studies of MMCD were undertaken following intravenous injection in rats of a ^{14}C-labeled MMCD (T-70) with the label located within the spacer moiety. At different time points after injection, the animals were sacrificed and various organs excised. The drug concentrations were determined radiometrically. Tissue distribution profiles were obtained both in the nonaccumulative organs and in the accumulative organs; the former includes lung and muscle into which MMCD distributes rapidly and does not accumulate, whereas the latter includes liver, lymph nodes, and spleen. Plasma concentrations decreased rapidly and accumulation of the conjugate was greatest in liver, followed ·by kidney, spleen and lymph nodes, suggesting the possibility of preferential drug delivery to such accumulative organs (Fig. 5). The higher and sustained concentration of radioactivity in the liver indicates that this organ plays an important role in the biotransformation of MMCD. MMCD distributed to the liver is converted to MMC, followed by rapid inactivation of the free drug. However, direct degradation of MMCD by hepatic enzymes cannot be disregarded. The distribution profiles in liver and kidney, two of the accumulative organs, vary according to the MMCD molecular weight. All of the prodrugs distribute well into the liver but

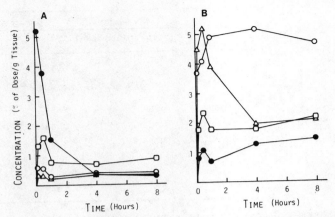

Figure 5. Tissue distribution of ^{14}C-labeled MMCD (T-70) after intravenous injection. A, nonaccumulative organs: filled circles, plasma; squares, lung; open circles, heart; triangles, muscle. B, accumulative organs: open circles, liver; squares, spleen; triangles, kidney; filled circles, lymph node. Each point represents the mean value of four rats.

only slight accumulation occurs in the kidney, except for the T-10 prodrug. Renal excretion of dextran, determined by the anthrone method, after intravenous injection of three types of MMCD, differed depending on the molecular size. However, no significant difference in excretion of free MMC was noted among the three types of MMCD. All conjugates produced slow but continuous excretion of free MMC for several days.

Dextran is used as a blood volume expander and is a safe water soluble polymer (17). Consequently, the conjugates are able to release MMC in the body by being retained in the circulation, or they remain in a specific locality for prolonged periods of time. In addition to decreased toxicity, these biopharmaceutical modifications may contribute to the efficacy of the drug.

LOCAL APPLICATION OF MITOMYCIN C PRODRUGS

In the surgical field, when a neoplasm is found and resected, the primary tumor is usually extirpated, along with its drainage lymph nodes. However, not all of the minute regional lymph nodes can be identified and some may be left behind; yet even the smallest node may contain metastatic emboli of cancer cells. Therefore, it is assumed that lymphatic metastases are sometimes left after surgical intervention. If certain drugs or drug products in an appropriate dosage form are injected locally and delivered into lymph nodes which are located adjacent to the primary tumor, they may suppress the lymphatic metastases.   In our previous investigations, increased lymphatic transfer of antineoplastic agents was successfully obtained using emulsion formulations as drug delivery systems (3-6, 10,11).   It has been reported that molecules having a lower molecular weight are absorbed primarily through the capillaries, while molecules having a higher molecular weight appear to be absorbed primarily by way of the lymph vessels (26). To explore the possibility of such selective lymphotropic delivery of dextran conjugates, experiments were carried out using rats. MMC and MMCD in saline solutions were injected with a microliter syringe into the left thigh muscle of rats.   At various time points after injection, the rats were sacrificed and the amount of drug at the injection site (thigh muscle), in the regional lymph node (left iliac node), and in the plasma was determined by bioassay.   As shown in Figure 6, MMCD remains at the site of injection for a longer period of time in contrast to the rapid disappearance of MMC.   Initial relatively rapid disappearance rates seem to depend on the prodrug molecular weight.   The parallel slower phases of concentration decline seem to reflect similar conversion rates to the parent drug.   Figure 7 shows the mean levels of MMC and three types of MMCD in the regional lymph nodes at various times following intramuscular administration.   MMCD levels in the node

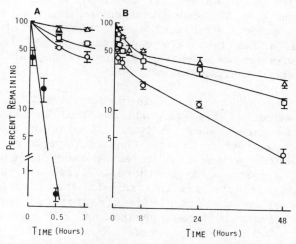

Figure 6. Disappearance of mitomycin C and mitomycin C-dextran
conjugates from the thigh muscle during the first hour
(A) and during 48 hours (B) after intramuscular injection.   Filled circles, MMC; open circles, MMCD (T-10);
squares, MMCD (T-70); triangles, MMCD (T-500).   Results
are expressed as the mean ± SE of at least four rats.

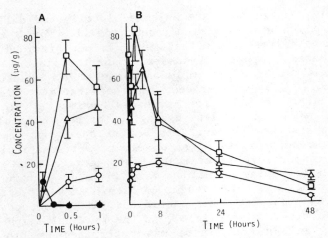

Figure 7. Concentration of mitomycin C and mitomycin C-dextran conjugates in the regional lymph node during the first hour (A) and during 48 hours (B) after intramuscular injection. Filled circles, MMC; open circles, MMCD (T-10); squares, MMCD (T-70); triangles, MMCD (T-500). Results are expressed as the mean ± SE of at least four rats.

remained high for about 48 hr. In contrast, after the administration of MMC, the free MMC concentration was only at a trace level even at 15 min after the injection. Intramuscular administration of MMC resulted in an immediate appearance of MMC in plasma followed by a rapid monoexponential disappearance, almost equal to that observed after intravenous adminstration (Fig. 3).

MMCD did not appear intact in plasma except as T-10, and only a trace amount of free MMC was detected in plasma following injection of the three types of MMCD. Cumulative amounts of free MMC and MMCD transferred to the thoracic lymph were determined after intramuscular administration using thoracic duct-cannulated rats. The MMC appearing in the thoracic lymph after injection of free MMC was apparently transported via the circulating blood, whereas MMCD reached the lymph directly from the local injection site. Larger amounts of intact prodrug and MMC appeared following administration of the T-10 prodrug. In contrast, for the T-500 prodrug, only free MMC was transported and the amount gradually increased up to 48 hours, suggesting that the carrier moiety affects the transport of the prodrugs. Figure 8 summarizes the transfer of MMC and its various molecular weight prodrugs after intramuscular injection. Local bioavailability of prodrugs and MMC is highly dependent on the size of the carriers. Most of the MMC is transported to the circulating blood, with only a small portion

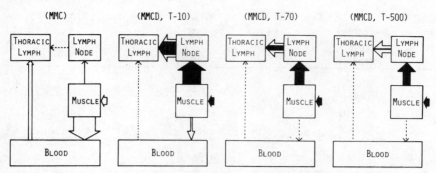

Figure 8. Schematic representation of lymphatic transfer patterns
of mitomycin C and mitomycin C—dextran conjugates after
intramuscular injection. Open arrows represent transfer
of free MMC; filled arrows represent transfer of
dextran—conjugated MMC.

of the dose reaching the thoracic lymph, and a trace amount
appearing in the lymph node (4,5).   In the case of high molecular
weight prodrugs, their lymphotropic nature is reflected in the
transport after injection and large amounts of prodrug are
transported to the lymph nodes.   Depending upon molecular weight,
the prodrugs accumulate in the lymph node and release the parent
compound there, which then may pass through the lymph node into the
thoracic lymph.

Finally, to test the advantages of using the dextran conjugate
of MMC for surgical chemotherapy against lymph node metastases, an
experimental model was set up using mice with L1210 leukemia cells
inoculated into the subcutaneous tissue of the left thigh (27).
Chemotherapy was given into the left thigh muscle on day 4.   On day
7, the mice were sacrificed and the lymph nodes were weighed.   As
shown in Table II, therapeutic activity against lymph node
metastases was enhanced by local injection of MMCD solutions.   It
appears, therefore, that high molecular weight carrier—mediated
drug delivery offers an interesting and potentially effective
method of cancer drug delivery by modifying the pharmacokinetics of
the parent drug in the case of local application.

PERSPECTIVES

Using MMC delivery as a model we have attempted to offer
approaches to the design of cancer drug delivery systems.   The
design of such drug delivery systems is still fraught with many
difficulties.   The importance of the role played by the host cannot
be overestimated in the design and rational utilization of drug

Table II. Inhibitory effect of mitomycin C and three types of mitomycin C-dextran conjugates on lymph node metastases of L1210 leukemia in mice[a].

Compound	Dose[b]	Weight of lymph node (mg)[c]	
		Left iliac node (Metastatic side)	Right iliac node (Reference side)
Control	---	20.05 ± 5.83	2.26 ± 0.77
MMC	0.5	16.10 ± 3.01	1.78 ± 0.25
	2.5	16.68 ± 4.62	2.58 ± 1.07
MMCD (T-10)	0.5	19.58 ± 5.76	2.04 ± 0.48
	2.5	16.32 ± 5.14	2.33 ± 1.60
MMCD (T-70)	0.5	14.58 ± 5.34	2.38 ± 0.26
	2.5	10.78 ± 2.99	2.33 ± 1.60
MMCD (T-500)	0.5	20.50 ± 7.07	2.98 ± 1.54
	2.5	13.38 ± 8.72	2.17 ± 0.73

[a]L1210 leukemia cells (1×10^6) were inoculated subcutaneously into the left thigh of BDF_1 mice on day 0.
[b]Drug (mg equivalent MMC/kg) in saline was injected into the left thigh muscle on day 4.
[c]On day 7, mice were sacrificed and the lymph nodes were weighed.

delivery systems. Changing pharmacokinetic events due to pathophysiological factors, multimodality of therapy, and immuno-logical and/or chronological considerations must be taken into account. It is not uncommon in cancer chemotherapy for each case to present unique problems requiring unique solutions. Neverthe-less, it is obvious that this domain of drug delivery is still open for future interdisciplinary collaborative research. The inte-grated use of information gained from an empirical approach as presented here, along with insights gained from other related fields, will point the way to optimization of drug therapy. Pharmacokinetics, from dosage regimen to cell kinetics, will undoubtedly contribute much.

REFERENCES

1. M.J. Cline and C.M. Haskell, "Cancer Chemotherapy," W.B. Saunders, Philadelphia (1980).
2. H. Sezaki, M. Hashida and S. Muranishi, Gelatin microspheres as carriers for antineoplastic agents, in: "Optimization of

Drug Delivery," H. Bundgaard, A.B. Hansen and H. Kofod, eds., Copenhagen (1982), pp. 316-329.

3. Y. Nakamoto, M. Fujiwara, T. Noguchi, T. Kimura, S. Muranishi, and H. Sezaki, Studies on pharmaceutical modification of anti-cancer agents. I. Enhancement of lymphatic transport of mitomycin C by parenteral emulsions, Chem. Pharm. Bull. 23:2232-2238 (1975).

4. M. Hashida, M. Egawa, S. Muranishi and H. Sezaki, Role of intramuscular administration of water-in-oil emulsions as a method for increasing the delivery of anticancer agents to regional lymphatics, J. Pharmacokin. Biopharm. 5:225-239 (1977).

5. M. Hashida, Y. Takahashi, S. Muranishi and H. Sezaki, An application of water-in-oil and gelatin-microsphere-in-oil emulsions to specific delivery of anticancer agent into stomach lymphatics, J. Pharmacokin. Biopharm. 5:241-255 (1977).

6. M. Hashida, S. Muranishi and H. Sezaki, Evaluation of water-in-oil and microsphere-in-oil emulsions as a specific delivery system of 5-fluorouracil into lymphatics, Chem. Pharm. Bull. 25:2410-2418 (1977).

7. M. Hashida, S. Muranishi, H. Sezaki, N. Tanigawa, K. Satomura and Y. Hikasa, Increased lymphatic delivery of bleomycin by microsphere-in-oil emulsion and its effect on lymph node metastasis, Int. J. Pharm. 2:245-256 (1979).

8. T. Yoshioka, M. Hashida, S. Muranishi and H. Sezaki, Specific delivery of mitomycin C to the liver, spleen, and lung: Nano-and microspherical carriers of gelatin, Int. J. Pharm. 8:131-141 (1981).

9. T. Kojima, M. Hashida, S. Muranishi and H. Sezaki, Antitumor activity of timed-release derivative of mitomycin C, agarose bead conjugate, Chem. Pharm. Bull. 26:1818-1824 (1978).

10. M. Hashida, T. Kojima, S. Muranishi and H. Sezaki, Antitumor activity of prolonged-release derivative of cytosine arabino-side, cytosine arabinoside-agarose conjugate, Gann 69:839-843 (1978).

11. N. Tanigawa, K. Satomura, Y. Hikasa, M. Hashida, S. Muranishi and H. Sezaki, Surgical chemotherapy against lymph node metas-tases: An experimental study, Surgery 87:147-152 (1980).

12. S. Wakaki, H. Marumo, K. Tomioka, G. Shimizu, E. Kato, H. Kamada, S. Kudo and Y. Fujimoto, Isolation of new fractions of antitumor mitomycins, Antibiotics and Chemotherapy 8:228-240 (1958).

13. K. Nakano, Synthesis and biological activities of mitomycin derivatives, Heterocycles 13:373-387 (1979).

14. S.T. Crooke, Mitomycin C: An overview, in: "Mitomycin C: Current Status and New Developments," S.K. Carter and S.T. Crooke, eds., Academic Press, New York (1979), pp. 1-4.

15. T. Kojima, M. Hashida, S. Muranishi and H. Sezaki, Mitomycin C-dextran conjugate: A novel high molecular weight pro-drug of mitomycin C, J. Pharm. Pharmacol. 32:30-34 (1980).

16. A. Kato, Y. Takakura, M. Hashida, T. Kimura and H. Sezaki, Physico-chemical and antitumor characteristics of high molecular weight prodrugs of mitomycin C., Chem. Pharm. Bull. 30:2951-2957 (1982).

17. L. Molteni, Dextrans as drug carriers, in: "Drug Carriers in Biology and Medicine," G. Gregoriadis, ed., Academic Press, London (1979), pp. 107-125.

18. E.P. Goldberg, Polymeric affinity drugs for cardiovascular, cancer, and urolithiasis therapy, in: "Polymeric Drugs," L.G. Donaruma and O. Vogl, eds., Academic Press, New York (1978), pp. 239-262.

19. M.J. Poznansky and L.G. Cleland, Biological macromolecules as carriers of drugs and enzymes, in: "Drug Delivery Systems: Characteristics and Biomedical Applications," R.L. Juliano, ed., Oxford University Press, New York (1980), pp. 253-315.

20. G. Wallenius, Some procedures for dextran estimation in various body fluids, Acta. Soc. Med. Upsalien. 59:69-75 (1953).

21. M. Hashida, A. Kato, T. Kojima, S. Muranishi, H. Sezaki, N. Tanigawa, K. Satomura and Y. Hikasa, Antitumor activity of mitomycin C-dextran conjugate against various murine tumors, Gann 72:226-234 (1981).

22. B. Barlogie and B. Drewinko, Lethal and cytokinetic effects of mitomycin C on cultured human colon cancer cells, Cancer Res. 40:1973-1980 (1980).

23. H.E. Skipper, F.M. Schabel, M.W. Trader and J.R. Thomson, Experimental evaluation of potential anticancer agents VI. Anatomical distribution of leukemic cells and failure of chemotherapy, Cancer Res. 21:1154-1164 (1961).

24. K. Yamaoka, Y. Tanigawara, T. Nakagawa and T. Uno, A pharmacokinetic analysis program (MULTI) for microcomputer, J. Pharm. Dyn. 4:879-885 (1981).

25. R.E. Notari, Prodrug design, Pharmac. Ther. 14:25-53 (1981).

26. B.E. Ballard, Biopharmaceutical considerations in subcutaneous and intramuscular drug administration, J. Pharm. Sci. 57:357-378 (1968).

27. S. Tsukagoshi and Y. Sakurai, Cancer chemotherapy screening with experimental tumors which metastasize to lymph nodes, Cancer Chemother. Rep. (Part 1) 54:311-318 (1970).

Chapter 26

ORGAN VARIATION IN TISSUE TO PLASMA PARTITION COEFFICIENTS OF ADRIAMYCIN, DAUNOMYCIN AND ACTINOMYCIN-D: CORRELATION TO TISSUE DNA CONCENTRATIONS

Tetsuya Terasaki, Tatsuji Iga, Yuicui Sugiyama and Manabu Hanano

Faculty of Pharmaceutical Sciences
University of Tokyo
Tokyo, Japan

The tissue distribution of adriamycin (ADR), daunomycin (DNR) and actinomycin-D (ACT-D), which are antitumor agents and intercalate the DNA double helix, has been studied in several animal species (1-6). These studies usually show that the antibiotics are extensively distributed in tissues and that there are large differences in drug concentrations in different tissues. Although it has been reported previously that ADR and DNR are localized in the cell nucleus (7,8), the cause of the organ variation in drug concentration has not yet been elucidated. ADR is able to bind to several tissue constituents in addition to DNA: phospholipids (9), actin and heavy meromyosin (10), tubulin (11), and mucopolysaccharides (12), for example. Moreover, it has been reported that there exist carrier mediated influx and active efflux mechanisms for these antibiotics in resistant tumor cell lines (13,14). Accordingly, the possible mechanisms of the extensive tissue distribution of ADR and reasons for the remarkable differences in tissue ADR concentration might include: differences in tissue DNA concentrations; differences in the concentration of tissue constituents other than DNA; differences in the affinity of ADR to tissue DNA; differences in the affinity of ADR to tissue constituents other than DNA; or the existence of different specific transport systems.

The purpose of this chapter is to elucidate the determinant organelle for the intracellular accumulation of ADR and to suggest possible mechanisms for the extensive tissue distribution and remarkable organ differences in the tissue concentration of ADR and its analogues, DNR, ADR-ol (adriamycinol), DNR-ol (daunorubicinol) and ACT-D. We investigated the tissue distribution of ADR in several rat tissues, the subcellular distribution of ADR in several rat tissues, the extent of ADR binding to homogenates prepared from rat tissues, and we compared the in vivo distribution of ADR, DNR, ADR-ol, DNR-ol and ACT-D to the concentrations of tissue DNA or phospholipids. These results have been reported elsewhere (15-18).

MATERIALS AND METHODS

Materials. Adriamycin hydrochloride (ADR) was generously supplied by Kyowa Hakko Kogyo Co. Ltd. (Tokyo). The antibiotic was stored in the dark in a desiccator at 4°C. The solution of ADR in buffer was freshly prepared before use. All other reagents were commercially available and of reagent grade.

ADR Assay. The ADR content of plasma, homogenates and subcellular fractions was determined by TLC scanning according to Watson and Chan (19) and Cradock et al. (20) in a Hitachi MPF-4 fluorospectrometer.

Blood to Plasma Concentration Ratio (R_B). Adult male Wistar rats (Nihon Ikagaku Dobutsu, Tokyo), weighing 250 ± 5 g and male albino rabbits (Ichikawaya, Tokyo), weighing 2.6-2.8 kg, were used after overnight fasting. After administration of heparin at a dose of 0.1 ml/100 g body weight (100 units), the whole blood was collected via a jugular artery at 30 minutes. After preincubation for 3 min at 37°C, small samples (10 µl) of isotonic solutions containing amounts of ADR (2.16×10^{-5} to 6.47×10^{-4} M for rats, 1.24×10^{-5} to 1.06×10^{-3} M for rabbits) were added to test tubes containing 1.5 ml of blood for the high concentrations and 5 ml for the low concentrations of ADR. The tubes were incubated with shaking (120 cycles/min) for 5 min at 37°C. The plasma was separated by centrifugation at 3000 rpm for 10 min and the concentration of ADR in plasma was determined. Metabolism during the incubation was negligible since no decrease was observed in the plasma concentration of ADR for 40 minutes.

Tissue to Plasma Concentration Ratio $(K_{p,app})$. ADR was dissolved in physiological saline and administered to rats via a femoral vein at a dose of 10 mg/kg under light ether anesthesia. After recovery from anesthesia, food and water were given ad libitum. At 6, 12, 24 and 48 hours after administration, blood samples were collected via a jugular artery and then the rat was killed by exsanguination. Each tissue was immediately excised, rinsed with physiological saline and stored at -40°C until assayed. ADR content in plasma and tissues was determined.

Hepatic and Renal Clearance in Rats. The urinary excretion of ADR was determined from the total amount excreted in the urine up to 48 hours after i.v. injection of 10 mg/kg. The apparent renal blood clearance ($CL_{B,app}^{KD}$) was calculated from the following equation:

$$CL_{B,app}^{KD} = \frac{X_u}{R_B \cdot AUC_p} \tag{1}$$

where X_u is the total amount of ADR excreted, R_B is the blood to plasma concentration ratio and AUC_p is the area under the plasma concentration versus time curve. In this study, X_u was calculated by the equation:

$$X_u = X_u^{48}(AUC_{p,0-\infty})/(AUC_{p,0-48}) \tag{2}$$

where 48 indicates the value at 48 hr.

The apparent hepatic blood clearance ($CL_{B,app}^{LV}$) was calculated from the following equation:

$$CL_{B,app}^{LV} = \frac{Dose}{R_B \cdot AUC_p} - CL_{B,app}^{KD} \tag{3}$$

The organ intrinsic clearance (CL_{int}) was calculated from the following equation:

$$f_p \cdot CL_{int} = \frac{CL_{B,app} \cdot Q_B R_B}{Q_B - CL_{B,app}} \tag{4}$$

where $CL_{B,app}$ is the apparent organ clearance, Q_B is the organ blood flow rate and f_p is the fraction of drug unbound in plasma.

<u>Tissue to Plasma Partition Coefficient</u> (K_p). The tissue to plasma partition coefficient which is commonly used in physiological pharmacokinetics and is defined as the ratio of drug concentration in tissue to that in the venous plasma, can be obtained by means of the equations proposed by Chen and Gross (19). Considering the distribution to blood cells, these equations have been further developed. The equations for K_p for lung, liver, kidney and noneliminating tissue or organ other than the lungs are, respectively:

$$K_p^{LU} = \frac{K_{p,app}^{LU}}{1 - (\beta V_{AB}/Q_B^{LU})} \tag{5}$$

$$K_p^{LV} = \frac{(R_B Q_B^{LV} + f_p CL_{int}^{LV}) K_{p,app}^{LV}}{\beta V_{LV} K_{p,app}^{LV} + R_B [(Q_B^{LV} - Q_B^{SP} - Q_B^{GT} - Q_B^{SM}) + (K_{p,app}^{SP}/K_p^{SP}) Q_B^{SP} +}$$

$$\overline{(K_{p,app}^{GT}/K_p^{GT}) Q_B^{GT} + (K_{p,app}^{SM}/K_p^{SM}) Q_B^{SM}]} \qquad (6)$$

$$K_p^{KD} = \frac{(1 + f_p CL_{int}^{KD}/R_B Q_B^{KD}) K_{p,app}^{KD}}{1 + (\beta V_{KD}/R_B Q_B^{KD}) K_{p,app}^{KD}} \qquad (7)$$

$$K_p^T = \frac{K_{p,app}^T}{1 + (\beta V_T K_{p,app}^T/R_B Q_B^T)} \qquad (8)$$

where LU, AB, LV, KD, SP, GT, SM and T represent lung, arterial blood, liver, kidney, spleen, gut, stomach and noneliminating tissue, respectively.

Subcellular Localization. ADR (10 mg/kg) was injected intravenously in rats as already described. At 12 hours after injection the rats were decapitated and the isolated tissues were immediately homogenized in buffer (pH 7.4) containing 340 mM sucrose, 15 mM Tris, 60 mM KCl, 15 mM 2-mercaptoethanol, 1 mM CaCl$_2$, 1 mM MgCl$_2$, 2 mM EDTA and 0.1 mM phenylmethylsulfonyl fluoride (20% w/v) at 4°C using a Potter-Elvehjem apparatus with a Teflon pestle. Subcellular fractionation of each homogenate was accomplished at 4°C by centrifugation at 600 x g for 10 min (nuclei and cell debris) and at 10,000 x g for 15 min (principally mitochondria). The amount of ADR in each fraction, including the 10,000 x g supernatant (principally microsomes and cytosol), was then determined.

Measurement of ADR Binding to Tissue Homogenates. The ADR binding to tissue homogenates was determined by a combination of ultracentrifuge and equilibrium dialysis methods (16). The tissue homogenate binding was calculated as:

$$C_{b,h}/C_f = C_{b,c}/C_f + C_{b,i,app}/C_f \qquad (9)$$

where $C_{b,h}$ and $C_{b,c}$ are the bound drug concentrations in the homogenate and cytosol fraction, respectively; $C_{b,i,app}$ is the apparent bound drug concentration in the insoluble fraction, and C_f is the unbound drug concentration.

The concentration ratio of the bound to unbound drug in cytosol, $C_{b,c}/C_f$, was determined by the method of equilibrium dialysis. After centrifugation of the tissue homogenate (5% w/v) at 100,000 x g for 60 min, the supernatant was used for the binding experiment as a cytosol fraction. Dialysis was performed at 4°C for 15 hr against 50 mM Tris buffer using a semipermeable membrane (Type 36/32, Visking Co., Tokyo, Japan). The concentrations of ADR on the buffer side and in the cytosol fraction were determined after dialysis.

Although the value of $C_{b,i,app}/C_f$ could not be directly determined, it was obtained by use of the following equation (16):

$$C_{b,i,app}/C_f = (1 + C_{b,c}/C_f) \times (C_{tot,i,app}/C_{tot,c}) \qquad (10)$$

where $C_{tot,i,app}$ is the apparent total drug concentration in the insoluble fraction and $C_{tot,c}$ is the total drug concentration in the cytosol fraction. The apparent total concentration ratio of ADR in the insoluble to cytosol fractions ($C_{tot,i,app}/C_{tot,c}$) was obtained using the following ultracentrifuge method: ADR was incubated with homogenate for 2 hr at 4°C. The cytosol and insoluble fractions were obtained in the same manner as in the dialysis study described above. The concentration of ADR in the cytosol fraction ($C_{tot,c}$) was experimentally determined. The apparent concentration of ADR in the insoluble fraction ($C_{tot,i,app}$) was calculated by subtracting the total ADR concentration in the cytosol fraction from the total concentration of ADR in the tissue homogenate.

Tissue DNA Concentration. The isolated tissues from rats and rabbits were homogenized in 50 mM Tris buffer, pH 7.4. Tissue DNA was extracted (20) and was determined by the method of Burton (23).

RESULTS

Tissue to Plasma Partition Coefficient (K_p).

The values of the apparent tissue to plasma concentration ratios ($K_{p,app}$) in the terminal elimination phase for rats, determined in the present study, are listed in Table I together with those for rabbits reported by Harris and Gross (2).

The results of determinations of the distribution of ADR to erythrocytes from rats and rabbits are shown in Figure 1. No concentration-dependence was observed over the plasma concentration range of ADR which corresponds to the <u>in vivo</u> plasma concentration range of the terminal elimination phase. The values of the blood to plasma concentration ratio (R_B) were 1.91 ± 0.18 (n = 18) for rats and 1.86 ± 0.08 (n = 9) for rabbits.

The physiological parameters for rats and rabbits which were used for the calculation of the intrinsic clearance (CL_{int}) and K_p values are listed in Table II.

Plasma disappearance and cumulative urinary excretion curves for 48 hr after intravenous administration of ADR (10 mg/kg) to

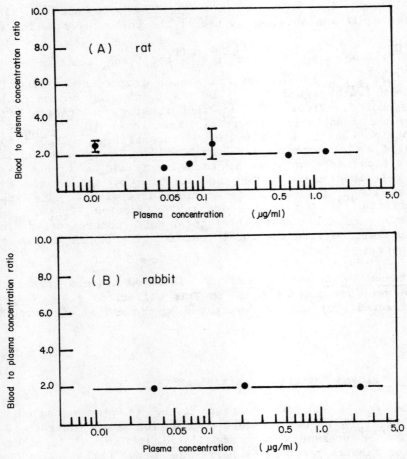

Figure 1. Blood to plasma concentration ratio (R_B) of adriamycin in rats (A) and rabbits (B). Each point represents the mean ± SE of three experiments.

Table I. Apparent tissue to plasma concentration ratio ($K_{p,app}$) in the terminal elimination phase after i.v. bolus injection of adriamycin.

Tissue	rabbits[a,b]	rats[a,c]
Adipose	19 ± 3.5	44 ± 7.6
Muscle	29 ± 3.6	74 ± 7.6
Liver	45 ± 8.3	148 ± 25
Gut	51 ± 7.7	168 ± 25
Heart	57 ± 5.0	232 ± 18
Stomach	--	282 ± 35
Kidney	512 ± 45	321 ± 26
Lung	155 ± 24	354 ± 54
Spleen	770	697

[a]Results are presented as the mean ± SE of each experiment.
[b]Body weight: about 2.33 kg; dose: 3 mg/kg; obtained from the literature (2).
[c]Body weight: 254 ± 5 g; dose: 10 mg/kg.

rats are shown in Figure 2. The pharmacokinetic parameters calculated from the biexponential curve fitting by an iterative least squares method (24) are listed in Table III. The estimated values of the organ clearance for rats determined in the present study are summarized in Table IV together with those for rabbits reported by Harris and Gross (2).

The K_p values of ADR for rats and rabbits were calculated by substituting the values listed in Tables I, II and IV into Equations (5-8); they are summarized in Table V.

Subcellular Distribution of ADR in Rat Tissues.

The results of the subcellular distribution study with ADR are shown in Table VI. In all tissues studied, a significant amount of ADR was found in the 600 x g pellet (the nuclear fraction).

ADR Binding to Tissue Homogenates Prepared From Rats.

ADR tissue binding was determined by ultracentrifugation and equilibrium dialysis. The direct results (5% homogenate) and results corrected to 100% homogenate are summarized in Table VII. There were large differences in ADR binding among tissues.

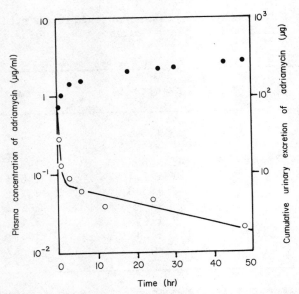

Figure 2. Plasma disappearance and cumulative urinary excretion time course after intravenous administration of 10 mg/kg adriamycin (ADR) in rats. Each urinary excretion point represents the mean of 3 rats, while the plasma concentrations were obtained from individual rats. The plasma disappearance curve was calculated by an iterative least squares method using a digital computer. Key: (open circles) plasma concentration; (filled circles) cumulative urinary excretion.

Correlation of the Tissue DNA Concentration With the Tissue to Plasma Partition Coefficient of ADR or With the Tissue to Plasma Concentration Ratio of DNR, ADR-ol DNR-ol and ACT-D in Rats and Rabbits.

The tissue DNA concentrations in rats and rabbits are listed in Table V. Figure 3 shows the relationship between the K_p value of ADR and the tissue DNA concentration (DNA amount per wet weight tissue) for each type of tissue from rats (upper panel) and rabbits (lower panel). In both species, good correlations were observed for most tissues studied. We also found good correlations between the tissue DNA concentration and the $K_{p,app}$ value for DNR in rats (Fig. 4, upper panel) and rabbits (Fig. 4, lower panel), for ADR-ol in rabbits (Fig. 5, panel A), for DNR-ol in rabbits (Fig. 5, panel B) and for ACT-D in rats (Fig. 5, panel C).

Table II. Physiological constants for adriamycin modeling.

Tissue	Volume (ml)		Blood flow (ml/min)	
	rats[a]	rabbits[b]	rats[a]	rabbits[b]
Arterial blood	6.2	66	39.0	460
Kidney	2.0	15	11.4	80
Heart	1.0	6	5.7	16
Muscle	125.0	1350	6.8	155
Adipose	10.0	120	0.4	32
Liver	11.0	100	14.7	177
Gut	11.1	120	11.0	111
Stomach	1.2	--	1.0	--
Spleen	1.0	1	0.9	9

[a] Obtained from the literature (25–28), based on 250 g rats.
[b] Obtained from the literature (2), based on 2.33 kg rabbits.

Table III. Pharmacokinetic parameters after intravenous administration of adriamycin in rats[a,b].

Parameters	Estimated values
A (μg/ml)	0.741 ± 0.0001
B (μg/ml)	0.081 ± 0.0124
α (min^{-1})	0.04254 ± 0.00292
β (min^{-1})	0.00050 ± 0.00021
AUC [(μg·min)/ml]	178.6

[a] Dose: 2.54 ± 0.05 mg/rat.
[b] Results are given as the mean ± SE. Parameters and respective SE were calculated from the biexponential curve fitting by a nonlinear iterative least squares method using a digital computer (see text).

Table IV. Pharmacokinetic parameters of adriamycin in rats and rabbits.

Parameters[a]		rabbit[b]	rat
Dose	$[\mu g]$	6.99×10^3	2.54×10^3
AUC_p	$[\mu g \cdot min \cdot ml^{-1}]$	—	1.79×10^2
$CL_{B,app}^{tot}$	$[ml \cdot min^{-1}]$	3.76×10^1	7.43
X_u^∞	$[\mu g]$	—	3.58×10^2
$CL_{B,app}^{KD}$	$[ml \cdot min^{-1}]$	—	1.05
$CL_{B,app}^{LV}$	$[ml \cdot min^{-1}]$	3.76×10^1	6.38
$f_p CL_{int}^{KD}$	$[ml \cdot min^{-1}]$	—	2.21
$f_p CL_{int}^{LV}$	$[ml \cdot min^{-1}]$	8.88×10^1	2.16×10^1
β	$[min^{-1}]$	7.00×10^{-4}	5.00×10^{-4}

[a] AUC_p = area under the plasma concentration versus time curve;

$CL_{B,app}^{tot}$ = apparent total blood clearance;

$CL_{B,app}^{KD}$ = apparent renal blood clearance;

$CL_{B,app}^{LV}$ = apparent hepatic blood clearance;

X_u^∞ = amount excreted in urine;

f_p = plasma unbound fraction;

CL_{int}^{KD} = renal intrinsic clearance:

CL_{int}^{LV} = hepatic intrinsic clearance;

β = the slope of the plasma concentration versus time curve during the terminal phase.

[b] Obtained from the literature (2).

Table V. Adriamycin K_p values and tissue DNA concentrations in rats and rabbits.

Tissue	K_p values		Tissue DNA concentration[a]	
	rat[b]	rabbit[c]	rat[d,f] (M, x 10^{-3})	rabbit[e,f] (M, x 10^{-3})
Lung	354	155	23.5 ± 0.4	20.0 ± 0.8
Kidney	349	494	12.5 ± 0.9	12.8 ± 1.2
Heart	230	57	4.59 ± 0.38	2.24 ± 0.08
Muscle	54	27	0.92 ± 0.16	0.26 ± 0.05
Adipose	33	19	1.35 ± 0.15	0.49 ± 0.09
Liver	242	56	6.43 ± 0.38	3.81 ± 0.51
Gut	161	50	20.5 ± 0.8	17.7 ± 1.0
Stomach	258	ND[g]	11.1 ± 0.4	7.77 ± 0.47
Spleen	697	746	54.1 ± 3.8	51.3 ± 2.7

[a]The mean ± SE of each experiment.
[b]n = 4
[c]From the literature (2).
[d]n = 4-7
[e]n = 3
[f]Calculated using calf thymus DNA (molecular weight 330.9; sodium salt of nucleotide) as the standard.
[g]Not determined.

Figure 6 shows the relationship between the K_p value of ADR and the concentration of diphosphatidylglycerol (cardiolipin) for several tissues in rats; no correlation was observed.

DISCUSSION

Previous investigations have found that ADR and its intercalative analogues distribute extensively into tissues and that there are remarkable differences in drug concentrations among tissues (1-6). In the present study, the tissue to plasma partition coefficient (K_p) of the physiological pharmacokinetic model or, for convenience, the apparent tissue to plasma concentration ratio, was used as an index of the tissue distribution of drugs. It was found that ADR has large K_p values (30-700) in rat tissues after i.v. bolus injection and that there are large variations in the K_p values for different organs and tissues (Table V). Since drugs

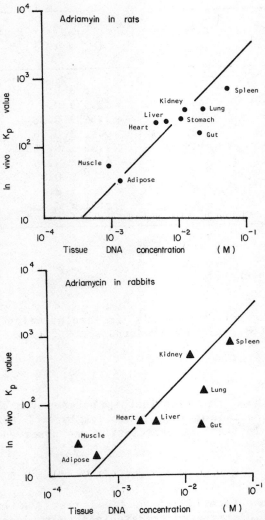

Figure 3. Correlation between the K_p value of adriamycin and the tissue DNA concentration in rats (upper panel) and rabbits (lower panel).

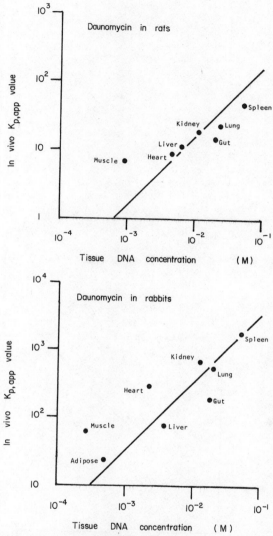

Figure 4. Correlation between the $K_{p,app}$ value of daunomycin and tissue DNA concentrations in rats (upper panel) and in rabbits (lower panel).

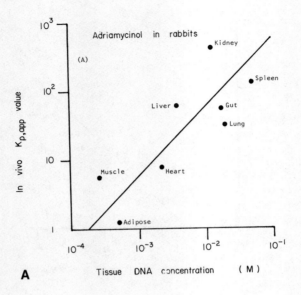

A

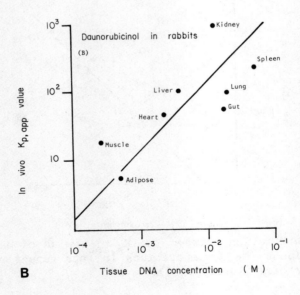

B

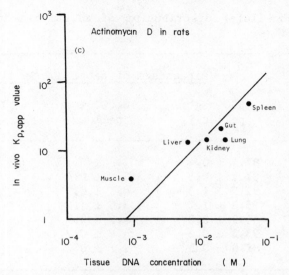

Figure 5. Correlation between the $K_{p,app}$ value and the tissue DNA concentration; facing page, panel A: adriamycinol in rabbits, B: daunorubicinol in rabbits; this page, C: actinomycin-D in rats.

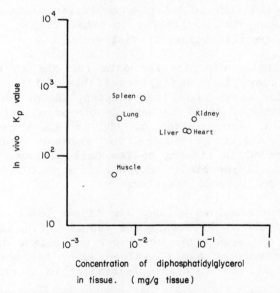

Figure 6. Relationship between K_p value of adriamycin and concentration of diphosphatidylgycerol in rats.

Table VI. Subcellular distribution of adriamycin in several rat tissues[a].

Tissue	Percentage of total ADR in tissue		
	600 x g pellet	10,000 x g pellet	10,000 x g supernatant
Muscle	97.4 ± 0.4	1.3 ± 0.1	1.3 ± 0.5
Liver	87.2 ± 0.5	12.0 ± 0.4	0.8 ± 0.1
Gut	92.9 ± 1.3	4.3 ± 0.9	2.8 ± 0.4
Heart	95.2 ± 1.2	3.6 ± 1.0	1.2 ± 0.2
Kidney	84.2 ± 0.8	14.9 ± 0.7	0.9 ± 0.1
Lung	93.3 ± 0.2	4.6 ± 0.2	2.1 ± 0.1
Spleen	87.0 ± 0.3	9.7 ± 0.2	3.3 ± 0.4

[a]Results are presented as mean ± SE of each experiment, (n = 3). Adriamycin (10 mg/kg) was administered by bolus injection through the femoral vein. The subcellular fractions were prepared at 12 hours post injection.

such as ADR, DNR, ADR-ol, DNR-ol and ACT-D have similar tissue distribution characteristics, it appears that there are common mechanisms for the intracellular accumulation of these drugs, such as nuclear binding and/or binding to other tissue constituents or involvement of specific transport systems.

The subcellular distribution data for ADR in muscle, liver, gut, heart, kidney, lung and spleen (Table VI) revealed that the nuclear fraction contained the largest amount of ADR. This observation suggested that the nucleus played an important role in the intracellular accumulation of ADR in all organs or tissues examined. In addition, binding to membrane phospholipids was negligible compared to binding to the cell nucleus. RNA could be ruled out as the tissue binder of ADR, since most RNA is located in the microsomal and cytosol fractions.

The good correlations between the tissue DNA concentration and the K_p value of ADR in both rats and rabbits (Fig. 3) suggest that differences in the amount of nuclei per wet weight of tissue cause extensive variations in the K_p values among tissues and that the binding affinity of ADR to nuclei is similar in all tissues.

We examined the tissue distribution of DNR, ADR-ol, DNR-ol and ACT-D which, like ADR, can also intercalate to DNA. Although the

Table VII. Comparison of ADR binding to tissue homogenate and cell nucleus in rats.

| Tissue | Binding to tissue homogenate | | Binding to nucleus | |
	$(\dfrac{C_{tot,i,app}}{C_{tot,c}})$ a,c	$(\dfrac{C_{b,c}}{C_f})$ b,c	$(\dfrac{C_{b,h}}{C_f})$ d	$\dfrac{nK_aC_N}{(1+K_aC_f)}$ e
Muscle	12.6 ± 0.95	0.975 ± 0.514	518	150
Heart	22.1 ± 2.85	0.793 ± 0.126	808	760
Liver	46.3 ± 3.79	1.271 ± 0.211	2130	1060
Stomach	35.9 ± 1.66	0.526 ± 0.109	1110	1830
Kidney	37.6 ± 2.44	1.866 ± 0.198	2190	2060
Gut	10.8 ± 1.43	10.36 ± 0.854	2660	3380
Lung	72.5 ± 10.65	1.12 ± 0.159	3090	3880
Spleen	114.8 ± 4.65	3.59 ± 0.322	10600	8970

[a] Concentration ratio of insoluble fraction to cytosol fraction.
[b] Ratio of bound drug concentration to that of unbound drug for cytosol fraction.
[c] Five percent homogenate at 4°C.
[d] Corrected to 100 percent homogenate.
[e] Calculated from Equation (11) (see text) using the values: $n = 6.70 \times 10^{-2}$, $K_a = 3.27 \times 10^6$ M^{-1} (obtained from reference 17), $C_f = 1 \times 10^{-7}$ M and C_N (tissue DNA concentration) listed in Table V.

K_p value is preferable as the index of tissue distribution, $K_{p,app}$ values were used for convenience as there was insufficient data for the determination of organ clearance; nor has the distribution of these drugs to erythrocytes been studied. There is a good correlation between the tissue DNA concentration and the $K_{p,app}$ values of DNR, ADR-ol, DNR-ol and ACT-D (Figs. 4 and 5). These results suggest that these drugs may have mechanisms similar to those responsible for the tissue distribution of ADR.

The results obtained from determinations of ADR binding to tissue homogenates suggested that remarkable intracellular binding accounts for the extensive tissue distribution and that the significant differences in tissue binding are responsible for the variation in K_p values for different organs (Table VII). Assuming that the nucleus is the only organelle involved in the intracellular binding of ADR, the concentration ratio of bound to unbound ADR in the tissue can be described by a Langmuir-type equation:

$$C_b/C_f = nK_a C_N/(1 + K_a C_f) \tag{11}$$

where n and K_a are the number of binding sites and the affinity constant to nuclei, respectively; C_N is the tissue DNA concentration and C_f is unbound drug concentration in the tissue.

We have also studied ADR binding to isolated liver nuclei from rats (17). The value of n was 6.70×10^{-2} at 37°C and no temperature dependence was observed in the value of this parameter. A significant temperature dependence was, however, observed in the value of K_a. Therefore, a correction was made for the K_a at 4°C by using the change in the enthalpy reported, $\Delta H° = -10$ kcal/mol (17). The value of K_a at 4°C was estimated to be 3.27×10^6 M^{-1}. We assumed that there was no difference in the nuclear binding of ADR among tissues. Substituting the binding parameters of the isolated nuclei from rat liver (n = 6.7×10^{-2}, K_a = 3.27×10^6 M^{-1}), the tissue DNA concentration (Table V) and the unbound concentration of ADR (C_f = 1×10^{-7} M) into Equation (11), the tissue binding parameters for ADR were calculated for the different organs or tissues. The results are listed in Table VII. There is good agreement between the calculated values of nuclear binding parameters and those determined using tissue homogenates. This suggests that the two stated assumptions are applicable to the estimation of the tissue binding of ADR in rats.

Since previous investigators reported that ADR binds to cardiolipin as strongly as it binds to DNA (9), we investigated whether cardiolipin plays an important role in the tissue accumulation of ADR. Examination of the relationship between the K_p value and the concentration of cardiolipin in tissues (29-31) suggests that the concentration difference of this tissue constituent is not a determinant of the variations in the K_p values (Fig. 6). Furthermore, there is no correlation between the K_p value of ADR and the concentrations of acidic phospholipid or total phospholipid (results not shown). These observations are consistent with the subcellular distribution of ADR (Table VI).

In conclusion, the extensive tissue distribution of ADR, DNR, ADR-ol, DNR-ol and ACT-D appears to be due mainly to nuclear binding. Differences in tissue distribution of these drugs correlate with differences in the amount of nuclei per unit of wet tissue weight.

REFERENCES

1.   N.R. Bachur, R.C. Hildebrand and R.S. Jaenke, Adriamycin and daunomycin disposition in the rabbit, J. Pharmacol. Exp. Ther. 191:331-340 (1974).

2. P.A. Harris and J. F. Gross, Preliminary pharmacokinetic model
    for adriamycin, Cancer Chemother. Rep. Part 1 59:819-825
    (1975).

3. N. Tavoloni and A.M. Guarino, Disposition and metabolism of
    adriamycin in the rat, Pharmacology 21:244-255 (1980).

4. D.S. Alberts, N.R. Bachur and J.L. Holtzman, The
    pharmacokinetics of daunomycin in man, Clin. Pharmacol. Ther.
    12:96-104 (1971).

5. A. Rusconi, G.D. Fronzo, and A.D. Marco, Distribution of
    tritiated daunomycin in normal rats, Cancer Chemother. Rep.
    52:331-335 (1968).

6. W.M. Galbraith and L.B. Mellett, Tissue disposition of ^{3}H-
    actinomycin D in the rat, monkey, and dog, Cancer Chemother.
    Rep. Part 1 59:1061-1069 (1975).

7. M.J. Egorin, R.C. Hildebrand, E.F. Cimino and N.R. Bachur,
    Cytofluorescence localization of adriamycin and daunorubicin,
    Cancer Res. 34:2243-2245 (1974).

8. A. Krishan, M. Israel, E.J. Modest and E. Frei, III,
    Differences in cellular uptake and cytofluorescence of
    adriamycin and N-trifluoroacetyl-adriamycin-14-valerate,
    Cancer Res. 36:2114-2116 (1976).

9. E. Goormaghtigh, P. Chatelain, J. Caspers and J.M.
    Ruysschaert, Evidence of specific complex between adriamycin
    and negatively-charged phospholipids, Biochim. Biophys. Acta
    597:1-14 (1980).

10. A. Someya, T. Akiyama, M. Misumi and N. Tanaka, Interaction of
    anthracycline antibiotics with actin and heavy meromyosin,
    Biochem. Biophys. Res. Commun. 85:1542-1550 (1978).

11. C. Na and S.N. Timasheff, Physical-chemical study of
    daunomycin-tubulin interactions, Arch. Biochem. Biophys.
    182:147-154 (1977).

12. M. Menozzi and F. Arcamone, Binding of adriamycin to sulphated
    mucopolysaccharides, Biochem. Biophys. Res. Commun. 80:313-318
    (1978).

13. T. Skovsgaard, Mechanisms of resistance of daunorubicin in
    Ehrlich ascites tumor cells, Cancer Res. 38:1785-1791 (1978).

14. T. Skovsgaard, Carrier-mediated transport of daunorubicin,
    adriamycin, and rubidazone in Ehrlich ascites tumor cells,
    Biochem. Pharmacol. 27:1221-1227 (1978).

15. T. Terasaki, T. Iga, Y. Sugiyama and M. Hanano, Experimental
    evidence of characteristic tissue distribution of adriamycin.
    Tissue DNA concentration as a determinant, J. Pharm. Pharma-
    col. 34:597-600 (1982).

16. T. Terasaki, T. Iga, Y. Sugiyama, Y. Sawada and M. Hanano,
    Nuclear binding as a determinant of tissue distribution of
    adriamycin, daunomycin, adriamycinol, daunorubicinol and
    actinomycin D, J. Pharm. Dyn. 7:in press (1984).

17. T. Terasaki, T. Iga, Y. Sugiyama and M. Hanano, Interaction of
    doxorubicin with nuclei isolated from rat liver and kidney, J.
    Pharm. Sci. 73:524-528 (1984).

18. T. Terasaki, T. Iga, Y. Sugiyama and M. Hanano, Pharmaco-
     kinetic study on the mechanism of tissue distribution of
     doxorubicin Interorgan variation and interspecies variation
     of tissue-to-plasma partition coefficients in rats, rabbits
     and guinea pigs, J. Pharm. Sci. 73:in press (1984).

19. E. Watson and K.K. Chan, Rapid analytic method for adriamycin
     and metabolites in human plasma by a thin-film fluorescence
     scanner, Cancer Treat. Rep. 60:1611-1618 (1976).

20. J.C. Cradock, M.J. Egorin and N.R. Bachur, Daunorubicin
     biliary excretion and metabolism in the rat, Arch. Int.
     Pharmacodyn. 202:48-61 (1973).

21. H.S.G. Chen and J.F. Gross, Estimation of tissue-to-plasma
     partition coefficients used in physiological pharmacokinetic
     models, J. Pharmacokin. Biopharm. 7:117-125 (1979).

22. W.C. Schneider, Phosphorus compounds in animal tissues, J.
     Biol. Chem. 164:747-751 (1946).

23. K. Burton, A study of the conditions and mechanism of the
     diphenylamine reaction for the colorimetric estimation of
     deoxyribonucleic acid, Biochem. J. 62:315-323 (1956).

24. T. Nakagawa, Y. Koyanagi and H. Togawa, "SALS, a computer
     program for statistical analysis with least squares fitting,"
     Library Program of the University of Tokyo Computer Center,
     Tokyo, Japan.

25. K.B. Bischoff, R.L. Dedrick, D.S. Zaharko and J.A. Longstreth,
     Methotrexate pharmacokinetics, J. Pharm. Sci. 60:1128-1133
     (1971).

26. R.L. Dedrick, D.S. Zaharko, and R.J. Lutz, Transport and
     binding of methotrexate in vivo, J. Pharm. Sci. 62:882-890
     (1973).

27. R.J. Lutz, R.L. Dedrick, H.B. Matthews, T.E. Eling and M.W.
     Anderson, A preliminary pharmacokinetic model for several
     chlorinated biphenyls in the rat, Drug Metab. Dispos. 5:386-
     396 (1977).

28. Y. Sasaki and H.N. Wagner, Measurement of the distribution of
     cardiac output in unanesthetized rats, J. Appl. Physiol.
     30:879-884 (1971).

29. C.F. Baxter, G. Rouser and G. Simon, Variations among
     vertebrates of lung phospholipid class composition, Lipids
     4:243-244 (1969).

30. G. Rouser, G. Simon and G. Kritchevsky, Species variation in
     phospholipid class distribution of organs: I. Kidney, liver
     and spleen, Lipids 4:599-606 (1969).

31. G. Simon and G. Rouser, Species variation in phospholipid
     class distribution of organs: II. Heart and skeletal muscle,
     Lipids 4:607-614 (1969).

Chapter 27

CLINICAL PHARMACOKINETICS IN THE THERAPEUTIC MANAGEMENT OF CANCER PATIENTS WITH METHOTREXATE AND ADRIAMYCIN

Eppo van der Kleijn[1], Robert Lippens[2] and Marijn Oosterbaan[1]

[1]Department of Clinical Pharmacy
[2]Department of Pediatrics
 Sint Radboud Hospital
 Catholic University of Nijmegen
 The Netherlands

Pharmacokinetic data has predictive value in establishing a treatment protocol, especially when clinical conditions influence the dose rate; this has been demonstrated with lidocaine, theophylline, and digoxin. The objective is to achieve amounts and concentrations in the body that produce the desired effect and avoid toxicity. This objective is particularly pertinent for oncochemotherapy. A few examples may illustrate the value of plasma concentration profile determination for the design and adaptation of drug treatment protocols in oncology.

TREATMENT OF MENINGEAL LEUKEMIA

Patients with acute lymphatic leukemia have a high probability for subclinical central nervous system leukemia. Treatment and prophylaxis is achieved by intrathecally (i.t.) administered oncochemotherapeutic agents. A commonly applied regimen uses methotrexate (MTX) and prednisolone combined with cranial irradiation. A frequently used scheme consists of five subsequent i.t. administrations of 0.1-0.2 mg MTX/kg body weight at 48-96 hour intervals (1). This procedure results in plasma concentration profiles for MTX that are different at subsequent administrations (Fig. 1). The maximum plasma concentration is higher and is reached at an earlier time when multiple i.t. injections are given. Following subsequent intravenous administrations, the pharmacokinetic parameters appear highly reproducible (2). The change in the time course of the plasma concentration following i.t. injection could therefore be attributed to a change in transfer rate: efflux rate from the cerebrospinal fluid compartment to the plasma compartment (Fig. 2). Because systemic toxicity often appears after the third and subsequent administrations and is more evident in patients with a so-called fast type efflux, it now appears useful to confirm the type of efflux (fast or slow) by obtaining one plasma concentration 18-24 hours after the last i.t. injection. Only patients with a plasma concentration over 3×10^{-8} mol/L are candidates for a subsequent i.t. injection, whereas for patients with a concentration lower than 3×10^{-8} mol/L, i.t. treatment is discontinued for two weeks when it appears that the slow type of efflux has been restored (3).

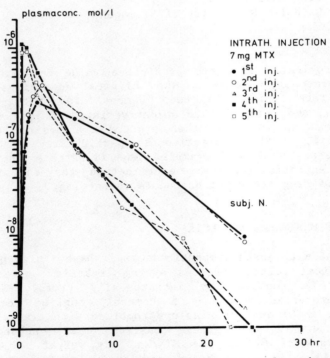

Figure 1. Plasma concentration-time profile of methotrexate following i.t. administration to a pediatric patient with acute lymphatic leukemia. In the course of subsequent administration the profile changes from a slow to a fast type.

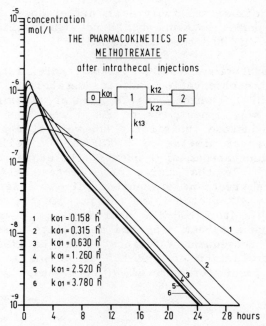

Figure 2. Simulated plasma concentration-time profiles in which the distribution and elimination constants remain constant and in which k_{01} (the efflux rate constant from the cerebrospinal fluid compartment to the plasma compartment) has been varied.

INTERPRETATION OF METHOTREXATE PLASMA CONCENTRATIONS

Methotrexate is used in a large variety of dosages, dosage forms, routes and time courses of administration, either alone or, more frequently, as part of a combination treatment. Based on reports of 50% inhibition of DNA synthesis in mouse bone marrow (4), a minimum therapeutic plasma concentration of $2-5 \times 10^{-8}$ M is maintained for a period long enough to obtain practically complete inhibition of mitosis of pathological cells in terms of the characteristic turnover time for these cells. The drug shows a relatively low direct toxicity. Delayed toxicity involves bone marrow depression and mucositis. Bone marrow toxicity can be prevented or treated by supplying the natural cofactor that is inhibited by MTX, 5-methyl-tetrahydrofolate (5-MTHF), through its precursor leucovorin or other folate derivatives. The cofactor 5-MTHF shows kinetic properties similar to MTX (5). This so-called "rescue" treatment appears effective only when the concentration of MTX is below 10^{-4} mol/L and the concentration of 5-MTHF is in the

same range.   Because of individual differences in the rate of
elimination, rescue treatment should not be instituted before the
concentration of MTX has been determined.

The interpretation of the plasma concentration of MTX is
complicated by the observation that its metabolite, 7-hydroxymetho-
trexate (7-OH-MTX), which has a longer intrinsic half-life
(9 hours) than MTX, appears to be 200 times less effective as a
dihydrofolate reductase inhibitor.   However, it appears to compete
with MTX in a manner similar to 5-MTHF at the cell membrane level
(5).   High concentrations of 7-OH-MTX, therefore, must be avoided
during therapy.   In the course of long-term MTX infusions, as
practiced in the treatment of choriocarcinoma (Fig. 3) and in so-
called high dose MTX protocols in the treatment of solid sarcomas,
the ratio of MTX to 7-OH-MTX decreases.   Theoretically, this
competition between parent drug and metabolite leads to decreased
effectiveness.   Subsequent infusions should be given at intervals
so that the accumulation of 7-OH-MTX in plasma is minimal.   However, clinical proof for reduced effectiveness has not yet been
obtained.

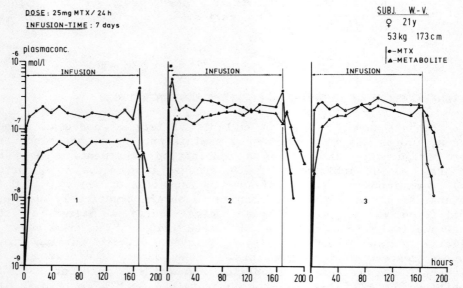

Figure 3. Plasma concentration-time profile of MTX and 7-OH-MTX
after three successive 7-day infusions. Whereas the MTX
concentration remains constant, increasing concentrations of the metabolite can be observed.

ADRIAMYCIN

After rapid i.v. administration of adriamycin (ADM), the plasma concentration declines one hundredfold during the first half hour. Distribution is claimed to be the major cause of this decline. However, only fluorescent metabolites having the same fluorescence spectrum as ADM have been measured, accounting for not more than 50% of the total drug dose. ADM metabolites in which fluorescent properties are lost or changed due to reactions that change the electron density of the aromatic rings are possible, but not yet identified. As can be seen in Figure 4, the metabolite adriamycinol (ADM-ol) can be identified directly after administration. The terminal half-life for both the parent drug and the metabolite is approximately 50 hours ($t_{1/2}$ γ).

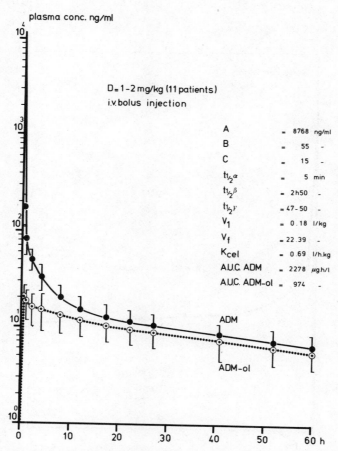

Figure 4. Plasma concentration-time profiles (mean ± SE) of ADM and ADM-ol obtained in 11 patients. The dosage varied from 1 to 2 mg/kg and was adjusted to 1.5 mg/kg.

The rate of metabolism appears to be different in different species. The ratio of ADM/ADM-ol is smaller in the rabbit due to a higher metabolic capacity. The intrinsic half-life of ADM-ol is, however, much smaller than that for the parent ADM (Fig. 5), as can be shown when ADM-ol is administered directly to the animal (Fig. 6); no ADM was measurable following ADM-ol dosing. The reduction of ADM to ADM-ol is an equilibrium reaction, yet presumably, the equilibrium favors the reduced side and the concentration of ADM remains below the limit of detection of the analytical procedure. The half-life of ADM-ol was 2.5 hours in this rabbit when the metabolite was dosed, while the apparent or measured half-life after ADM administration was 25 hours. When ADM was dosed, the plasma concentration of the metabolite declined with the same half-life as its precursor. The reduction of ADM to ADM-ol requires a reductase enzyme, which depends upon the presence of the cofactor NADPH. The reaction can be influenced by simultaneous administration of

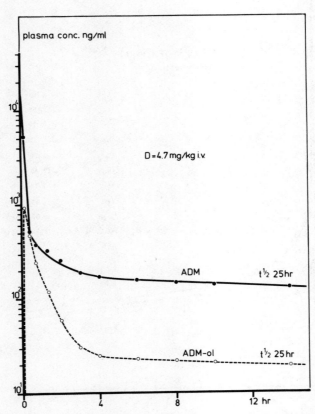

Figure 5. Plasma concentration-time profiles of ADM and ADM-ol after administration of 4.7 mg/kg ADM to a rabbit. The terminal half-life of both ADM and ADM-ol is 25 hours.

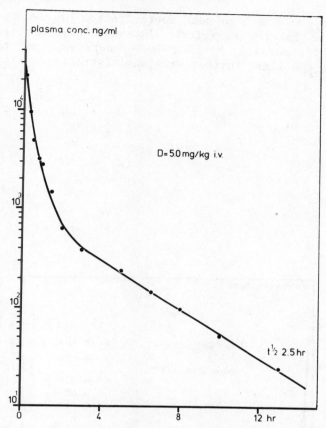

Figure 6. Plasma concentration-time profile of ADM-ol after administration of 5 mg/kg ADM-ol to a rabbit. The terminal half-life is 2.5 hours. No ADM could be identified.

ethanol, which increases the availability of the cofactor. If this reduction is a rate-limiting step in the metabolism of ADM, alteration in the half-life of both ADM and ADM-ol should be observed. In Figure 7, it can be seen that the half-lives of ADM and ADM-ol are reduced from 11 to 4 hours when ethanol is simultaneously administered.

Treatment of patients with adriamycin is limited by the occurrence of irreversible cardiac toxicity of the congestive heart failure type. Following the traditional bolus injection protocol of two to three administrations on successive days, the maximum amount of ADM should not exceed 450-500 mg/m^2 body surface area. Long-term zero-order drug infusion appears able to limit this cardiac toxicity, allowing the drug to accumulate to higher amounts before congestive heart failure becomes apparent (6) (Fig. 8).

Therefore, only a high peak concentration of ADM seems to be responsible for cardiac toxicity. However, long-term peripheral i.v. infusion for possibly as long as 96 hours may lead to serious phlebitis that can limit further drug administration.

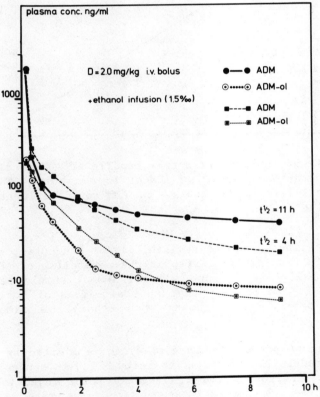

Figure 7. Plasma concentration-time profile of ADM and ADM-ol in a rabbit with and without simultaneous administration of ethanol. The terminal half-lives for both ADM and ADM-ol change from 11 to 4 hours.

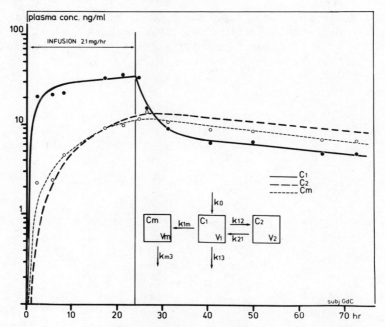

Figure 8. Plasma concentration-time profile of ADM and ADM-ol after a 24-hour infusion. The concentration in fictive comparment two is also shown.

REFERENCES

1. W.A. Bleyer, The clinical pharmacology of methotrexate, Cancer 41:36–51 (1978).
2. J. Lankelma, E. van der Kleijn and E.F.S. Termond, Assay of methotrexate and 7-hydroxymethotrexate by high pressure liquid chromatography and its application to clinical pharmacokinetics, in: "Clinical Pharmacology of Anti-Neoplastic Drugs," H.M. Pinedo, ed., Elsevier/North-Holland Biomedical Press, Amsterdam (1978), pp. 13–28.
3. R.J.J. Lippens, Methotrexate in the central nervous system prophylaxis of children with acute lymphoblastic leukemia, Ph.D. Thesis, Medical School, Catholic University of Nijmegen, The Netherlands, (1981).
4. B.A. Chabner and R.C. Young, Threshold methotrexate concentration for in vivo inhibition of DNA synthesis in normal and tumorous target tissues, J. Clin. Invest. 52:1804–1811 (1973).
5. J. Lankelma and E. van der Kleijn, The role of 7-hydroxymethotrexate during methotrexate anti-cancer therapy, Cancer Letters 9:133–142 (1980).

6.   R.S. Benjamin, S. Legha, B. Mackay, M. Ewer, S. Wallace, M.
      Valdevieso, S. Rasmussen, G. Blumenschein and E. Freireich,
      Reduction of adriamycin cardiotoxicity using prolonged contin-
      uous infusion, Proc. 17th Ann. Meeting Am. Soc. Clin. Oncol.
      22:179 (1981).

Chapter 28

THE IMMUNOPHARMACOKINETICS OF PREDNISONE/PREDNISOLONE

Leslie Z. Benet, Udo F. Legler, Brigitte M. Frey,
Felix J. Frey and Sue Y. Tsang

Department of Pharmacy
School of Pharmacy
University of California
San Francisco, California

Although immunosuppressive agents have been utilized extensively in a number of patient populations, little pharmacokinetic information has been available concerning the absorption and distribution of these compounds, and even less information has been available relating the efficacy and toxicity of these drugs to pharmacokinetic measurements. Studies in this area may be subsumed under the title immunopharmacokinetics which may be defined as the study of the rate processes of absorption, distribution, metabolism and excretion of immunoregulating (immunosuppressive and immunostimulating) drugs and their corresponding immunologic efficacious or toxic responses (1). Studies in our laboratory over the past few years have concentrated on defining the immunopharmacokinetics of prednisone and prednisolone, the most commonly used immunosuppressive agents. Before attempting to relate the kinetics of these exogenous glucocorticoids to their immunosuppressive effects, we felt that it was necessary to accurately define the pharmacokinetics of these agents in both normal volunteers and the patient populations receiving the drug.

Three unique problems must be addressed before one is able to accurately define the pharmacokinetics of prednisone and prednisolone. First, prednisone and prednisolone are interconverted by the microsomal enzyme 11-β-hydroxysteroid dehydrogenase. This interconversion process causes difficulties in accurately defining the clearance of either prednisone or prednisolone, as discussed by Professor Wagner in Chapter 16. The second major problem relates to the presence of the endogenous corticosteroids, cortisone and cortisol, which also are interconverted by the microsomal enzyme 11-β-hydroxysteroid dehydrogenase and which are thought to compete with prednisolone for specific binding sites on transcortin. This interaction is further complicated by the fact that the administration of exogenous glucocorticoids such as prednisone and prednisolone normally leads to the suppression of endogenous cortisol production. As depicted in Figure 1, the synthetic corticosteroids prednisone and prednisolone differ from the endogenous cortisone and cortisol only by the double bond at the 1,2 position. The third difficulty in accurately defining prednisolone pharmacokinetics is the fact that this compound appears to show saturable binding over the concentration range observed in patients following the usual doses of this drug. Human corticosteroid-binding globulin (CBG, transcortin) binds prednisolone with a high affinity but low capacity, due to the relatively low concentrations ($\approx 10^{-7}$ M) in plasma. However, albumin, although it has a lower affinity for prednisolone, has a larger capacity for binding due to its higher plasma concentrations, approximately 10^{-4} M. The saturable binding of prednisolone is represented in Figure 2 where bound versus free concentrations of prednisolone in a patient are depicted. Note that the binding relation is curvilinear over a concentration range of approximately 0–300 ng/ml.

Cognizant of the three problems listed above, we chose to develop a specific and sensitive assay method which would allow us

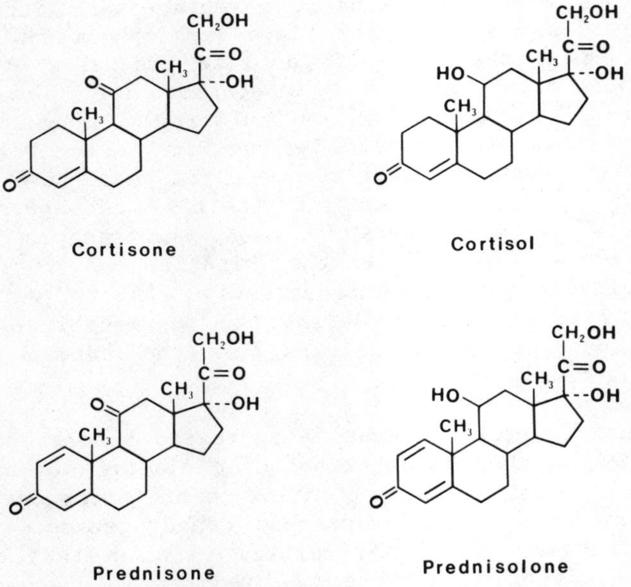

Figure 1. Structures of prednisone, prednisolone, cortisone and cortisol.

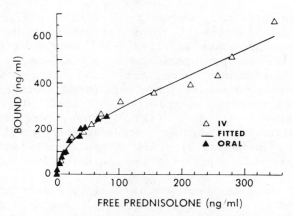

Figure 2. Plot of bound versus unbound prednisolone concentrations obtained for plasma samples in a patient. The solid line indicates the computer fit of the measurements following both intravenous and oral dosing where the binding relation assumes a high affinity, low capacity site (transcortin) and a low affinity, high capacity site (albumin). Reproduced with permission of the publisher (20).

to simultaneously measure the concentrations of cortisone, cortisol, prednisone and prednisolone in plasma using high pressure liquid chromatography (2). The steroids, together with an internal standard, dexamethasone, are extracted from 1 ml of plasma with methylene chloride/ether, washed with acid and base, and separated isocratically on a normal phase silica column with a mobile phase consisting of methylene chloride/tetrahydrofuran/methanol/glacial acetic acid (96.85/1/2.1/0.05 by volume) at a flow rate of 1.3 ml/min. The steroids are detected at 254 nm and quantitated by peak-height measurements; their retention times range from 6 to 20 minutes. The lower limit for routine detection of all four compounds is 8 ng/ml. Analytical recoveries are about 75%; the intraday variability (CV) is 1-9% and the interday variability 2-11%. The free fraction of prednisolone is determined by equilibrium dialysis of each plasma sample. Since prednisolone exhibits concentration-dependent changes in binding, as noted above, free prednisolone plasma concentrations were calculated allowing for dilution during the dialysis process (3). Corrections were also made for volume shifts during dialysis (4).

The pharmacokinetics of prednisolone and prednisone were reviewed through 1979 by Pickup (5) and Gambertoglio et al. (6). These reviewers concluded that the available studies (7-10) indicated that prednisolone and prednisone appear to exhibit dose-dependent kinetics, as might be expected for a compound showing nonlinear protein binding. However, a recent publication (11) concludes that the kinetics of total prednisolone are not dose-dependent. All of the above studies (7-11) have been carried out using single doses of prednisone or prednisolone. Thus, the concentration measurements were not made at steady state. Furthermore, none of the studies have determined whether the inter-conversion of prednisolone and prednisone is saturable, as we have recently demonstrated in dogs (12). Thus, we undertook to determine unambiguously whether prednisolone exhibits dose-dependent kinetics in humans by studying ten normal individuals at two different steady-state prednisolone concentrations (13).

Each of the ten volunteers was infused to steady state over a seven-hour period at a low (5.5 µg/hr · kg) and a high (64 µg/hr · kg) rate with prednisolone. The results of this study are summarized in Table I. Steady-state prednisolone concentrations differed by a factor of 5 when the infusion rate was increased approximately twelvefold, indicating a marked increase in the apparent clearance of total prednisolone with increasing dose. The fraction of unbound prednisolone increased from 0.12 ± 0.02 to 0.24 ± 0.02 with increasing dose. Since the increase in the free fraction (twofold change) was not as great as the increase in apparent clearance of total prednisolone, there was a slight but significant ($p < 0.05$) increase in the apparent clearance of unbound prednisolone (see Table I). The interconversion between prednisolone and prednisone appears to be such as to approach a maximum prednisone concentration as was previously noted by us in dogs (12). In humans, we found this maximum prednisone concentration to be 52 ng/ml when prednisolone was infused. Thus, the ratio of concentrations, prednisolone to prednisone, also increased with increasing prednisolone dose. These results unambiguously indicate that prednisolone exhibits dose- and concentration-dependent kinetics and that the great majority of the change in kinetics may be attributed to saturable protein binding of prednisolone. Although there is an increase in the apparent clearance of unbound prednisolone with increasing concentration, these results are confounded by the interconversion process between prednisone and prednisolone. We are presently synthesizing radiolabeled prednisone so that we may be able to determine unbound concentrations of this compound. These future studies will allow us to determine whether in fact the metabolic elimination of unbound prednisolone changes with increasing dose.

Two of the ten subjects in the above study appeared to show kinetic results which differed from those of the other eight volun-teers. Cortisol levels obtained at time zero for the two subjects were approximately twice the levels found for the remaining subjects. In addition, these two volunteers exhibited higher total prednisolone levels, lower total prednisolone apparent clearance values and higher concentration ratios of total prednisolone to

Table I. Mean parameters and ratio of values obtained during 7-hour infusions with low and high dose prednisolone sodium phosphate in ten healthy volunteers[a].

Parameter	Low Dose	High Dose	High Dose / Low Dose
Infusion rate (ng/min · kg)	91.8 ± 8.3	1067 ± 115	11.7 ± 1.45
Total prednisolone steady-state concentration (ng/ml)	91 ± 25	437 ± 116	4.9 ± 0.3
Unbound prednisolone steady-state concentration (ng/ml)	11 ± 2	103 ± 27	9.5 ± 2.0
Apparent total prednisolone clearance (ml/min · kg)	1.06 ± 0.24	2.54 ± 0.50	2.47 ± 0.29
Apparent unbound prednisolone clearance (ml/min · kg)	8.69 ± 1.58	10.9 ± 2.4	1.29 ± 0.24
Total prednisone steady-state concentration (ng/ml)	13 ± 2	37 ± 4	2.8 ± 0.4
Ratio of concentrations: total prednisolone/ total prednisone	6.8 ± 1.3	12.0 ± 3.3	1.8 ± 0.2

[a]Data represents mean ± SD (see reference 13).

total prednisone. Upon reviewing the medical history of these two subjects, we noted that both of these female volunteers had previously been receiving oral contraceptive preparations, although neither subject was taking these preparations at the time of the study. It is well known that exogenous estrogen therapy increases transcortin levels and thereby increases the protein binding of cortisol and decreases the clearance of total cortisol (14). Since prednisolone and cortisol share a common binding site on transcortin, decreased total clearance of prednisolone would also be expected. We have recently evaluated the influence of oral progestational agents on the time course of exogenous and endogenous glucocorticoids.

Twelve healthy female volunteers were studied (15). Six women had been taking low dose oral contraceptives for at least six months. Each subject received a 0.53 mg/kg intravenous dose of prednisolone at 7:45 a.m. during days 15 to 28 of her menstrual cycle. As noted in Table II, a marked difference in the apparent total prednisolone clearance was found between the two groups of women. This could be due in part to the increased transcortin concentrations which result from exogenous estrogen therapy. However, when the apparent unbound prednisolone clearances were calculated, it was obvious that the oral contraceptives had affected the metabolic processes involved. An approximate threefold difference in unbound clearance was noted between the two groups of women. Apparently, the presence of the ethynyl estrogens results in irreversible binding to cytochrome P-450 and a subsequent decrease in the amounts of this hepatic oxidative drug metabolizing enzyme system (16,17).

Two previous studies (18,19) suggested that the clearance rate of prednisolone may be lower in patients exhibiting cushingoid side

Table II. Mean parameters found following intravenous administration of prednisolone to six women taking low dose oral contraceptives for at least six months and six age and weight matched controls[a].

Parameter	Controls	Women Receiving Oral Contraceptive Steroids
Apparent total prednisolone clearance (mg/min · kg)	3.44 ± 1.10	0.92 ± 0.25
Apparent unbound prednisolone clearance (ml/min · kg)	10.2 ± 1.50	3.76 ± 0.66
Transcortin binding capacity (ng/ml)	111 ± 58	721 ± 291

[a]Data represents mean ± SD; the dose was 0.53 mg/kg (see reference 15).

effects from glucocorticoid dosing. We investigated the pharmacokinetics of prednisone/prednisolone and the time course of
endogenous cortisol in 15 stable renal transplant patients and 12
patients with oral mucocutaneous vesiculoerosive diseases; of the
27 volunteers studied, 14 patients were without cushingoid side
effects and 13 had this steroid toxic side effect (20,21). All 27
patients were given their usual prednisone dose orally on one occasion and an equivalent amount of prednisolone intravenously on
another occasion. Following dosing, 8 to 14 plasma samples were
obtained for the determination of total prednisolone, prednisone
and cortisol concentrations by HPLC (2) and unbound prednisolone
concentrations by equilibrium dialysis. The bioavailability of
prednisone, the interconversion of prednisone to prednisolone, the
total and unbound prednisolone apparent clearances, the prednisolone binding capacity of albumin and transcortin, and the affinity
of albumin for prednisolone were not different when the 14 patients
without cushingoid side effects were compared with the 13 cushingoid patients. Patients who developed side effects had a higher
affinity constant for prednisolone binding to transcortin, more
frequently exhibited higher peak cortisol levels and more often had
measurable (> 10 ng/ml) cortisol in the plasma samples collected
during the kinetic studies, as compared with those not showing side
effects. The data suggest that endogenous cortisol production is
not as suppressed in patients with visible cushingoid signs as in
noncushingoid patients, and that there is no significant difference
in the pharmacokinetics of exogenous glucocorticoids between
patients with and without cushingoid side effects.

When we began our immunopharmacokinetic studies, we were
confident that we could develop sensitive and specific analytical
methodology which would allow us to measure immunoregulating drugs
at the concentrations usually found in biological fluids following
dosing to patients. We were less sure of our ability to develop
indices of immunosuppressive activity which could be correlated
with drug pharmacokinetics. The most frequently described
immunologic effects of the corticosteroids are those related to
lymphocyte function. Although it has been well established that
corticosteroids can suppress lymphocyte blastogenic responses in
vitro (22), it is still debated whether direct suppression of
lymphocyte proliferation is a major mechanism of immunosuppressive
action for in vivo corticosteroids. Recent observations, as
reviewed by Fauci (23), however, suggest that corticosteroid
induced suppression of blastogenic responses may have important
immunoregulatory implications. Ilfeld et al. (24) have demonstrated that physiologic concentrations of corticosteroids markedly
suppress the autologous mixed lymphocyte reaction between T cells
and B cell enriched suspensions without any suppression of the
allogeneic mixed lymphocyte reaction (MLR). This suggests that
corticosteroids may have a physiologic role in the in vivo regulation of T cell autoreactivity.

To quantify the inhibition of T cell function by immunosuppressive drugs, Bach (25) studied and described the inhibition of rosette formation using a mouse system. However, we believe that an in vitro test of human T cell function would be a more desirable and probably more relevant tool for assessing immunosuppressive activity in human plasma. Our collaborators, Cochrum et al. (26), have previously demonstrated a good relation between the intensity of the MLR and the survival of renal allografts. Thus, we believe that the inhibition of this MLR should be a rational model for quantifying immunosuppressive activity in plasma, especially in renal allograft recipients. Laborde and Bach (27) and Bach (25), using macro-mixed lymphocyte cultures (MLC), have attempted to describe the kinetics of immunosuppressive activity in human plasma after doses of prednisolone and azathioprine. Bach et al. (28) state that the method is technically difficult to perform and the interpretation of results is complicated by what they call the appearance of a metabolite which inhibits the immunosuppressive effect on the MLR. To avoid this kind of stimulatory effect on the MLR, dilutions of up to 1,028 times were proposed so as to obtain a standardized 50% inhibition (27). We have described (29) a simple and reproducible in vitro measure of immunosuppressive activity which varies as a function of time following administration of prednisolone to patients. This modification of the two-way MLC evaluates drug inhibition of MLRs utilizing 50% plasma and a three-day incubation period (29). The major finding, which allowed us to develop a reasonable measure of immunosuppression, was the fact that maximum inhibitory effects for prednisolone on tritiated thymidine incorporation occurred at day three of the MLC incubation as opposed to day five, the time for maximum tritiated thymidine incorporation. The most probable explanation may be that at various time points during the MLR, different subpopulations of lymphocytes are active, with different sensitivities to plasma containing immunosuppressive compounds. This finding may also explain why previous workers were unable to obtain reproducible measures of immunosuppression using the usual procedures for the MLR.

To gain a better understanding of the kinetics of T cell subsets as well as the influence of prednisolone, we studied the induction kinetics of human suppressor cells in the MLR (30). In this work, we found that suppressor cells are apparently generated in the MLCs between days 1 and 4, and, as expected, their genesis is not affected by usual therapeutic concentrations of prednisolone.

Our recent work has been related to developing measures of immunosuppression. We first were able to show the expected relation between a pharmacodynamic measure (% MLC inhibition) and plasma concentrations of total as well as unbound prednisolone in patient plasma following prednisolone or prednisone administration.

Figure 3 depicts the steep hyperbolic concentration-response curve found when percent MLC inhibition is plotted versus unbound prednisolone concentration (31). From studies in 12 patients receiving chronic prednisone dosing, we calculated 50% effective concentrations with respect to MLR inhibition for both total and unbound prednisolone following oral and intravenous dosing (31). The following mean (± SD) values were found for the EC_{50} (ng/ml): oral dosing – 10.0 ± 5.0 unbound concentrations and 86.5 ± 30.0 total concentrations; intravenous dosing – 12.4 ± 12.6 unbound concentrations and 66.3 ± 26.7 total concentrations.

The EC_{50} values found for total prednisolone following i.v. and oral dosing to the patient population studied here are higher than those found when the inhibition of the MLC is determined following spiking of serial amounts of prednisolone to plasma obtained from a normal volunteer. Tsang and Benet (unpublished results) found an EC_{50} of 29.7 ± 5.7 ng/ml for prednisolone in such spiked samples. This difference emphasizes the importance of carrying out the correlation using plasma samples (and preferentially lymphocytes) from the patient populations being treated, since a variety of suppressive and/or stimulatory humoral factors may be released by treated lymphocyte subpopulations in vivo.

We have recently examined the differences between the effects of prednisone, prednisolone and cortisol on the MLR (32). Micro-MLCs were cultured in the presence of 15% pooled serum spiked with drug. Cultures were harvested on day 3. As measured by the

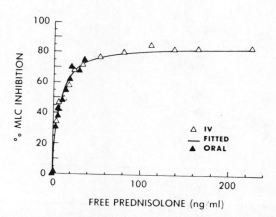

Figure 3. Concentration-response curve for free prednisolone in a patient receiving oral prednisone and i.v. prednisolone. The best computer fit line for the intravenous data is shown. Both the intravenous and oral data points are plotted. Reproduced with permission of the publisher (31).

inhibition of the MLR, prednisolone is 2 to 2.5 times more potent
than cortisol (see Fig. 4). Despite their differences in potency,
both prednisolone and cortisol yield the same maximal inhibition.
This maximal inhibition varies with different donor pairs, ranging
from 55 to 100%. Prednisone, on the other hand, shows no significant immunosuppressive activity despite the significant slow
conversion of prednisone to prednisolone in the MLR by 11-hydrox-
ylation: 28 ng/ml prednisolone in a 92 ng/ml culture and 44 ng/ml
in a 460 ng/ml culture after 3 days of incubation. This finding
indicates the importance of the duration and timing of prednisolone's presence in the culture to the overall immunosuppressive
activity. The presence of prednisone has no effect on the inhibition due to prednisolone or cortisol.

Since assessment of immunosuppressive capacity in a single
plasma sample provides little information concerning the magnitude
of immunosuppression over an entire day, we believe that an
integrated measure, area under the inhibition curve (AUIC), may be
more meaningful. Figure 5 represents the plot of area under the
inhibition-time curve versus area under the unbound prednisolone
concentration-time curve following i.v. prednisolone and oral prednisone administration in the 12 patients discussed above (31). We

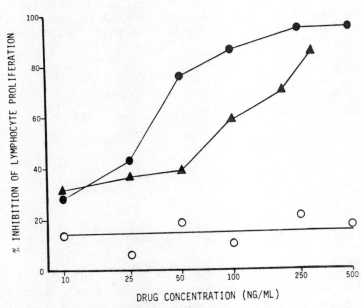

Figure 4. The effect of different concentrations of prednisolone
(filled circles), prednisone (open circles) and cortisol
(filled triangles) on inhibition of the mixed lymphocyte
reaction.

find no simple linear relationship between these values of AUIC and the integrated prednisolone concentrations (AUC). With increasing AUC of prednisolone, the increment of immunosuppression (AUIC) decreases. Provided our model is relevant to the clinical situation, doses of prednisone which yield an AUC for free prednisolone greater than 40,000 ng min/ml will cause little increase in AUIC (see Fig. 5). In most of our subjects, this AUC corresponds to an available prednisone dose of 50 mg. Thus, doses of prednisone higher than 50 mg may add little to therapeutic efficacy. To our knowledge, there is no controlled study available at present which demonstrates that prednisone doses higher than 50 mg/day add anything to the therapeutic efficacy, both for prevention and treatment of kidney allograft rejections.

We are aware that the MLR inhibition measurement which we have developed is only an intermediate index of immunosuppressive activity. Our long range goal is to extend this correlation between the intermediate index and pharmacokinetics to actual measures of efficacy and toxicity. We are encouraged by our ability to develop a simple, reproducible intermediate measure. In addition, there is a rationale for the method chosen since Cochrum

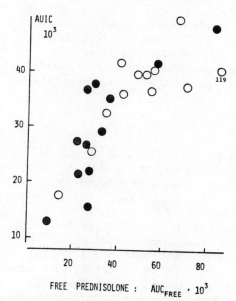

Figure 5. Plot of area under inhibition-time curve (AUIC) versus the area under the unbound prednisolone concentration-time curve (AUC_{free}) following oral prednisone (filled circles) and i.v. prednisolone (open circles) dosing in 12 patients. Reproduced with permission of the publisher (31).

and co-workers (26) did show a correlation of graft survival with a measure of the MLR.

The field of immunopharmacokinetics is in its infancy. Not only are measures of clinical efficacy and toxicity for immunoregulating agents poorly defined but, in addition, sensitive and specific assays for the drugs are just being developed, thereby allowing the investigator to measure immunoregulating drugs in the biological fluids of patients following doses usually administered to those patients. The future of this subdiscipline seems promising since there is a definite need to define rational therapeutic dosage regimens for immunopharmacologic agents. The work described here, limited to prednisolone/prednisone, is obviously only a beginning.

Acknowledgements. Preparation of this manuscript and the studies in the authors' laboratories were supported by National Institutes of Health grants GM 26691 and GM 26551. During the course of this work, Dr. Udo Legler was supported by the Deutsche Forschungsgemeinschaft. Drs. Brigitte M. and Felix J. Frey were supported by the Swiss National Foundation for Scientific Research. Ms. Sue Y. Tsang was supported as an NIH Predoctoral Scholar on NIH Training Grant GM 07175. The authors are indebted to a number of scientists and clinical collaborators who served as willing consultants during the course of the studies described. We wish to express our sincere thanks to Drs. W.J.C. Amend, Jr., K.C. Cochrum, J.G. Gambertoglio, M.R. Garovoy, N.H.G. Holford, E.T. Lin, F. Lozada, O. Salvatierra, Jr. and S. Silverman, Jr. Special thanks to Ms. Maria Rosen for her aid in preparing the manuscript.

REFERENCES

1. L.Z. Benet, B.M. Frey, T.L. Ding and F.J. Frey, The pharmacokinetics of immunoregulating drugs: Immunopharmacokinetics, in: "Advances in Immunopharmacology," J. Hadden, L. Chedid, P. Mullen and F. Spreafico, eds., Pergamon Press, Oxford (1981), pp. 29-36.

2. F.J. Frey, B.M. Frey and L.Z. Benet, Liquid-chromatographic measurement of endogenous and exogenous glucocorticoids in plasma, Clin. Chem. 25:1944-1947 (1979).

3. H.L. Behm and J.G. Wagner, Errors in interpretation of data from equilibrium dialysis protein binding experiments, Res. Commun. Chem. Path. Pharmacol. 26:145-160 (1979).

4. T.N. Tozer, J.G. Gambertoglio, D.E. Furst, D. Avery and N.H.G. Holford, Volume shifts during equilibrium dialysis and protein binding estimates - application to prednisolone binding in man, J. Pharm. Sci. 72:1442-1446 (1983).

5. M.E. Pickup, Clinical pharmacokinetics of prednisone and prednisolone, Clin. Pharmacokin. 4:111-128 (1979).

6. J.G. Gambertoglio, W.J.C. Amend and L.Z. Benet, Pharmaco-
    kinetics and bioavailability of prednisone and prednisolone in
    healthy volunteers and patients: A review, J. Pharmacokin.
    Biopharm. 8:1-52 (1980).

7. A.W. Meikle, J.A. Weed and F.H. Tyler, Kinetics and intercon-
    version of prednisolone and prednisone studied with new radio-
    immunoassays, J. Clin. Endocrinol. Metab. 41:717-721 (1975).

8. M.E. Pickup, J.R. Lowe, P.A. Leathan, V.M. Rhind, V. Wright
    and W.W. Downie, Dose-dependent pharmacokinetics of prednisone
    and prednisolone, Eur. J. Clin. Pharmacol. 12:213-219 (1977).

9. J.C.K. Loo, I.J. McGilveray, N. Jordan, J. Moffatt and R.
    Brien, Dose-dependent pharmacokinetics of prednisone and pred-
    nisolone in man, J. Pharm. Pharmacol. 30:736 (1978).

10. A. Tanner, F. Bochner, J. Caffin, J. Halliday and L. Powell,
    Dose-dependent prednisolone kinetics, Clin. Pharmacol. Ther.
    25:571-578 (1979).

11. S. Al-Habet and H.L. Rogers, Pharmacokinetics of intravenous
    and oral prednisolone, Br. J. Clin. Pharmacol. 10:503-508
    (1980).

12. F.J. Frey, B.M. Frey, A. Greither and L.Z. Benet, Prednisolone
    clearance at steady state in dogs, J. Pharmacol. Exp. Ther.
    215:287-291 (1980).

13. U.F. Legler, F.J. Frey and L.Z. Benet, Prednisolone clearance
    at steady state in man, J. Clin. Endocrinol. Metab. 55:762-767
    (1982).

14. I.H. Mill, H.P. Schedl, P.S. Chen and F.C. Bartter, The effect
    of estrogen administration on the metabolism and protein bind-
    ing of hydrocortisone, J. Clin. Endocrinol. Metab. 20:515-528
    (1960).

15. U.F. Legler and L.Z. Benet, Marked alteration in prednisolone
    kinetics in women taking oral-contraceptive steroids, Clin.
    Pharmacol. Ther. 31:243 (1982).

16. P.R. Ortiz de Montellano, K.L. Kunze, G.S. Yost and B.A. Mico,
    Self-catalyzed destruction of cytochrome P-450: Covalent
    binding of ethynyl sterols to prosthetic heme, Proc. Natl.
    Acad. Sci. 76:746-749 (1979).

17. P.R. Ortiz de Montellano and K.L. Kunze, Self-catalyzed inac-
    tivation of hepatic cytochrome P-450 by ethynyl substrates, J.
    Biol. Chem. 255:5578-5585 (1980).

18. M. Kozower, L. Veatch and M.M. Kaplan, Decreased clearance of
    prednisolone, a factor in the development of corticosteroid
    side effects, J. Clin. Endocrinol. Metab. 38:407-412 (1974).

19. J. Gambertoglio, F. Vincenti, N. Feduska, J. Birnbaum, O.
    Salvatierra and W. Amend, Prednisolone disposition in cush-
    ingoid and noncushingoid kidney transplant patients, J. Clin.
    Endocrinol. Metab. 51:561-565 (1980).

20. F.J. Frey, W.J.C. Amend, F. Lozada, B.M. Frey, N.H.G. Holford
    and L.Z. Benet, Pharmacokinetics of prednisolone and endoge-
    nous hydrocortisone levels in cushingoid and non-cushingoid
    patients, Eur. J. Clin. Pharmacol. 21:235-242 (1981).

21. F.J. Frey, W.J.C. Amend, Jr., F. Lozada, B.M. Frey and L.Z. Benet, Endogenous hydrocortisone, a possible factor contributing to the genesis of cushingoid habitus in patients on prednisone, J. Clin. Endocrinol. Metab. 53:1076-1080 (1981).

22. A.S. Fauci, D.C. Dale and J.E. Barlow, Glucocorticosteroid therapy: Mechanisms of action of steroid hormones, Ann. Intern. Med. 84:304-315 (1976).

23. A.S. Fauci, Mechanisms of the immunosuppressive and antiinflammatory effects of glucocorticoids, J. Immunopharmacol. 1:1-25 (1978-79).

24. D.N. Ilfeld, R.S. Krakauer and R.M. Blaese, Suppression of the human autologous mixed lymphocyte reaction by physiologic concentrations of hydrocortisone, J. Immunol. 119:428-434 (1977).

25. J.F. Bach, "The Mode of Action of Immunosuppressive Agents," North Holland, Amsterdam (1975).

26. K.C. Cochrum, O. Salvatierra, Jr., H.A. Perkins and F.O. Belzer, MLC testing in renal transplantation, Transplant. Proc. 7:659-662 (1975).

27. A. Laborde and J.-F. Bach, Immunologie-inhibition et stimulation par l'incorporation de thymidine par les lymphocytes en culture mixte, C.R. Acad. Sci., Paris, D. 272:509-512 (1971).

28. J.-F. Bach, M. Dardenne and M.-A. Bach, Dosage des metabolites actifs des immunosuppresseurs dans le serum, La Nouvelle Presse Medicale 1:2293-2298 (1972).

29. B.M. Frey, F.J. Frey, L.Z. Benet and K.C. Cochrum, Modification of the mixed lymphocyte reaction for pharmacokinetic assessment of immunosuppressive activity in human plasma, Int. J. Immunopharmac. 2:129-134 (1980).

30. B.M. Frey, F.J. Frey, K.C. Cochrum and L.Z. Benet, Induction kinetics of human suppressor cells in the mixed lymphocyte reaction and influence of prednisolone on their genesis, Cellular Immunol. 56:225-234 (1980).

31. B.M. Frey, F.J. Frey, N.H.G. Holford, F. Lozada and L.Z. Benet, Prednisolone pharmacodynamics assessed by inhibition of the mixed lymphocyte reaction, Transplantation 33:578-584 (1982).

32. S.Y. Tsang, B.M. Frey and L.Z. Benet, Effects of corticosteroids on the in vitro proliferative response of human lymphocytes to allogeneic cells, Abstracts of APhA Academy of Pharmaceutical Sciences 11(2):143 (1981).

Communication 1

THE INTERPRETATION OF IN VIVO MEAN DISSOLUTION TIME DATA

Paul S. Collier

Department of Pharmacy
The Queen's University of Belfast
Northern Ireland, United Kingdom

Of the various published methods for determining rates of absorption or in vivo dissolution of drugs, only the method of Riegelman and Collier (1) is not unduly affected by changes in clearance (CL) between successive doses. The estimation of in vivo mean dissolution time ($MDT_{in\ vivo}$) requires that drug be administered on two separate occasions, once as a solution and once as the drug product under investigation:

$$MDT_{in\ vivo} = (MRT_{prod} - 1/\lambda z_{prod}) - (MRT_{soln} - 1/\lambda z_{soln}) \qquad (1)$$

where λz represents the terminal elimination rate constant and MRT is the mean residence time. The $MDT_{in\ vivo}$ was shown to correspond to 63.2% dissolution for a first-order process and 50% for a zero-order process. However, in vitro dissolution rarely corresponds to either pure first- or zero-order kinetics. The Weibull function, which can be expressed as:

$$\text{Amount remaining to be dissolved} = D \exp[-(\frac{t}{td})^S] \qquad (2)$$

has therefore been used to describe sigmoidal in vitro dissolution curves where td is the in vitro mean dissolution time (e.g., see reference 2). Although $MDT_{in\ vitro}$ for a first-order dissolution process described by Equation (2) (S = 1) can be obtained from AUMC/AUC, this approach is invalid when dissolution is nonlinear (S ≠ 1). The method of von Hattingberg et al. (3) applied to in vitro dissolution curves plotted as amount remaining to be absorbed versus time:

$$MDT_{in\ vitro} = AUC/D \qquad (3)$$

403

gives values which correspond to $MDT_{in\ vivo}$ for first- and zero-order dissolution calculated by the method of Riegelman and Collier (1).

Simulations have been performed to study the effect of differing dissolution profiles on the estimation of $MDT_{in\ vivo}$. The following equation was assumed to describe plasma concentrations following oral administration of a solution containing 100 mg of drug:

$$Cp = 7.12\ e^{-0.688t} + 3.92\ e^{-0.072t} - 11.04\ e^{-5.0t} \qquad (4)$$

By means of convolution (the reverse of the deconvolution method of Chiou, see reference 4), simulated plasma concentration data were obtained for three types of dissolution profiles (described by Eq. (2) when S = 0.5, 1 or 2). From these data, values for $MDT_{in\ vivo}$ and the corresponding percentage dissolution were calculated.

From the results presented in Table I, the importance of frequent sampling during the early stages can be seen. The error increases as td (the time for 63.2% dissolution) decreases relative to the frequency of sampling. When S = 1 or 2, the percentage dissolution at $MDT_{in\ vivo}$ (Eq. (1)), corresponds well to that at $MDT_{in\ vitro}$ (Eq. (3)). Minor differences can be explained in terms of the measurement of AUMC and AUC. However, the reason for the poor correlation when S = 0.5 is that as td becomes longer, not only is there an increased risk of a flip-flop situation developing when it is no longer possible to compensate for a change in CL between doses, but since a cutoff for absorption at 24 hours was assumed, bioavailability is reduced and $MDT_{in\ vivo}$ corresponds to the MDT of the absorbed drug. As stated by Riegelman and Collier (1), the MRT can be defined as the mean time for the transit of intact drug molecules through the body and involves a composite of all kinetic processes including release from the dosage forms, absorption into the body and all disposition processes.

The use of AUMC/AUC to determine MRT is only appropriate when the disposition processes obey first-order kinetics. The first in a series of contributing kinetic processes, e.g., dissolution, may be nonlinear and in this case the $MDT_{in\ vivo}$ is equivalent to the AUC for drug at the site of dissolution divided by the total amount of drug absorbed, and can be obtained using Equation (1).

When the shape parameter (S) of the Weibull function describing in vivo dissolution is less than one, the $MDT_{in\ vivo}$ will correspond to greater than 63.2% dissolution. Because $MDT_{in\ vivo}$ is a single time value, it does not give any indication of the shape of the in vivo dissolution curve and it is therefore impossible to relate the parameter to any given percentage dissolution. Therefore, when a range of products with differing dissolution

Table I. Simulations to determine in vivo mean dissolution time, percent dissolved at MDT and bioavailability as a function of the Weibull shape factor (S) and the in vitro mean dissolution time[a].

S	td(hr) in vitro	MDT(hr) in vivo	Percent Dissolved at MDT in vivo	in vitro	Bioavailability
0.5	0.125	0.34	80.6	75.7	100
	0.25	0.55	77.4	75.7	100
	0.5	1.07	76.8	75.7	100
	2.0	2.94	70.3	75.7	96.7
	6.0	4.78	59.0	75.7	86.5
1.0	0.125	0.2	80.4	63.2	100
	0.25	0.27	66.0	63.2	100
	0.5	0.55	66.4	63.2	100
	2.0	2.02	63.6	63.2	100
	6.0	5.74	61.6	63.2	98.1
2.0	0.125	0.19	91.1	54.4	100
	0.25	0.20	48.1	54.4	100
	0.5	0.45	55.1	54.4	100
	2.0	1.78	54.8	54.4	100
	6.0	5.35	54.9	54.4	100

[a]Sampling every 30 minutes during the early stages.

profiles for the same drug is studied it is unlikely that there will be a good correlation between $MDT_{in\ vivo}$ and a parameter such as the time for 50% or 63.2% dissolution in vitro. The value of $MDT_{in\ vivo}$ is that it is a model independent parameter which is not unduly affected by changes in CL between successive doses and which should correlate well with $MDT_{in\ vitro}$ (AUC/D) when an appropriate in vitro dissolution system is used.

REFERENCES

1. S. Riegelman and P.S. Collier, The application of statistical moment theory to the evaluation of in vivo dissolution time and absorption time, J. Pharmacokin. Biopharm. 8:509–534, (1980).

2. S. Riegelman and R. Upton, Studies on in vitro and in vivo drug release correlation, in: "Drug Absorption - Proceedings

of Edinburgh International Conference,", L.F. Prescott and W.S. Nimmo, eds., ADIS Press, New York (1980), pp. 297-312.

3. H.M. von Hattingberg, D. Brockmeier and D. Voegele, A method for in vivo - in vitro correlation using the additivity of mean times in biopharmaceutical models, Proceedings of International Symposium on Methods in Clinical Pharmacology, Frankfurt (1979).

4. W.L. Chiou, New compartment- and model-independent method for rapid calculation of drug absorption rates, J. Pharm. Sci. 69:57-62 (1980).

Communication 2

APPLICATION OF STATISTICAL MOMENT ANALYSIS TO THE EVALUATION OF CONTROLLED RELEASE FORMULATIONS

J.C.K. Loo, C. Charette, N. Jordan and I.J. McGilveray

Bureau of Drug Research
Health Protection Branch
Health and Welfare Canada
Ottawa, Ontario

Riegelman and Collier have recently reviewed (1) the application of first moment analysis, also termed the mean residence time (MRT) method, to the evaluation of in vivo absorption time using plasma concentration data following single dose administration. The object of the present report is to apply the MRT method, as well as conventional pharmacokinetic techniques, and to evaluate data derived from comparative bioavailability trials of controlled release formulations versus conventional products. The analyses were performed on data from single dose as well as from multiple dose studies conducted in our laboratories.

METHODS

Single Dose Studies

Quinidine. Twelve normal volunteers participated in this trial. The test product was a prolonged release formulation and the reference a conventional tablet, both containing 166 mg of "quinidine base equivalent." Following both treatments, blood was sampled at appropriate intervals over a period of thirty hours.

Theophylline. Eight normal volunteers participated in this study. The test product was a sustained release product containing 180 mg of theophylline as well as ephedrine and phenobarbital; the reference tablet contained 130 mg of theophylline as well as other ingredients. Following both treatments, blood was sampled at appropriate intervals over a 24-hour period.

Multiple Dose Study

Twelve normal volunteers participated in this study. The subjects were given either a single dose of a controlled release tablet containing 1 mg betamethasone disodium phosphate in the outer core and an equivalent "delayed release" dose of betamethasone disodium phosphate in the inner core, or two separate (2 x 0.5 mg) tablets containing betamethasone, 4 hours apart, according to a cross-over design. Following both treatments, blood was sampled at appropriate times over a period of 27 hours.

Mathematical and Statistical Analysis of the Data

MRT values were derived by the linear trapezoidal rule and percent absorbed ($At/A\infty$) at one hour values were calculated by the method of Wagner and Nelson. Analysis of variance (ANOVA) was performed on the $\log_{10}$ transformed data and the 95% confidence limits (CI) are expressed as mean ± percent mean.

The following equations are used for the interpretation of the MRT values derived from the multiple dose study:

$$MRT_o^\infty = \frac{1}{2} (MRT)D_1 + \frac{1}{2} (MRT)D_2 \tag{1}$$

where D_1 corresponds to the first dose of the conventional tablet or the dose on the outer core of the controlled release product and D_2 corresponds to the second dose or the dose of the inner core. It is assumed that $D_1 = D_2$ and:

$$MRT_{D_2} = \frac{\int_{t_o}^{\infty} (Cp - Cp_{t_o} e^{-kt^1})t^1 dt}{\int_{t_o}^{\infty} (Cp - Cp_{t_o} e^{-kt^1})dt} \tag{2}$$

where $t^1 = t - t^o$.

RESULTS AND DISCUSSION

The results of the analyses of the three trials are summarized in Table I. For the single dose studies, the 95% CI for MRT values are much narrower than those for the percent absorbed values as calculated by the conventional pharmacokinetic technique. For both the quinidine and the theophylline studies, the MRT for the test is significantly longer than for the reference. The MRT analysis of betamethasone data derived from the multiple dose study indicated that the mean ($MRT D_2/MRT\infty$) ratio is 0.995 for the reference and in agreement with the theoretical value of one, whereas the ratio for

Table I. Pharmacokinetic analyses of three bioavailability studies by different methods.

	Quinidine[a]		Theophylline[b]		Betamethasone[a]	
	MRT_0[30] (hr)	(A_t/A_∞)[c] % at 1 hr	MRT_0[24] (hr)	(A_t/A_∞) % at 1 hr	MRT_0[27] (hr)	$\dfrac{MRTD_2}{MRT_\infty}$
Reference	7.9 (9.8)[d]	64.2 (55.8)	7.9 (6.2)	98.8 (13.6)	10.2 (6.1)	0.995
Test (prolonged release)	9.1 (5.4)	34.1 (44.3)	8.8 (5.0)	81.9 (23.4)	11.1 (7.6)	1.14
Geometric mean ratio (%)	115.0[e]	54.3[e]	111.5[e]	81.1	108.0[e]	–
95 % CI						
U.L.	μ +4.8 % μ	+44.8 % μ	μ +10.0 % μ	+37.2 % μ	μ +3.8 % μ	–
L.L.	μ −5.1 % μ	−81.2 % μ	μ −11.1 % μ	−59.1 % μ	μ −4.0 % μ	–

a $N = 12$.

b $N = 8$.

c (A_t/A_∞) % at 1 hr, percentage absorbed of total (asymptotic) at specific time calculated according to Wagner-Nelson equation.

d % CV appears in parentheses.

e Significantly different at $\alpha = 0.05$ level based on 2-tailed T test.

the tested product is 1.14 which indicates that the "second dose" exhibits slower release characteristics.

In conclusion, the narrow 95% CI obtained for MRT values in this limited study indicate that the first moment analysis method is suited for the evaluation of controlled release formulations.

REFERENCE

1. S. Riegelman and P. Collier, The application of statistical moment theory to the evaluation of in vivo dissolution time, and absorption time, J. Pharmacokin. Biopharm. 8:509-533 (1980).
2. J.C.K. Loo, N. Jordan, C. Charette, R. Brien and I.J. McGilveray, Pharmacokinetic evaluation of a conventional and controlled release product of betamethasone, Biopharm. Drug Dispos. 5:97-100 (1984).

Communication 3

CONCEPT OF TIME-AVERAGED TOTAL CLEARANCE AND MEAN RESIDENCE TIME IN MICHAELIS-MENTEN ELIMINATION SYSTEMS

A.E. Staubus and D.F. Smith

Division of Pharmaceutics and Pharmaceutical Chemistry
College of Pharmacy and The Clinical Pharmacology/
Pharmacokinetic Laboratory
The OSU Comprehensive Cancer Center
Ohio State University
Columbus, Ohio

In contrast to first-order elimination systems, time-averaged clearance (Dose/$AUC_{0\to\infty}$) in Michaelis-Menten elimination systems is considered to be meaningless since the instantaneous clearance [Vmax/(Km + Cp)] in such systems changes as a function of time and concentration. The mean residence time is also not considered to be meaningful in Michaelis-Menten systems since it is normally calculated using the first-order assumption for the area under the first moment curve. However, computer simulations demonstrate the applicability of the time-averaged total clearance to multiple-compartment model systems with Michaelis-Menten elimination. Such simulations show that useful Michaelis-Menten parameters and mean residence times can be obtained from plasma concentration-time data.

Numerical integration of the differential equations describing the particular model was performed via the 4th order Runge-Kutta numerical integration technique on an IBM 4331 VM/CMS system. Computer simulations were performed for both the one- and two-compartment open model systems having Michaelis-Menten elimination or parallel first-order and Michaelis-Menten elimination from the central compartment.

Time-averaged clearance (Dose/$AUC_{0\to\infty}$) was calculated for each dose ranging from 0.01 to 2700 mg. First moment plots (t·Cp versus t) were also constructed for each dose (Fig. 1). Although the <u>area</u> under the first moment of the plasma curve ($AUMC_{0\to\infty}$) requires the assumption of first-order kinetics, the <u>peak time</u> of the first

411

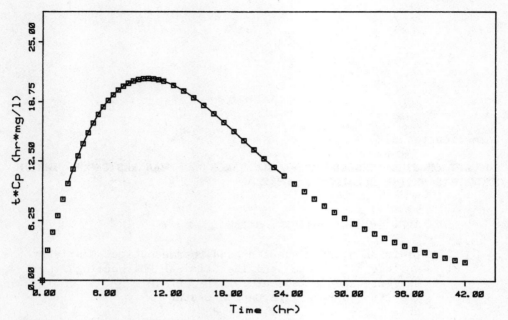

Figure 1. First moment plot of a 100 mg i.v. bolus administered into a two-compartment open model system where
Vmax = 0.234 mg/min, Km = 5.12 mg/L and Vd_{ss} = 19.84
L.   Peak time ($\bar{t}$) for this dose corresponds to 10.8
hours.   Peak time can be obtained by graphical analysis
or by polynomial curve fitting of the upper portion of
the plot, followed by setting the first derivative of
the fitted equation to zero and then selecting the root
corresponding to the peak time.

moment of the plasma curve (tmax) does not require such an assumption.   Peak time of the first moment curve corresponds to the
mean residence time ($\bar{t}$) whenever the elimination rate constant
($\bar{C}L/V_1$) is rate-limiting with respect to the distribution rate
constant k_{21}; that is, when k_{21} = 10 $\bar{C}L/V_1$, $\bar{t}$ = tmax – (0.25 →
2.56%); when k_{21} = 5 $\bar{C}L/V_1$, $\bar{t}$ = tmax – (0.31 → 5.22%).

The mean residence time for Michaelis-Menten eliminated drugs
ranges from the time corresponding to the elimination of 50%
(pseudo-zero-order) to 63.2% (pseudo-first-order) of a given dose.
Noncompartmental determination of the steady-state volume of
distribution (Vd_{ss}) for either first-order or Michaelis-Menten
elimination can be obtained from the peak time of the first moment
curve and the time-averaged total clearance:

$$Vd_{ss} = \bar{t}\ \overline{CL} \tag{1}$$

A new term, $\hat{C}p$, can be defined as the "mean distribution concentration" for a given dose. For i.v. bolus administration:

$$\hat{C}p = \frac{Dose}{2\ Vd_{ss}} \tag{2}$$

For i.v. infusion administration:

$$\hat{C}p = \frac{Ro\ \tau}{2\ Vd_{ss} + \overline{CL}\ \tau} \tag{3}$$

where Ro is the infusion rate and τ is the infusion time. As τ approaches infinity, $\hat{C}p$ approaches the value of Cp_{ss}. For oral administration:

$$\hat{C}p = \frac{F\ Dose}{2\left[(\overline{CL}/ka) + Vd_{ss}\right]} \tag{4}$$

where F is the extent of bioavailability and ka is the apparent first-order absorption rate constant.

For model systems having only Michaelis-Menten elimination, the Michaelis-Menten parameters, Vmax and Km, can be determined from examination of $\overline{CL}$ and $\hat{C}p$ for two or more doses:

$$\overline{CL} = \frac{Vmax}{Km + \hat{C}p} \tag{5}$$

For model systems having parallel first-order and Michaelis-Menten elimination, the Michaelis-Menten parameters and the first-order clearance component (CL') can be determined from examination of $\overline{CL}$ and $\hat{C}p$ for three or more doses:

$$\overline{CL} = \frac{Vmax}{Km + \hat{C}p} + CL' \tag{6}$$

For a single i.v. bolus dose of a drug eliminated solely with Michaelis-Menten kinetics, the Michaelis constant, Km, can theoretically be determined from the ratio of $AUC_{0 \to \bar{t}}/AUC_{0 \to \infty}$ and $\hat{C}p$. The value of $AUC_{0 \to \bar{t}}/AUC_{0 \to \infty}$ ranges from 0.632 (pseudo-first-order) to 0.750 (pseudo-zero-order) and is a linear function of the degree of saturation ($\hat{C}p/(Km + \hat{C}p)$):

$$Km = \frac{\hat{C}p}{m(AUC_{0 \to \bar{t}}/AUC_{0 \to \infty}) + b} - \hat{C}p \tag{7}$$

where m = 8.4746 and b = -5.3559. Having calculated Km from Equation (7), Vmax can be obtained from Equation (8):

$$\text{Vmax} = \overline{CL} \ (Km + \hat{Cp}) \tag{8}$$

Therefore by examination of the apparent time-averaged clearances and mean residence times for multiple compartment Michaelis-Menten eliminated drugs, calculations of Vd_{ss}, Cp, Km and Vmax can now be more readily performed.

Communication 4

A GENERAL METHOD OF OPTIMIZING INDIVIDUAL DRUG DOSAGE

Keith T. Muir

School of Pharmacy
University of Southern California
Los Angeles, California

For many drugs there is a high correlation between the concentration of drug in serum and clinical reponse. Optimal therapy with these drugs requires exceeding a minimal effective concentration (below which no adequate response is seen) while remaining below a maximal allowable concentration (above which drug toxicity becomes evident). Thus, a dose may be chosen quite rationally by the use of a desired serum concentration as the "therapeutic" end point. However, it is not possible to give the same dosage to all patients; a dose which proves effective in one patient will be ineffective in some and even toxic in others. This is because the dosage required to achieve serum concentrations within a certain, frequently narrow, range is confounded by variations in the way in which different individuals distribute and eliminate drugs.

The prediction of individual dosage requires a knowledge of individual pharmacokinetic characteristics. Population average pharmacokinetic parameters can be obtained from the literature (prior information) and can be adjusted for certain indirect but clinically relevant features (such as age, weight and renal/cardiac/hepatic function) in order to arrive at an estimate of an individual patient's pharmacokinetic parameters. However, this approach is rarely adequate due to substantial interindividual variations which still persist. Blood concentration measurements are therefore obtained in order to check and, if necessary, adjust the dosage regimen. Frequently such measurements are then regarded as the only important pharmacokinetic information and individual parameters are chosen which minimize (squared) deviations between the predicted and observed blood concentrations. Prior information regarding the population from which the individual comes is frequently discarded at this point despite the fact that only a small number of error-containing measurements may be available.

A Bayesian approach to the estimation of these pharmacokinetic parameters also considers the minimization of deviations between the predicted and observed concentrations (see Chapter 22). In addition, however, the likelihood of very unusual kinetic parameters (in the form of significant deviations from the population average values) is also minimized. Thus, the parameter estimates chosen must strike a balance between the probability of the deviation from the population mean parameter (a function of the interindividual standard deviation) and the uncertainty in the measured concentrations (primarily, though not exclusively, a function of the assay error standard deviation). If these standard deviations are known, then an optimally weighted average parameter estimate can be obtained (that is, a weighted average of the prior expectation – the population average, and the observed outcome – parameter estimates which would be obtained by minimizing only deviations between the observed and predicted concentrations). This procedure requires the minimization of a function which is nonlinear in the parameters. Until recently, the implementation of such an algorithm was thought possible only on large and expensive computers and, consequently, the method was unappealing. However, if a first-order approximation is made of this nonlinear function, then the algorithm can be implemented on a programmable calculator with only a minimal loss of information. This was the version utilized in the present analysis. Even a single measured concentration can be used in the Bayesian method to estimate any number of pharmacokinetic parameters (additional information being present in the form of the population average parameter values, their interindividual standard deviations, and the error standard deviation of the assay procedure). On the other hand, classical methods require at least as many measured concentrations as parameters to be estimated and ideally more.

The Bayesian method has been tested by its application to the estimation of theophylline pharmacokinetic parameters (clearance and volume of distribution) during a simulated intravenous infusion of aminophylline. In practice, this would allow early adjustment of the infusion rate in order to avoid toxic or ineffective steady-state plasma concentrations of the drug. Unfortunately, only small differences between successive blood concentration determinations may exist and these small differences may be exceedingly sensitive to error in the measurement. Random values for clearance and volume of distribution (based on the generally well documented distributions of these values in typical populations) were generated and used to simulate two plasma concentrations of theophylline during an intravenous infusion. A realistic degree of error was then added to these simulated concentrations (mean error = 0, error standard deviation = 2.0 mg/L). The original parameters were then

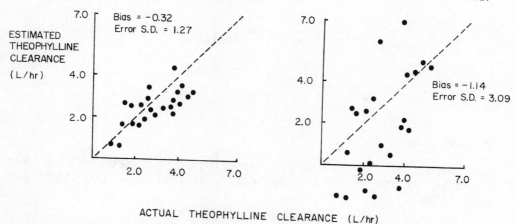

Figure 1. Comparison of Bayesian versus classical methods to estimate theophylline clearance for two plasma concentration measurements during an intravenous infusion.

re-estimated using the Bayesian technique described above and by a classical method in which the volume of distribution is assumed to be known and the deviations between predicted and observed concentrations are minimized by setting these deviations to zero; that is, by assuming that no error exists (1). Both the bias and precision of the Bayesian estimation procedure were significantly improved when compared to the classical method of parameter estimation when two data points, three to six hours apart, were used to estimate each individual's parameters (Fig. 1). The relative simplicity of the classical method (a short and simple arithmetic calculation) has undoubted appeal when compared to the more complex Bayesian algorithm. However, the classical method (as with any least squares approach) sometimes produces impossible (negative) estimates for clearance, attesting to the problems which might be encountered when trying to estimate pharmacokinetic parameters in a clinically constrained environment. The "buffering effect" of the Bayesian method in essentially preventing unrealistic parameter estimates is convincingly displayed.

REFERENCE

1. W.L. Chiou, M.A.F. Gadalla and G.W. Peng, Method for the rapid estimation of total body drug clearance and adjustment of dosage regimens in patients during a constant rate intravenous infusion, J. Pharmacokin. Biopharm. 6:135-151 (1978).

Communication 5

ESTIMATION OF POPULATION PHARMACOKINETIC PARAMETERS WITH THE COMPUTER SYSTEM NONMEM: PATIENTS TREATED WITH LIDOCAINE AND MEXILETINE

S. Vozeh and F. Follath

Division of Clinical Pharmacology
Department of Medicine, University Hospital
Kantonsspital
Basel, Switzerland

Estimation of pharmacokinetic parameters in a patient population in which a drug is used therapeutically is often difficult
because the experimental design of pharmacokinetic studies may not
be suitable for patients who are treated with the drug. Consider,
for example, the widely used antiarrhythmic lidocaine. Although
its pharmacokinetics have been extensively investigated by several
groups, no study has been reported, to our knowledge, in which all
four parameters describing the two-compartment pharmacokinetic
model have been reliably estimated in a larger group of patients.
This is not surprising considering the elaborate experimental
design that must be employed to describe the parameters of the full
two-compartment open model that characterizes lidocaine pharmacokinetics.

Sheiner and co-workers have recognized this handicap of
classical pharmacokinetic studies and proposed a novel approach
which can use unsystematically sampled serum concentrations with
few measurements per individual to determine the mean population
parameters and their interindividual variability (1). We used
NONMEM, a computer program recently developed by Beal and Sheiner
(2), for the analysis of the nonlinear mixed effects regression
model to analyze data from patients treated with the antiarrhyth-
mics lidocaine and mexiletine. Three hundred and twenty-seven
serum concentration measurements in 42 patients receiving lidocaine
for treatment of ventricular arrhythmias after an acute coronary
episode were available for the analysis. Seven patients were women
and 22 had congestive heart failure (CHF). In 22 patients at least

418

one blood sample was obtained within 15 minutes after the initiation of therapy, yielding information about the "distribution phase." In 10 patients the serum concentration of lidocaine was followed for 24 hours after the infusion had been stopped. In no instance was the dosing regimen changed because of the study.

The deterministic model used to describe the pharmacokinetics of lidocaine was the two-compartment open model with a zero-order input. To describe the interindividual variability of the serum concentrations in the population studied, each parameter to be estimated (the total body clearance $(CL), V_1, k_{12}, k_{21}$) is expressed as the population mean $(\bar{P})$ and the random deviation (η). The population average and the variance of η are estimated by NONMEM. The statistical model used in NONMEM allows one to investigate the effect of different factors on the pharmacokinetic parameters. Of the four factors tested (sex, age, time in therapy and CHF), only CHF could be shown to have a significant effect on lidocaine's pharmacokinetics. The average CL was decreased in CHF by 46% and V_1 was decreased by 23%. Clearance in patients without CHF was 0.6 L/hr/kg, V_1 was 0.61 L/kg, k_{12} was 1.6 hr^{-1} and k_{21} was 0.62 hr^{-1}. The interindividual variability was large, even after adjusting for CHF (coefficient of variation 64% for CL and 34% for V_1). Our estimate of CL compares well with the results of Zito et al. (3) who found an average CL in patients without CHF of 0.65 L/hr/kg.

The larger average decrease in the presence of CHF may be due to the fact that some of their patients were more severely ill than ours. It was difficult to compare our estimates of the remaining pharmacokinetic parameters with the findings of others because, as mentioned before, most studies in patients do not describe the full two-compartment model. We took, therefore, another approach. Woosley and Shand reported the average serum lidocaine concentration in 13 patients without CHF receiving a rapid infusion (120 µg/kg/min) for 25 minutes, followed by a maintenance infusion of 32.7 µg/kg/min (4). Figure 1 shows the measured serum concentrations in these 13 patients and the average concentration predicted with the parameter estimates obtained in our study. A good agreement between the predicted and measured values is apparent.

Four hundred and fifty-two serum concentrations in 58 patients were available for the determination of the population pharmacokinetic parameters of oral mexiletine. Twenty-seven patients had evidence of CHF, 8 had a liver function impairment including 4 severe cases. No effect of CHF on the pharmacokinetics of oral mexiletine was found. In patients with liver disease, the oral mexiletine clearance was lower, but the effect was not statistically significant, probably because of the small number of patients with severe liver function impairment. The estimates of the population average and the interindividual variability (CV) of the

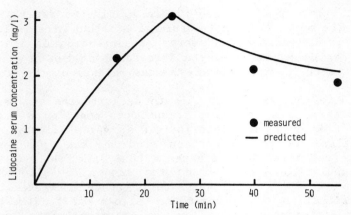

Figure 1. Average serum concentration of lidocaine in 13 patients
receiving a two-infusion dosing regimen as reported by
Woosley and Shand (4). The solid line represents the
concentration predicted with the parameters estimated in
our study.

pharmacokinetic parameters were CL = 0.38 (42%) L/hr/kg, Vd = 5.3
(40%) L/kg, ka = 3.1 (205%) hr^{-1}, time lag = 0.3 hr. Our estimates
are in very good agreement with the results reported by Prescott et
al. (5), who found an average oral clearance of 0.34 L/hr/kg in 101
patients at steady state on maintenance therapy.

In conclusion, our experience with NONMEM confirms the theoretical advantages of this new method. We believe that because of
its unique features, which allow one to estimate pharmacokinetic
parameters and their interindividual variability from fragmentary
patient data, the NONMEM system has great potential in clinical
pharmacokinetics.

Acknowledgment. Supported in part by the Swiss National Research
Foundation.

REFERENCES

1. L.B. Sheiner, B. Rosenberg and V.V. Marathe, Estimation of
    population characteristics of pharmacokinetic parameters from
    routine clinical data, J. Pharmacokin. Biopharm. 5:445–479
    (1977).
2. L.B. Sheiner and S.T. Beal, Evaluation of methods for esti-
    mating population pharmacokinetic parameters. I. Michaelis-
    Menten model: routine pharmacokinetic data, J. Pharmacokin.
    Biopharm. 8:553–571 (1980).

3. R.A. Zito and P.R. Reid, Lidocaine kinetics predicted by indocyanine green clearance, N. Engl. J. Med. 298:1160–1163 (1978).
4. R.L. Woosley and D.G. Shand, Pharmacokinetics of antiarrhythmic drugs, Am. J. Cardiol. 41:986–995 (1978).
5. L.F. Prescott, J.A. Clements and A. Pottage, Absorption, distribution and elimination of mexiletine, Postgrad. Med. J. 53 (Suppl. 1):50–55 (1977).

Communication 6

CONSIDERATIONS OF LINEAR REGRESSION WITH ERRORS IN BOTH VARIABLES AS APPLIED TO CLINICAL PHARMACOKINETICS

M.R. Blum, S.H.T. Liao and G. Hajian

Wellcome Research Laboratories
Research Triangle Park
North Carolina

The straight line equation $y = \alpha + \beta x$ is often used in the biological sciences to describe the relationship between two measured variables. In clinical pharmacokinetics, a linear model is used in many different situations (to describe the relationship between renal function and drug half-life or for correlating plasma drug concentrations with concentrations in other biological fluids, for example). During the pharmacokinetic analysis of a new anti-viral agent, acyclovir, a linear model was sought to correlate the total body clearance (CL_{tot}) with the endogenous creatinine clearance (CL_{cr}). Such a linear model is useful in developing dosage recommendations for patients with varying degrees of renal insufficiency. The almost exclusive approach of finding the "best fit" solution to the straight line equation is by linear least squares regression analysis of y on x. It is not widely recognized that this analysis assumes that only y is subject to error and that α and β are estimated by minimizing the sum of squared deviations of y only. When both x and y are subject to error, the usual least squares regression underestimates the slope and overestimates the intercept.

The linear regression problem has recently been the subject of a thorough examination by Riggs et al. (1). Several methods have been extensively evaluated by these investigators using Monte Carlo simulations. "Weighted perpendicular least squares" or weighted orthogonal regression was found to be generally the most satisfactory method to use, whereas "geometric mean" or geometric regression was found to be a good method when the relative size of the errors in x and y is in a limited range.

422

Dolby (2) has also presented a maximum likelihood solution to the linear regression problem. The relative sizes of the errors must be known, and the slope β is a root of a quintic polynomial equation. The relative sizes of the errors are hard to obtain in clinical pharmacokinetics and the maximum likelihood solution is too complex to be of practical application in clinical pharmacokinetics.

In the present study, Monte Carlo simulations of the linear model were carried out with data which were more representative of parameters and anticipated error terms encountered in our problem of finding the linear relationship between CL_{tot} and CL_{cr}. Orthogonal and geometric regressions, the most promising methods from Riggs' study, were evaluated along with the usual least squares regression of y on x. Orthogonal regression minimizes the sum of the squared perpendicular deviations from the observed points to the line while least squares regression minimizes the sum of the squared vertical deviations from the points to the line. Unweighted orthogonal regression is a solution to the special case where the error terms in x and y are equal. Weighted orthogonal regression can be applied when they are not equal. The slope of geometric regression, β_G, is calculated by the following equation:

$$\beta_G = (\beta_{yx} \cdot \beta_{xy})^{1/2}$$

(1)

where β_{yx} and β_{xy} are the slopes of the least squares regression of y on x and x on y, respectively. Geometric regression does not require an estimate of the relative sizes of the errors in x and y, while weighted orthogonal regression does.

The Monte Carlo simulation model applied in this study differs from Riggs' study in two ways: x values are random numbers from a normal distribution instead of equally spaced numbers in a given range, and the errors in both x and y are random numbers from a normal distribution $N(0,\sigma^2)$ where σ is a _constant_ _fraction_ of x or y (i.e., 10%, 20% or 30%) instead of a constant, independent of x and y values. In the Monte Carlo simulations, a linear model was defined with a given α and β. N points of x_i were generated from a normal distribution with mean μ_x and variance σ_x^2. N points of y_i were generated for each x_i based on the linear model. Random errors δ and ε were added to x_i and y_i, respectively, to generate n "observed" points for an "experiment." δ and ε are generated from normal distributions with the mean equal to zero and the variance of σ_δ^2 and σ_ε^2, respectively. Two hundred replicate "experiments" were generated with a given α, β, σ_ε^2 and λ, where $\lambda = \sigma_\varepsilon^2/\sigma_\delta^2$. λ is dependent on the relative scales of x and y. A linear "star" transformation (1) was applied to reduce x and y dimensionless. K^2 defines the variance ratio after transformation:

$$K^2 = \sigma_{\varepsilon*}^2/\sigma_{\delta*}^2 = \lambda \cdot S_{xx}/S_{yy} \tag{2}$$

where S_{xx} and S_{yy} are sums of squared deviations of x and y. When the percent errors in x and y are equal, $K^2 = 1$ and weighted orthogonal and geometric regressions will result in the same β. Simulated experiments with a combination of $\sigma_\delta = 10$, 20 and 30% of x and $K^2 = (1/9)^2$, $(1/6)^2$, $(1/3)^2$, $(2/3)^2$, 1, $(4/3)^2$, 2^2, 3^2 and 10^2 were employed to evaluate the reliability of estimates of α and β by each of the three methods using 10, 25 and 50 data points.

Our evaluation of the linear regression methods with a different simulation model confirms the following of Riggs' findings. Weighted orthogonal regression proves generally to be the most satisfactory method; however, it tends to give highly unreliable estimates of β when errors in x and y are large and N is small. Also, geometric regression is a good method when $0.5 < K < 2$, but it tends to overestimate β when $K > 2$ and underestimate β when $K < 0.5$. Geometric regression tends to give a more reliable estimate of β when errors in x and y are large and N is small.

When $\lambda = \infty$, least squares regression of y on x yields the best estimate of β, and when $\lambda = 0$, least squares regression of x on y yields the best estimate of β. For any given set of data, the best estimate of β falls between the two slopes, depending on the λ value. When λ is not known, geometric regression is recommended when K is anticipated to be close to 1. Least squares regression of y on x or x on y is recommended when $K \gg 1$ or $K \ll 1$, respectively. As an example, when the linear relationship between CL_{tot} of acyclovir and CL_{cr} was examined, information about the relative size of the errors in these two parameters was not available. The values of CL_{tot} were approximately 3 times the values of the corresponding CL_{cr}. It was anticipated that these two parameters were subject to approximately the same percent error (e.g., $\lambda \cong 9$) and result in $K = [(S_{xx}/S_{yy})\lambda]^{1/2} \cong 1$. Geometric regression was applied under these circumstances and the relationship $CL_{tot} = 28.7 + 3.37\ CL_{cr}$ was derived, whereas usual least squares regression gave $CL_{tot} = 123 + 1.96\ CL_{cr}$. The predicted CL_{tot} by geometric regression for anuric patients was subsequently confirmed in a study of acyclovir pharmacokinetics in end stage renal disease (3).

REFERENCES

1. D.S. Riggs, J.A. Guarnieri and S. Addelman, Fitting straight lines when both variables are subject to error, Life Sci. 22:1305-1360 (1978).
2. G.R. Dolby, The ultrastructural relation: A synthesis of the functional and structural relations, Biometrika 63:39-50 (1976).

3.   M.R. Blum, S.H.T. Liao and P. de Miranda, An overview of
      acyclovir pharmacokinetic disposition in adults and children,
      Am. J. Med. 73:1A, 186–192 (1982).

Communication 7

INTESTINAL DRUG METABOLISM – PRESYSTEMIC AND SYSTEMIC MECHANISMS AND IMPLICATIONS

W.H. Barr[1], M. Chung[2] and M. Shukur[3]

[1]Department of Pharmacy and Pharmaceutics
Medical College of Virginia
Virginia Commonwealth University
Richmond, Virginia

[2]Schering-Plough Corporation
Bloomfield, New Jersey

[3]Fairview State Hospital
Costa Mesa, California

INTRODUCTION

The purpose of this communication is to briefly review a series of studies, initiated with Sid Riegelman and carried on by a second generation of graduate students, on mechanisms involved in the intestinal conjugation of drugs.

Some general conclusions regarding mechanisms involved in the metabolism of drugs in the presystemic (absorptive) phase are briefly reviewed, followed by experimental evidence that these principles may also apply to the intestinal metabolism of drugs in the systemic circulation.

Dose-Dependent Intestinal Metabolism During the Presystemic, Absorptive Phase ("First-Pass")

Early studies on salicylamide in animals and humans and subsequent studies on cortisol and cortisone in humans in which both parent drug and metabolites were studied simultaneously at different dosage levels, indicate that the intestinal sites of metabolism are usually saturated before the hepatic sites (1-3). The intestinal cell has unique structural features which facilitate

in vitro studies on the kinetics and the biochemical and physiologic mechanisms involved in capacity limited metabolism and drug
interactions. These mechanisms appear to be different for glucuronide and sulfate conjugation. In vitro studies using intestinal
everted sacs have shown that sulfate conjugation is saturated at
very low concentrations. Glucuronide conjugation shows a biphasic
curve in which higher concentrations of parent drug result in
decreased glucuronide production. Interaction between salicylic
acid and salicylamide during intestinal conjugation is competitive
for the glucuronide pathway and noncompetitive for the sulfate
conjugation pathway.

Evidence for the Contribution of Intestinal Metabolism to Systemic Elimination of a Drug

It is usually assumed that intestinal drug metabolism occurs
only during absorption through the gastrointestinal mucosa. We
have found that the contribution of the intestine to drug metabolism is not limited to the absorptive phase. The intestinal mucosa
can, in fact, contribute to the metabolism and elimination of drugs
from the systemic circulation, even when the drug has been administered intravenously.

Studies in the rabbit have shown that the intestinal mucosa
can metabolize intravenously administered salicylamide to both the
glucuronide and sulfate conjugates which are subsequently transported bidirectionally from the intestinal mucosa back to the
systemic circulation and to the intestinal lumen. Thus the intestine can behave both as a "liver" in metabolizing systemic drug and
a "kidney" in eliminating the conjugate via the intestinal lumen.

METHODS

After pentobarbital anesthesia, salicylamide was infused into
the jugular vein of 2 to 3 lb New Zealand White rabbits at a
constant rate of 2 mg/min for a period of time sufficient to reach
steady state (approximately 60 min). Blood samples were taken from
the portal vein, the inferior vena cava and the carotid artery at
35, 50, 65 and 80 minutes after the infusion was started. These
samples were analyzed for free (unmetabolized) salicylamide and the
glucuronide conjugate by a minor modification of the fluorometric
method used in earlier studies (1,2). Samples of intestinal lumen
fluid were also taken at the end of the study and analyzed for free
drug and salicylamide glucuronide and sulfate conjugates.

RESULTS AND DISCUSSION

To determine the contribution of a particular tissue or organ system to the production of a substance it is necessary only to show that an arterio-venous concentration gradient exists across the system at steady state. When the concentration of a metabolite in the venous effluent (C_{Mv}) is higher than the concentration in the arterial input to the system at steady state (C_{Ma}), then there is a net rate of production of the metabolite (dM/dt) as described by the equation:

$$dM/dt = Q_a(C_{Mv} - C_{Ma}) \tag{1}$$

where it is assumed that the blood flow into the system is the same as flow out of the system (Q_a).

Since the drug and metabolite concentrations are assumed to be the same throughout the arterial system, any convenient artery (such as the carotid) can be used as the input for all tissue or organ systems. The contribution of the intestine to glucuronidation of systemic salicylamide is shown in Figure 1. A 20% increase in the plasma concentration of salicylamide glucuronide in the portal blood (intestinal output) compared to the carotid arterial concentration (intestinal input) is seen.

As a control, blood from the inferior vena cava was also sampled since the lower extremities would be expected to behave as a nonmetabolizing system. This was found to be the case. As shown in Figure 1, there is no difference between the arterial and vena caval glucuronide concentrations.

Samples of fluid from the intestinal lumen and intestinal tissue showed significant amounts of both glucuronide and sulfate conjugates of salicylamide. Preliminary studies at higher infusion rates (4 mg/min) indicated that systemic intestinal conjugation appears to be capacity limited which is consistent with previous studies on conjugation during the absorptive phase.

These results show that the intestine can participate in the systemic elimination of drugs through metabolism by the intestinal mucosa. Several important questions remain to be explored such as the relative contribution of the intestinal site compared to other sites of metabolism (hepatic, for example). We plan also to compare mechanisms of systemic intestinal metabolism with the capacity limited conjugation mechanisms that we have observed in our previous studies on presystemic intestinal metabolism during the absorptive phase.

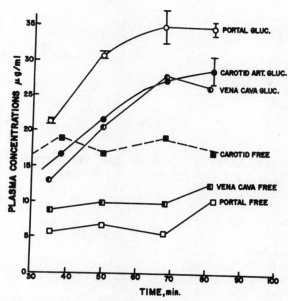

Figure 1. Evidence for systemic intestinal metabolism as shown by plasma concentrations of salicylamide (free) and salicylamide glucuronide (gluc.) in the portal vein (output of the metabolizing intestinal system), the vena cava (output of the nonmetabolizing tissue system) and the carotid artery (input to both systems) following a constant infusion of 2 mg/min of salicylamide.

REFERENCES

1. W.H. Barr and S. Riegelman, Intestinal drug absorption and metabolism I. Comparison of methods and models to study physiological variables of in vitro and in vivo intestinal absorption, J. Pharm. Sci. 59:154-163 (1970).
2. W.H. Barr and S. Riegelman, Intestinal drug absorption and metabolism II. Kinetic aspects of intestinal glucuronide conjugation, J. Pharm. Sci. 59:164-168 (1970).
3. W.H. Barr, T. Aceto, M. Chung and M. Shukur, Dose-dependent drug metabolism during the absorptive phase, Rev. Can. Biol. 32:21-42 (1973).

Communication 8

PHARMACOKINETICS OF ASPIRIN: TOTAL AND PRESYSTEMIC CLEARANCE BY
RATS AND HYDROLYSIS IN BLOOD OF RATS AND HUMANS

M. Guillaume Wientjes

Department of Pharmaceutics
School of Pharmacy
State University of New York
Amherst, New York

In the last decade, aspirin has been examined for its efficacy
as a blood platelet anti-aggregatory agent in the prevention of
secondary myocardial infarction and transient cerebral ischemia.
The anti-aggregatory effect of aspirin is due to its inhibition of
the enzyme cylco-oxygenase in platelets by irreversible acetylation. However, inhibition of this enzyme in the blood vessel wall
stimulates platelet aggregation (1). These two opposing effects of
aspirin are concentration-dependent, and it has been hypothesized
that a narrow range of aspirin plasma concentrations, or areas
under the aspirin concentration-time curve (AUC), is required to
produce optimal therapeutic effects (1). In view of the more than
threefold variation in the AUC's following oral administration of
aspirin in humans (2), it is necessary to establish the factors
which determine the systemic availability of unhydrolyzed aspirin.
In this study, the pharmacokinetics of aspirin in rats, the hydrolysis of aspirin by rat and human blood, and the correlation
between in vivo and whole blood hydrolysis of aspirin were
investigated.

Male Sprague-Dawley rats (400-500 g) received single 200 mg/kg
doses of aspirin orally and i.v. according to a cross-over design.
Blood samples were withdrawn through an indwelling jugular vein
catheter, and were extracted with acetonitrile. The organic layer
was concentrated and analyzed by reversed phase HPLC for aspirin
and its metabolite salicylic acid. 4-Methoxysalicylic acid was
used as the internal standard.   Blood concentration-time curves
of aspirin and salicylic acid in a representative rat are shown
in Figure 1. Blood concentrations of aspirin in 9 rats declined

430

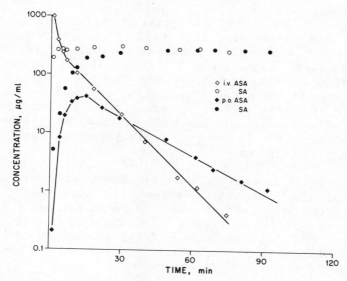

Figure 1. Concentration-time profiles of unhydrolyzed aspirin and its metabolite salicylic acid after oral and parenteral administration of 200 mg/kg aspirin to a rat.

biexponentially with time. The α and β half-lives were 1.0 ± 0.2 and 7.6 ± 0.9 minutes (mean $\pm$ SD), respectively. The blood clearance was 45.5 ± 11.4 ml/min/kg which approximates hepatic blood flow. The bioavailability of the oral aspirin solution (equimolar aspirin and sodium bicarbonate in water, 2.0 ml/kg) was $23.0 \pm 14.0\%$. Urinary recoveries of aspirin and salicylic acid after oral and i.v. doses of aspirin were essentially identical, indicating that absorption is complete. The AUC_{po} ranged from 531 to 2014 μg/min/ml with a mean $\pm$ standard deviation of 960 ± 433 μg/min/ml.

Aspirin is hydrolyzed to salicylic acid mainly by enzymatic action catalyzed by esterases which are widely distributed in the body tissues, including the liver and blood (3). The <u>in vitro</u> blood hydrolysis rate of aspirin was determined using blood samples collected from the rats two weeks after completion of the pharmacokinetic studies. Heparinized blood was incubated with aspirin at 37°C for 1-2 hours with minimal exposure to air. Changes in pH during the experiments were less than 0.2 units. Nonlinearity in aspirin hydrolysis kinetics was observed using pooled rat blood. Apparent hydrolysis half-lives ranged from 3 to 84 minutes for starting concentrations of 12 and 3800 μg/ml, respectively. The assumption of two concurrent Michaelis-Menten processes was required to describe the <u>in vitro</u> aspirin hydrolysis in rat blood. Mean parameter values were: $Km_1 = 23.8$ μg/ml, $Vm_1 = 4.8$ μg/ml/min, $Km_2 = 625$ μg/ml and $Vm_2 = 28.6$ μg/ml/min. At a starting concentration of 660 µg/ml, the apparent hydrolysis half-life in individual rats ranged from 26.2 to 36.6 minutes with a mean of 30.6 minutes (n = 9). The inter-rat variability was relatively small (coefficient of variation = 12.1%). If one assumes that the blood esterase activity correlates with liver esterase activity and that the liver is the major metabolizing organ, then a relatively large blood hydrolysis rate constant may be expected to be associated with a relatively small AUC_{po}. However, the correlation between AUC_{po} and in vitro hydrolysis constant was not statistically significant.

Hydrolysis of aspirin in human blood was determined with blood samples from eight healthy volunteers (6 males and 2 females) obtained on two or more occasions. Exponential decay of aspirin concentrations was found between 1 and 200 µg/ml, with half-lives ranging from 19.2 to 28.5 (mean = 24.6) minutes in 19 determinations. The intersubject variability (CV = 9.4%) and intrasubject variability (CV = 10.8%) were comparable.

In summary, the elimination of aspirin in rats after i.v. injection is apparently biexponential. The average systemic availability of aspirin after an oral dose of 200 mg/kg in solution was 23% (range: 9.7 to 57%); the intersubject variability of AUC_{po} in rats is comparable to that previously observed in humans. In vitro aspirin hydrolysis was nonlinear in rat blood and apparently exponential in human blood. There was little intersubject variability of the blood hydrolysis rate of aspirin in rats and humans. Whole blood hydrolysis kinetics are not a suitable indicator of oral bioavailability of aspirin in rats.

REFERENCES

1. E.F. Ellis, K.F. Wright, P.S. Jones, D.W. Richardson and C.K. Ellis, Effect of oral aspirin dose on platelet aggregation and vascular prostacyclin (PGI_2) synthesis in humans and rabbits, J. Cardiovasc. Pharmacol. 2:387-397 (1980).
2. G. Levy, Clinical pharmacokinetics of aspirin and other salicylates: Implications for research and therapy, New Engl. Soc. Allergy Proc. 2:68-71 (1981).
3. M. Rowland, S. Riegelman, P.A. Harris and S.D. Sholkoff, Absorption kinetics of aspirin in man following oral administration of an aqueous solution, J. Pharm. Sci. 61:379-385 (1972).

Communication 9

DO PLASMA CONCENTRATIONS OF ACETAMINOPHEN AND ITS CONJUGATED METABOLITES REFLECT CONCENTRATIONS IN VARIOUS TISSUES?

Lawrence J. Fischer

The Toxicology Center
Department of Pharmacology
University of Iowa
Iowa City, Iowa

The mild analgesic drug acetaminophen (N-acetyl-p-aminophenol, APAP) is hepatotoxic in large doses (1). The major pathways for elimination of APAP are by conjugation to glucuronic acid and sulfate. A smaller fraction of the drug is converted in the liver via cytochrome P-450(s) to a reactive, potentially toxic metabolite (1). This metabolite is detoxified by conjugation to glutathione, (α-L-glutamyl-L-cysteinylglycine) in liver cells (2). When the glutathione concentration in the liver is low, increased amounts of the reactive metabolite(s) of APAP bind covalently to cellular macromolecules and this apparently leads to hepatic necrosis. The glutathione conjugate of acetaminophen (A-GSH) formed in the liver is excreted primarily in the bile (3). This conjugate is then converted to the cysteine (A-Cys) and mercapturic acid (A-Mercap) conjugates of APAP and these substances are excreted in urine. The sites in the body for the catabolism of A-GSH to form A-Cys and the conversion of A-Cys to A-Mercap have not been entirely identified.

Tissue and plasma concentrations of APAP and its conjugates after administration of a toxic dose to mice have recently been reported by this laboratory (4). The data, collected for several reasons, also allowed us to determine whether the appearance and disappearance of the unchanged drug and metabolites in plasma reflected the kinetics of drug related substances in some major tissues of the body. It is the aim of the present report to show that the pharmacokinetics of APAP and some of its metabolites in liver, kidney and brain cannot always be assessed by following plasma concentrations after hepatotoxic doses.

Male Swiss Webster mice were given a 500 mg/kg oral dose of ^{14}C-APAP (ring labeled) and at 0.5, 1, 2, 4 and 12 hours the animals were killed for measurement of tissue and plasma concentrations of drug related substances. The radiolabeled drug and its glucuronic acid (A-Gluc), sulfate (A-Sulf), glutathione (A-GSH), cysteine (A-Cys) and mercapturic acid (A-Mercap) conjugates were extracted from tissue and separated by high performance liquid chromatography (4). Mean concentrations (± SE) of drug and metabolites in each tissue have been reported elsewhere (4).

Figure 1 shows tissue and plasma concentrations of APAP and the conjugates of APAP arising from glutathione conjugation of reactive metabolites. (For ease in comparing tissue and plasma concentrations of APAP and some of its metabolites, mean values reported previously have been replotted and are presented here.) Unchanged APAP (Fig. 1a) reached high concentrations in plasma, liver and kidneys at 0.5 hour and declined with an apparent half-life of one hour. Brain concentrations were somewhat lower at 0.5 hour but did not start to decline until after one hour. These somewhat lower and delayed peak concentrations of unchanged drug in the brain probably reflect the influence of the blood-brain barrier. It is apparent, however, that the kinetics of the disappearance of the unchanged drug in these tissues reflect its disappearance from plasma.

A comparison of tissue and plasma concentrations of the glutathione conjugate of APAP (A-GSH) reveals a different pattern than that shown for the unchanged drug (see Figure 1b). A-GSH was found in relatively high concentrations in liver when compared to its concentrations in kidneys and plasma. Its appearance in liver reached a peak at one hour and then declined. There was no visible peak of A-GSH in plasma or kidneys and low concentrations persisted in those tissues throughout the experimental period. It is apparent that plasma concentrations of A-GSH did not reflect liver concentrations of this conjugate. No A-GSH was found in the brain.

The cysteine conjugate (A-Cys) was concentrated in the kidneys of the mouse (see Figure 1c). Relatively low and constant concentrations of this conjugate were found in liver and plasma. The appearance and disappearance of kidney concentrations of A-Cys were not reflected in concentrations of this conjugate in plasma. Like A-GSH, A-Cys was not found in the brain.

The mercapturate (A-Mercap) was concentrated in the liver and reached peak concentrations at one hour (Fig. 1d). Kidney and plasma concentrations of this conjugate were low and relatively constant. It was apparent that peak liver concentrations of A-Mercap were not reflected by corresponding peak concentrations of the conjugate in plasma. A-Mercap also did not reach measurable concentrations in the brain.

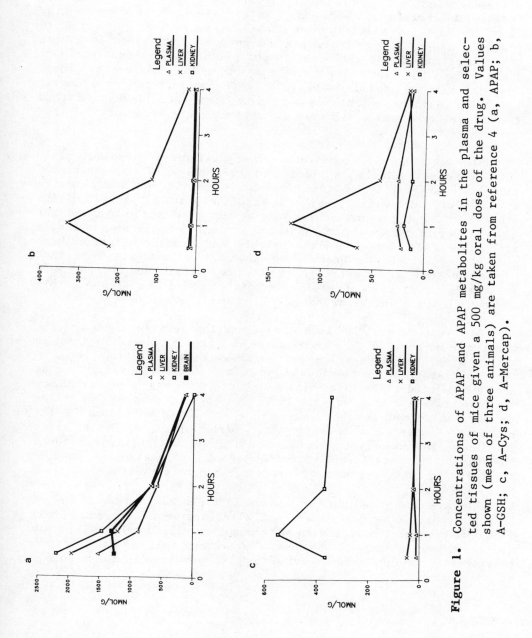

Figure 1. Concentrations of APAP and APAP metabolites in the plasma and selected tissues of mice given a 500 mg/kg oral dose of the drug. Values shown (mean of three animals) are taken from reference 4 (a, APAP; b, A-GSH; c, A-Cys; d, A-Mercap).

The data in Figure 1 indicate that the kinetics in tissues of APAP metabolites derived from glutathione conjugation are not always reflected in plasma concentrations of the metabolite. Certain metabolites (A-GSH and A-Mercap) reached peak concentrations in the liver but low constant concentrations persisted in plasma. A-Cys, in contrast, reached peak concentrations in kidney but this also was not reflected in the plasma. Not shown in Figure 1 are plasma and tissue concentrations of A-Gluc and A-Sulf. These conjugates were found to be relatively concentrated in kidneys, but their appearance and disappearance from that tissue and from the liver were reflected by the plasma concentrations of the conjugates.

The water soluble conjugates of APAP, including A-Gluc and A-Sulf, were essentially excluded from the brain. This undoubtedly reflects the ability of the blood-brain barrier to restrict the movement of hydrophilic substances into the brain by passive diffusion. Active transport of the conjugates into the brain was not apparent even though the metabolites contained endogenous moieties linked to APAP. The more lipid soluble unchanged drug reached high concentrations in the brain even though its entrance into that organ appeared to be delayed. Plasma concentrations of APAP were reasonably predictive of brain concentrations of the drug but this was not the case for water soluble drug conjugates.

The reasons for the lack of correlation between blood concentrations of certain APAP conjugates and their concentrations in either liver or kidneys are not entirely clear. Current work in this laboratory and a previously published report (5) indicate that the amino acid-containing conjugates of APAP may concentrate in certain tissues connected with their synthesis. Thus, A-GSH and A-Mercap are formed in the liver while A-Cys may be formed in the kidneys. Removal from these organs, however, must be slow relative to their clearance from the blood. That situation would produce low blood concentrations which were not responsive to changes occurring in tissues responsible for metabolite formation.

The results shown here emphasize that plasma concentrations of drug metabolites are not necessarily reflective of concentrations in tissues connected with drug action and/or elimination. This may contribute to a lack of success when attempting to use a simple pharmacokinetic approach to solve complex problems in pharmacology and toxicology.

REFERENCES

1.   J.R. Mitchell, D.J. Jollow, W.Z. Potter, D.C. Davis, J.R. Gillette and B.B. Brodie, Acetaminophen-induced hepatic

necrosis. I. Role of drug metabolism, J. Pharmacol. Exp. Ther. 187:185-194 (1973).

2. J.R. Mitchell, D.J. Jollow, W.Z. Potter, J.R. Gillette and B.B. Brodie, Acetaminophen-induced hepatic necrosis. IV. Protective role of glutathione, J. Pharmacol. Exp. Ther. 187:211-217 (1973).

3. L.T. Wong, L.W. Whitehouse, G. Solomonraj, C.J. Paul and B.H. Thomas, Separation and quantitation of acetaminophen and its metabolites in bile of mice, J. Anal. Toxicol. 3:260-263 (1979).

4. L.J. Fischer, M.D. Green and A.W. Harman, Levels of acetaminophen and its metabolites in mouse tissues after a toxic dose, J. Pharmacol. Exp. Ther. 219:281-286 (1981).

5. P. Moldeus, D.P. Jones, K. Ormstad and S. Orrenius, Formation and metabolism of a glutathione-S-conjugate in isolated rat liver and kidney cells, Biochem. Biophys. Res. Comm. 83:195-200 (1978).

Communication 10

INTERSPECIES VARIATIONS IN PHARMACOKINETICS: A PERSPECTIVE

H. Boxenbaum[1] and R. Ronfeld[2]

[1]School of Pharmacy
University of Connecticut
Storrs, Connecticut

[2]Pfizer, Inc.
Groton, Connecticut

As part of the pharmacokinetic ground plan, interspecies variations are considered and treated as a property and consequence of body size (allometry) and longevity. In 10 mammalian species other than man, antipyrine intrinsic clearance of unbound drug (CLu_{int}, liters/min) is given (1) by the following allometric relationship:

$$CLu_{int} = 0.00816\ B^{0.885} \tag{1}$$

where the coefficient takes on appropriate units and B is body weight in kg. In these same species, liver weight (L, kg) is given by (1):

$$L = 0.0370\ B^{0.849} \tag{2}$$

Combining Equations (1) and (2), one obtains:

$$CLu_{int} = 0.00816\ (L/0.0370)^{0.885/0.845} \sim 0.22\ L \tag{3}$$

This relationship indicates that antipyrine CLu_{int} may be approximated as 0.22 liters/min/kg liver weight (invariant number) in all 10 mammalian species. The CLu_{int} for man is 0.028 liters/min/kg liver weight, or about one-eighth that of other species. Similar liver weight-adjusted CLu_{int} ratios between animals and man have been noted for phenytoin, clonazepam and propranolol. Multiplying CLu_{int} by species maximum lifespan potential (MLP, years) gives the volume cleared per MLP, assuming constant drug exposure. The

438

appropriate equation for antipyrine (2) is:

$$(CLu_{int}) \, (MLP) \; = \; (0.33 \cdot 10^5) \; B^{1 \cdot 09} \tag{4}$$

Approximating $B^{1 \cdot 09}$ as $B^{1 \cdot 0}$., and assuming constant drug exposure, Equation (4) indicates that all mammalian species, including man, clear the same volume of drug per kg body weight over their lifetimes (MLP). Drug metabolism rates are models for species' capacities to dispose of naturally occurring xenobiotics (plant secondary metabolites). Chemotherapy is an invention of civilization; species were never designed or intended by nature to take synthetic substances. Relationships such as Equation (4) suggest that most mammalian species are genetically endowed with an equivalent (per kg body weight) amount of phase I hepatic "pharmacokinetic stuff." Comparative pharmacokinetics is simply the study of the rates of depletion (Abnützung) of pharmacokinetic stuff, as regulated by the pharmacokinetic clock. The situation can be complicated by internal and external perturbations to the pharmacokinetic clock, such as drug interactions, disease states, enzyme induction, wear and tear on the body and so forth.

To achieve superimposability of intravenous plasma concentration-time curves among species, either an elementary or complex Dedrick plot may be used (2,3). In the elementary Dedrick plot, plasma concentrations on the ordinate are normalized by dividing by mg/kg dose. Chronologic time on the abscissa is converted to "pharmacokinetic space-time" (kallynochrons) by dividing by B^{1-x}. Here, x is the allometric exponent relating CL to B, that is, CL $\propto$ B^x, where B^x represents the number of "working body" units, or ergosomes. In one kallynochron, all species will have cleared the same volume of drug per kg body weight. When volume of distribution is not a constant fraction of body weight, the complex Dedrick plot is used. The ordinate is plasma concentration divided by mg/kg^y, where y is the allometric exponent relating volume of distribution to body weight. Chronologic time on the abscissa is converted to "pharmacokinetic space-time" (apolysichrons) by dividing by B^{y-x}. In one apolysichron, all species will have eliminated the same fraction of the dose from their bodies.

Figure 1 illustrates an elementary Dedrick plot for antipyrine disposition in the dog and human. Using the appropriate data transformations, superimposability is achieved; one disposition half-life (mesochron) is 5.53 kallynochrons in both species. Human chronologic time in this plot is accelerated relative to the dog, whereas human data points are contracted in interspecies space. This apparent simultaneous time expansion and space contraction is redundant, since time expansion and space contraction are identical. The perspective achieved is dependent upon the reference

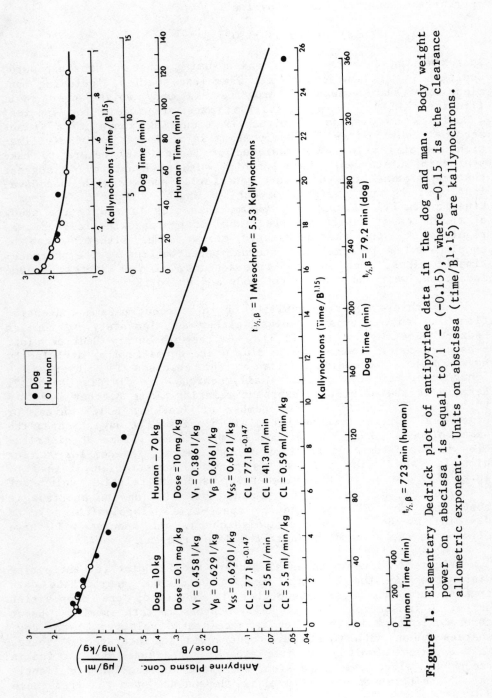

Figure 1. Elementary Dedrick plot of antipyrine data in the dog and man. Body weight power on abscissa is equal to 1 − (−0.15), where −0.15 is the clearance allometric exponent. Units on abscissa (time/B[1.15]) are kallynochrons.

system one adopts within the context of the pharmacokinetic space-time continuum, as conceptualized from the elementary Dedrick plot.

REFERENCES

1. H. Boxenbaum, Interspecies variation in liver weight, hepatic blood flow, and antipyrine intrinsic clearance: extrapolation of data to benzodiazepines and phenytoin, J. Pharmacokin. Biopharm. 8:165-176 (1980).
2. H. Boxenbaum, Interspecies scaling, allometry, physiological time, and the ground plan of pharmacokinetics, J. Pharmacokin. Biopharm. 10:201-226 (1982).
3. H. Boxenbaum and R. Ronfeld, Interspecies pharmacokinetic scaling and the Dedrick plots, Am. J. Physiol. 245:R768-R775 (1983).

Communication 11

NONRENAL ELIMINATION, EXTENSIVE RENAL TUBULAR REABSORPTION AND SECRETION OF CREATININE IN HUMANS AND ANIMALS

Win L. Chiou

Department of Pharmacodynamics
University of Illinois Medical Center
Chicago, Illinois

The nonrenal elimination (NE), tubular reabsorption (TR) and tubular secretion (TS) of creatinine (CR) in humans and animals, especially those with normal kidney function, are often assumed to be negligible (1-6). Recent preliminary studies (4-7) indicate that the magnitude of NE, TR and TS of CR might be much greater than commonly recognized. For example, plots of renal clearance (CLr) versus the reciprocal of the (pseudo-) steady-state serum creatinine concentration yielded nonrenal clearances (CLnr) of 1.4, 8.1, 35 and 42 ml/min in 4 adult chronic renal patients studied within 6 years (4). High CLnr values were also suggested from analysis of other human studies (4).

The CLnr in 5 normal New Zealand White rabbits was evaluated (6) by the i.v. steady-state CR infusion method, using a specific HPLC assay (8,9). Total body clearance (CL) and CLr were experimentally determined. The CLnr was estimated to represent a mean of 15.3% (3.6-22%) of the CL (7). A mean of about 10% in NE was also found in 5 normal rabbits after an i.v. bolus injection of exogenous creatinine.

The minimum extent of TR or TS was estimated by the secretion inhibitor method (5). Assuming that TS is completely blocked by the administration of a secretion inhibitor or competitor, the fraction (f) of filtered CR (no protein binding) reabsorbed by renal tubules can be estimated by: f = 1 - Ri, where Ri is the creatinine renal clearance to GFR ratio after inhibitor treatment, and GFR is measured by inulin, iothalmate or EDTA. Assuming TR is passive, and the fraction (f) of filtered and secreted CR reabsorbed is not significantly affected by the inhibitor, the extent of TS in terms of percent of GFR can be estimated by the relationship: $TS\% = TS \cdot 100/GFR = (R - R_i)100/R_i$, where R is the creatinine renal clearance to GFR ratio determined in the absence of secretion inhibitor. Results of some "normal" human (5) and rabbit (6) studies are summarized in Table I.

The data indicate that CR might be extensively secreted and reabsorbed by the renal tubules. Both acids and bases could inhibit the TS, reflecting the amphoteric nature of CR (10). The evidence for extensive TR was apparent in dogs, sheep and goats because their CLr/GFR ratios could be (reversibly) reduced to well below unity (0.2 - 0.5) by decreasing GFR by hexamethonium produced hypotension, hemorrhage or partial aortic occlusion (11,12). At a reduced GFR (40% of control), diuresis alone could increase the CLr/GFR ratio from 0.4 to 1.0 in a dog (11). The clinical and pharmacokinetic implications of potentially significant NE, TS or TR are discussed elsewhere (4-7).

Table I. Summary of some human (H) and rabbit (R) studies.

Subject	GFR (ml/min)	R	Inhibitor	R_i	100f	TS%
H1	~ 134	1.24	caronamide	0.60	40	107
H2	70	1.40	trimethoprim	0.76	24	84
H3	76	1.14	trimethoprim	0.78	22	46
H4	116	1.05	salicylate	0.46	54	128
H5	122	1.24	salicylate	0.44	56	177
H6	126	0.82	salicylate	0.54	46	52
H7	138	0.88	salicylate	0.61	39	44
H8	127	1.06	cimetidine	0.80	20	33
H9	153	1.21	cimetidine	0.94	6	29
R1	—	0.93	probenecid	0.86	14	8
R2	—	1.16	probenecid	0.65	35	79
R3	—	1.34	probenecid	0.58	42	131
R4	—	1.00	probenecid	0.80	20	25

REFERENCES

1. W.L. Chiou and F.H. Hsu, A new simple and rapid method to monitor the renal function based on pharmacokinetic consideration of endogenous creatinine, Res. Commun. Chem. Pathol. Pharmacol. 10:315-330 (1975).

2. W.L. Chiou and F.H. Hsu, Pharmacokinetics of creatinine in man and its implications in the monitoring of renal function and in dosage regimen modifications in patients with renal insufficiency, J. Clin. Pharmacol. 15:427-432 (1975).

3. T.D. Bjornsson, Use of serum creatinine concentrations to determine renal function, Clin. Pharmacokinet. 4:200-222 (1979).

4. Y.C. Huang, S.M. Huang and W.L. Chiou, Creatinine X. Potential nonrenal elimination of endogenous creatinine in humans and its clinical significance, Int. J. Clin. Pharmacol. Ther. Toxicol. 20:343-345 (1982).

5. W.L. Chiou, Creatinine XI. Extensive renal tubular reabsorption and secretion in man and its clinical significance, Res. Commun. Chem. Pathol. Pharmacol. 36:349-352 (1982).

6. Y.C. Huang, S.M. Huang and W.L. Chiou, Creatinine XII. Renal excretion mechanism of the endogenous creatinine in rabbits studied with a specific HPLC assay, submitted.

7. Y.C. Huang, S.M. Huang and W.L. Chiou, Creatinine XIII. Pharmacokinetics of endogenous and exogenous creatinine in normal rabbits studied with a specific HPLC assay, J. Pharmacokin. Biopharm., submitted.

8. W.L. Chiou, G.W. Peng, M.A.F. Gadalla and S.T. Nerenberg, Comparison of plasma creatinine levels in patients determined by the high pressure liquid chromatographic, autoanalyzer and boiling alkaline picrate methods, J. Pharm. Sci. 67:292-293 (1978).

9. W.L. Chiou and F.S. Pu, Creatinine VIII. Saliva levels of endogenous "true" creatinine in normal subjects, Clin. Pharmacol. Ther. 25:777-782 (1979).

10. B.R. Rennick, Transport mechanisms for renal tubular excretion of creatinine in the chicken, Amer. J. Physiol. 212:1131-1134 (1967).

11. M. Ladd, L. Liddle and J.A. Gagnon, Renal excretion of inulin, creatinine and ferrocyanide at normal and reduced clearance levels in the dog, Amer. J. Physiol. 184:505-514 (1956).

12. M. Ladd, L. Liddle, J.A. Gagnon and R.W. Clarke, Glomerular and tubular functions in sheep and goats, J. Appl. Physiol. 10:249-255 (1957).

Communication 12

PHENOBARBITAL PHARMACOKINETICS WITH PARTICULAR EMPHASIS ON THE TREATMENT OF OVERDOSED PATIENTS

J. Robert Powell
Schools of Pharmacy and Medicine
University of North Carolina
Chapel Hill, North Carolina

Phenobarbital has been used for many years as an anticonvulsant and sedative. Although phenobarbital is a relatively safe drug when used appropriately, iatrogenic or intentional phenobarbital overdosage is relatively common and dangerous without proper management. If untreated, patients may die from respiratory depression. Conservative treatment of an intoxicated patient includes correction of life-threatening symptoms which may include assisted ventilation, prevention of further drug absorption from the gastrointestinal tract, alkaline diuresis to increase the rate of phenobarbital removal from the body and to decrease drug distribution into the brain, and general supportive care. The aim of alkaline diuresis in adults is to produce a urine flow of 300–500 ml/hr and a urine pH approaching 8. More aggressive forms of therapy include charcoal hemoperfusion and hemodialysis.

Goodman et al. (1) reported the complications encountered in treating 185 barbiturate intoxicated patients. They found that the pneumonia, which was the major cause of morbidity and mortality, was best correlated with the initial depth of coma and the use of an endotracheal tube for assisted ventilation. The second leading cause of morbidity and mortality was cardiovascular instability manifesting as pulmonary edema. This was best correlated with the initial depth of coma and the volume of i.v. fluids administered. Hence, contrary to the conservative management of phenobarbital intoxication previously outlined, more severely intoxicated patients may benefit from more efficient extracorporeal drug clearance procedures. In fact, fluid overload induced by excessive doses of sodium and water during alkaline diuresis should be avoided.

445

The two objectives of this study were to determine the absolute bioavailability of phenobarbital and to quantitate the increase in phenobarbital clearance induced by alkaline diuresis. Six healthy male volunteers received three treatments in a randomized sequence: 2.6 mg/kg phenobarbital i.v. (sodium salt), 2.9 mg/kg phenobarbital orally as 60 mg tablets and 2.6 mg/kg phenobarbital i.v. followed by alkaline diuresis from 48 to 60 hours after receiving the phenobarbital dose. The alkaline diuresis treatment consisted of a 50 mEq sodium bicarbonate loading dose and a 500 ml/hr constant infusion of 5% dextrose in water with 100 mEq/L sodium bicarbonate. Plasma samples were collected for 21 days and urine for 96 hours after phenobarbital doses. Over the 12-hour alkaline diuresis period, blood and urine were collected hourly. Phenobarbital was analyzed by an HPLC technique (2). Other blood and urine measurements included electrolytes and pH.

Based on the i.v. phenobarbital dose, mean pharmacokinetic parameters were calculated: total body clearance = 3.0 ml/hr/kg, renal clearance = 0.8 ml/hr/kg, volume of distribution = 0.6 L/kg, and elimination half-life = 139 hr. The oral dose produced a peak plasma concentration of 5.5 mg/L at 2.3 hours after the dose. The percentage absorbed adjusted for variation of the elimination rate constant was 95% (2).

During the alkaline diuresis period all subjects achieved and maintained a urine pH of 7.8 and a urine flow of 500 ml/hr. Venous blood pH never exceeded 7.48. This is in contrast to the control phenobarbital dose during which urine pH was always less than 7.0 and urine flow rarely exceeded 60 ml/hr. Alkaline diuresis increased phenobarbital renal clearance to 5.1 ml/hr/kg which is a 6.4-fold increase in renal clearance over the control value. If it is assumed that phenobarbital nonrenal clearance is unaffected by alkaline diuresis, then total body clearance during alkaline diuresis can be estimated by adding renal clearance from the alkaline diuresis period (5.1 ml/hr/kg) to the nonrenal clearance from the control dose (2.2 ml/hr/kg). Hence, this alkaline diuresis regimen can be expected to increase phenobarbital total body clearance from a control value of 3.0 to an alkaline diuresis value of 7.3 ml/hr/kg. That is, alkaline diuresis increases phenobarbital renal clearance 6.4-fold, but increases total body clearance only 2.4-fold (3).

Alkaline diuresis does increase phenobarbital clearance and should decrease the duration of intoxication. Systemic alkalinization should also be beneficial by ion-trapping phenobarbital in the blood, thereby decreasing distribution into the brain. In mild to moderate phenobarbital intoxication when assisted ventilation is not necessary, alkaline diuresis should decrease the duration of intoxication. However, in the comatose patient who requires assisted ventilation and who has a very high initial phenobarbital concentration (>120 mg/L), a more efficient method of facilitated drug removal (e.g., hemoperfusion) may produce a more favorable effect on patient recovery.

The efficiency of charcoal hemoperfusion in removing phenobarbital from an intoxicated patient is illustrated in Figure 1. This 26-year-old female was admitted to the hospital with an initial phenobarbital plasma concentration of 183 mg/L. She was placed on assisted ventilation and alkaline diuresis was begun. Four hours later charcoal hemoperfusion was performed over a three-hour period. The post-hemoperfusion concentration was 94 mg/L without signs of an increase from redistribution. She was extubated 12 hours later and was discharged from the intensive care unit the next day.

If it is assumed that this patient would have been comatose until the phenobarbital concentration declined to 95 mg/L, the projected duration of coma would have been about 4 days had no method of enhanced clearance been used. At most, alkaline diuresis would decrease this period by half. In this patient, charcoal hemoperfusion may have decreased the risks of pneumonia from prolonged intubation and cardiovascular instability from prolonged alkaline diuresis.

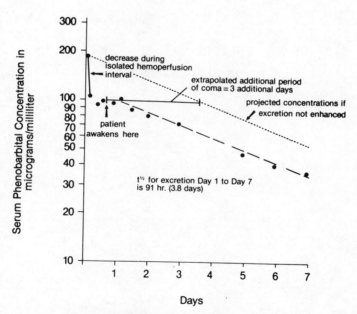

Figure 1. Serum phenobarbital concentrations during alkaline diuresis and hemoperfusion and for the following 6 days compared to projected concentrations if excretion had not been enhanced.

Pharmacokinetic techniques are clinically useful in predicting the duration of intoxication and, in the case of several poisons, may be useful in determining the most appropriate treatment.

REFERENCES

1. J.M. Goodman, M.D. Bischel, P.W. Wagers and B.H. Barbour, Barbiturate intoxication: Morbidity and mortality, West. J. Med. 124:179-186 (1976).
2. E.A. Nelson, J.R. Powell, K. Conrad, K. Likes, J. Byers, S. Baker and D. Perrier, Phenobarbital pharmacokinetics and bioavailability in adults, J. Clin. Pharmacol. 22:605-612 (1982).
3. J.R. Powell, E.A. Nelson, K. Conrad, K. Likes, J. Byers and D. Perrier, Phenobarbital disposition as influenced by alkaline diuresis, in preparation.

Communcation 13

RENAL ELIMINATION IN ALCOHOLIC CIRRHOSIS

J. P. Cello and S. Øie

Departments of Medicine and Pharmacy
University of California
San Francisco, California

Renal elimination is usually considered to be insignificantly altered in patients having alcoholic cirrhosis because the creatinine clearance remains within normal limits until the onset of the hepato-renal syndrome in end stage cirrhosis. However, it is interesting to note that recent electron microscopy studies have demonstrated varying degrees of cellular injury to the epithelial cells in the kidney (1). Two groups of investigators recently reported that although the total renal clearance of a drug remained relatively unchanged, the unbound renal clearance was substantially decreased in patients with alcoholic cirrhosis (2,3). This observation may bear importantly on drug therapy in this patient population.

To investigate this phenomenon, the renal elimination of two compounds (cimetidine, a base, and sulfisoxazole, an acid) was studied in 11 and 6 patients, respectively, with biopsy-proven Laennec's alcoholic cirrhosis. Cimetidine was studied under multiple dose steady-state conditions during a regular oral dosing interval and again during another dosing interval when an equal amount of drug given as an intravenous injection was substituted for the oral dose. Plasma and urine were collected and the concentration of drug was determined during the dosing intervals. Sulfisoxazole was studied after a 500 mg intravenous bolus dose. Plasma and urine concentrations were determined for 48 hr after administration of the dose. Four of the 6 patients receiving sulfisoxazole were restudied after clinical improvement of their conditions. Of the remaining two, one did not improve clinically and subsequently expired, while the other was lost to follow-up.

449

The renal elimination of cimetidine in this patient population was, on the average, not statistically significantly different from normal values. The renal clearance was proportional to the creatinine clearance in all subjects, regardless of whether they had normal or decreased creatinine clearance for age and weight. The correlation was found to be described by the relationship:

$$CL_R = 3.95 \ CL_{cr} - 48.8 \ (ml/min) \tag{1}$$

and is statistically significant ($r^2 = 0.923$, $p < 0.001$). No correlation between renal urine flow or urine pH and renal clearance was observed.

In 3 of 6 subjects receiving sulfisoxazole, a decreased creatinine clearance for age and weight was observed. While the 3 subjects with normal creatinine clearance had normal renal clearance of unbound sulfisoxazole, the 3 subjects with decreased creatinine clearance had a disproportionate decrease in their renal clearance of unbound sulfisoxazole (see Table I.) Although sulfisoxazole is both urine pH- and urine flow-sensitive, the observed changes were larger than could be expected from the observed renal

Table I. Renal parameters in cirrhotic patients receiving sulfisoxazole.

Subject Number	Study Number	Renal Clearance of Unbound Sulfisoxazole (ml/min)	Creatinine Clearance (ml/min)	Urine Flow (ml/hr)	Urine pH
1	1	181	108	90	7.0
1	2	131	95	72	7.5
2	1	6.3	55	45	5.2
2	2	67	105	28	5.8
3	1	184	104	121	7.6
3	2	97	90	24	7.2
4	1	8.4	63	40	5.7
4	2	68	115	107	5.6
5	1	3.4	21	18	6.4
6	1	94	103	48	6.0

pH and renal flow values in these patients. Two of the 3 patients with a decreased renal clearance were restudied after having been judged to be clinically improved. Their creatinine clearance returned to expected values (approximately a twofold increase; see Table I) and the renal clearance of unbound sulfisoxazole increased 8- to 10-fold. The sulfisoxazole increase was more than what normally could be expected from creatinine clearance, urine pH and urine flow changes.

Upon restudy after clinical improvement, two subjects who had normal renal clearance values of unbound sulfisoxazole and normal creatinine clearance values showed changes that were within normal variability in the renal clearance of unbound sulfisoxazole.

These results suggest that determination of renal function on the basis of creatinine clearance will not always reliably indicate the ability of patients with alcoholic cirrhosis to renally eliminate sulfisoxazole. Furthermore, caution should be exercised when estimating the ability of this patient population, with decreased creatinine clearance, to renally secrete drugs.

REFERENCES

1. D.H. Van Thiel, W.D. Williams, Jr., J.S. Gavaler, J.M. Little, L.W. Estes and B.S. Rabin, Ethanol. Its nephrotoxic effects in the rat, Am. J. Path. 89:67-84 (1977).

2. V.K. Sawhney, P.B. Gregory, S.E. Swezey and T.F. Blaschke, Furosemide disposition in cirrhotic patients, Gastroenterology 81:1012-1016 (1981).

3. K.-H. Breuning, H.-J. Gilfrich, T. Meinertz, U.-W. Wiegand and E. Jähnchen, Disposition of azapropazone in chronic renal and hepatic failure, Eur. J. Clin. Pharmacol. 20:147-155 (1981).

Communication 14

ALTERED DISPOSITION OF NAPROXEN BY CIRRHOTIC AND BY ELDERLY INDIVIDUALS

R.A. Upton, R.L. Williams, J.G. Kelly and J.P. Cello

Schools of Pharmacy and Medicine
University of California
San Francisco, California

Naproxen is a drug almost exclusively eliminated by metabolism
(1) and widely used for the treatment of arthritis, an ailment
commonly afflicting the elderly. Thus, with practical as well as
scientific objectives, naproxen pharmacokinetics were studied in 3
groups of 10 men each; normals, cirrhotics and elderly. Normal
(22-39 years) and elderly (65-81 years) subjects were in good
health (physical examination, blood screen, urinalysis) taking no
medication. Cirrhotic subjects (31-58 years) had Stage I or II
encephalopathy and Status A or B cirrhosis (Laennec's) by Child's
classification (2), 6 with biopsy confirmation. Three took other
drugs (aldactone, allopurinol, lactulose). In other respects (such
as weight and ethnic mix) the 3 groups were similar. All
volunteers took a single oral 375 mg naproxen dose on day 1 and
blood was sampled serially for 48 hours. Doses were then taken
every 12 hours for 6 days ending with the 13th dose at 8 a.m. on
day 9, when serial blood sampling was reinstituted for 48 hours.
Naproxen plasma protein binding was studied by equilibrium dialysis. Plasma and dialysate concentrations of naproxen were measured
by a specific HPLC assay sensitive down to 2 ng/ml (3). Pharmacokinetic parameters were estimated by standard noncompartmental
analyses.

The data are shown in Table I. Despite in vitro (4) and in
vivo data showing saturable plasma protein binding, total plasma
concentration-time profiles from all groups closely approximated
those from drugs obeying single-compartment first-order kinetics,
with no obvious differences between the profiles of normal,
cirrhotic or elderly individuals. In all individuals from all
groups, plasma concentrations in all day 9 (steady-state) samples

452

Table I. Disposition of naproxen by normal, cirrhotic and elderly subjects.

	Normals(N)	Cirrhotics(C)	Elderly(E)
% Free at 2 hr, day 1	0.13 ± 0.05	0.70 ± 0.80	0.33 ± 0.17
% Free at 24 hr, day 1	0.074 ± 0.056	0.21 ± 0.13	0.11 ± 0.03
% Free at 1 hr, day 9	0.24 ± 0.14	0.84 ± 0.66	0.39 ± 0.15
% Free at 24 hr, day 9	0.067 ± 0.035	0.20 ± 0.16	0.10 ± 0.04
$CL_{unbound}/F$ (L/hr)[a]	396 ± 155	149 ± 68	213 ± 64
$\bar{C}p_{unbound}^{ss}$ (mg/L)	0.086 ± 0.02	0.27 ± 0.16	0.16 ± 0.04
CL/F, day 1 (L/hr)[b]	0.42 ± 0.06	0.34 ± 0.11	0.32 ± 0.08
CL/F, day 9 (L/hr)[c]	0.55 ± 0.08	0.56 ± 0.10	0.50 ± 0.08
	day 1 ≠ day 9	day 1 ≠ day 9	day 1 ≠ day 9
$\bar{C}p^{ss}$ (mg/L)	58 ± 8	58 ± 10	64 ± 9
V_{area}/F, day 1[c]	9.3 ± 1.0	10.8 ± 2.1	9.6 ± 1.6
V_{area}/F, day 9[d]	12 ± 2	17 ± 5	14 ± 2
	day 1 ≠ day 9	day 1 ≠ day 9	day 1 ≠ day 9
Cpeak, day 1 (mg/L)[d]	63 ± 11	48 ± 8	62 ± 14
Interdose Cp swing (mg/L)[c]	48 ± 11	38 ± 14	41 ± 12

[a] C ≠ N ≠ E
[b] C = N ≠ E
[c] C = N = E
[d] C ≠ N = E

were higher than in the sample taken at the same time after the day 1 dose. The average accumulation factor was 1.6, approximately that expected from a first-order drug with an average 15-hour half-life dosed every 12 hours. Elderly subjects had only 76% of normal naproxen clearance on day 1 but no other differences in clearance between subject groups were statistically significant. Day 9 clearances for each group were higher than day 1 clearances, almost certainly due to the above-mentioned accumulation to steady state coupled with nonlinear protein binding. Unbound clearances were calculated from AUC based on the unbound concentration at each sampling time for day 9. (This information was not available for day 1.) Cirrhotic individuals had unbound clearances which

averaged 60% less and elderly individuals 50% less than normals.
It is noteworthy that while on day 1 and 9 the elderly appear to be
more discrepant from normals in total clearance than cirrhotics,
with respect to unbound clearance it is the cirrhotics who are
further removed from normal.   In determining total clearance,
reduced intrinsic clearance in cirrhotics and, to a lesser extent,
in the elderly is offset by an increased fraction of drug free from
plasma proteins (4 times normal in cirrhotics, 2 times normal in
the elderly at peak total concentrations).   In consequence, while
there were no detectable intergroup differences in mean steady-
state total plasma concentrations, the elderly reached twice and
cirrhotics three times normal unbound steady-state concentrations.
It is this latter measure which is the more likely to relate to
effect.   While unbound clearance gives a concentration-independent
index of clearance, there is no concentration-independent index of
volume of distribution in the face of nonlinear protein binding.
Using V_{area} as a relative measure, however, there was a trend
towards higher apparent volumes with less protein binding on both
days 1 and 9 (V_{area} for cirrhotic > elderly > normal) and between
days 1 and 9 (V_{area} on day 9 > day 1 for each subject group).   As
might be expected, there was the inverse trend in both Cpeak from a
single dose and interdose Cp swing upon multiple dosing (cirrhotic
< elderly < normal).

Thus, there is less binding of naproxen to plasma proteins in
cirrhotics and the elderly than in normal young adults, a decrease
in unbound clearance in these two groups and an apparent increase
in volumes of distribution although these are concentration-dependent.   None of these data address differences in bioavailability.
The reduction in unbound clearance probably results from impaired
hepatic function but might also reflect impaired renal elimination
of conjugates, their accumulation and subsequent ready hydrolysis
to regenerate the parent drug (5).   As a response to either mechanism, it may be desirable to reduce the dosing rate in cirrhotic
and elderly patients to as little as one-third or one-half of that
given normally.   It is interesting that the effects of disease
states can be manifold and may appear to compete with one another.

REFERENCES

1.   R.A. Upton, J.N. Buskin, R.L. Williams, N.H.G. Holford and S.
     Riegelman, Negligible excretion of unchanged ketoprofen,
     naproxen and probenecid in urine, J. Pharm. Sci. 69:1254-1257
     (1980).
2.   J.P. Cello, Gastroesophageal variceal hemorrhage - Pathogene-
     sis and management, West. J. Med. 130:531-539 (1979).
3.   R.A. Upton, J.N. Buskin, T.W. Guentert, R.L. Williams and S.
     Riegelman, Convenient and sensitive high-performance liquid

chromatography assay for ketoprofen, naproxen and other allied drugs in plasma or urine, J. Chromatgr. 190:119-128 (1980).

4.   V.H. Held, Serumproteinbindung und Eliminationshalbwertszeiten von Naproxen bei Patienten mit hepatozellulärem bzw. obstruktivem Ikterus, Arzneim. Forsch. 30:843-846 (1980).

5.   R.A. Upton, R.L. Williams, J.N. Buskin and R.M. Jones, Effects of probenecid on ketoprofen kinetics, Clin. Pharmacol. Ther. 31:705-712 (1982).

Communication 15

DRUG–DRUG INTERACTIONS: PROTEAN MANIFESTATIONS

R.L. Williams and R. A. Upton

Drug Studies Unit
School of Pharmacy
University of California
San Francisco, California

Clinicians and clinical investigators have sometimes assumed that an interaction between drugs occurs through one specific, discrete mechanism, such as displacement of a drug from plasma protein binding sites by an interacting drug or by inhibition of the metabolism of one drug by another. While this may sometimes be true, more detailed and accurate methods of pharmacokinetic analysis have suggested that drug–drug interactions may occur through several mechanisms. The final outcome will depend on the degree to which one mechanism or another is predominant. In a series of investigations assessing an interaction between a nonsteroidal anti-inflammatory agent and two potentially interacting drugs, we had the opportunity to observe in detail the multiple ways by which the disposition of one drug can be altered by another.

This study was designed to assess the influence of aspirin and probenecid on the pharmacokinetics and protein binding of ketoprofen, a nonsteroidal anti-inflammatory agent undergoing clinical trials in the United States. The study was performed as two separate clinical trials of two periods each, with six healthy male subjects assigned to each trial. In one period, ketoprofen was administered as a 50 mg oral dose every six hours for 13 doses, ending at 8:00 a.m. on the fourth day. In the second period, subjects received the same regimen of ketoprofen together with either 500 mg of probenecid or 975 mg of aspirin every six hours, given concurrently with the doses of ketoprofen. Both aspirin and probenecid were continued for an additional three doses following the final dose of ketoprofen. Blood and urine samples were collected over a six-hour (interdose) interval at steady state following the last dose of ketoprofen and analyzed for ketoprofen

456

and ketoprofen conjugates in plasma, ketoprofen binding to plasma constituents and ketoprofen conjugates in urine (1,2). Previous investigations have shown that little or no ketoprofen is excreted unchanged in the urine (3). Total ketoprofen clearance (CL) was calculated as Dose/AUC, assuming complete absorption, using noncompartmental methods for calculation. Assuming elimination of ketoprofen conjugates only into the urine, ketoprofen clearance to conjugates ($CL_{K \to C}$) was calculated by multiplying the fraction of dose appearing in urine as conjugates by the total drug clearance. Clearance to nonconjugated metabolites ($CL_{K \to NC}$) was calculated by subtracting $CL_{K \to C}$ from CL. Conjugate, nonconjugate and total plasma clearances were corrected for protein binding to give unbound clearance (CLu) by dividing the appropriate clearance by fu, the fraction of drug unbound in plasma. Renal clearance of ketoprofen conjugates ($CL_{R,KC}$) was calculated by dividing the amount of conjugates in urine in the steady-state interdose interval by the interdose conjugate AUC. The results appear in Table I.

Both aspirin and probenecid decreased ketoprofen plasma binding, reduced ketoprofen unbound clearance to conjugates, and decreased renal clearance of ketoprofen conjugates. Probenecid appeared to decrease while aspirin appeared to increase nonconjugate unbound clearance, although these results did not achieve statistical significance. In comparison to aspirin, probenecid was a much more potent inhibitor of ketoprofen conjugation and of renal elimination of ketoprofen conjugates. The net effect of aspirin on ketoprofen disposition was to increase total ketoprofen clearance without changing clearance based on the unbound concentration. The net effect of probenecid was to markedly decrease both ketoprofen

Table I. Influence of aspirin and probenecid on the disposition of ketoprofen.

Variable	(−) Aspirin	(+) Aspirin	(−) Probenecid	(+) Probenecid
fu	0.705 ± 0.104	1.28 ± 0.22[a]	0.662 ± 0.079	0.849 ± 0.107[a]
CL[b]	4.69 ± 0.28	7.74 ± 0.63[a]	6.37 ± 2.3	1.95 ± 0.44[a]
CLu	677 ± 103	623 ± 144	974 ± 370	233 ± 69[a]
$CLu_{K \to C}$	529 ± 52	381 ± 56[a]	726 ± 309	55.1 ± 29[a]
$CLu_{K \to NC}$	147 ± 63	241 ± 94	284 ± 82	178 ± 44
$CL_{R,KC}$	49.9 ± 3.37	22.8 ± 13.8[a]	32.3 ± 11.6	2.11 ± 1.57[a]

[a] Statistically significant ($p < 0.05$).
[b] Units of clearances are L/hr.

total and unbound clearance. We believe aspirin and probenecid interact with ketoprofen in similar ways, namely by interfering with ketoprofen conjugation at intrahepatic and other sites of conjugation and by reducing the renal elimination of conjugated metabolites. The influence of each drug on nonconjugate metabolism is dissimilar and less pronounced for both. We speculate that the greater lipophilicity of probenecid in comparison to aspirin allows the former drug similar access to intrahepatic and renal sites of elimination as ketoprofen and thus accounts for the demonstrably greater influence of probenecid on ketoprofen disposition than aspirin.

REFERENCES

1.   R.L. Williams, R.A. Upton, J.N. Buskin and R.M. Jones, Keto-profen-aspirin interactions, Clin. Pharmacol. Ther. 30:226-231 (1981).
2.   R.A. Upton, J.N. Buskin, T.W. Guentert, R.L. Williams and S. Riegelman, Convenient and sensitive high performance liquid chromatography assay for ketoprofen, naproxen and other allied drugs in plasma or urine, J. Chromatogr. 190:119-128 (1980).
3.   R.A. Upton, J.N. Buskin, R.L. Williams, N.H.G. Holford and S. Riegelman, Negligible excretion of unchanged ketoprofen, naproxen, and probenecid in urine, J. Pharm. Sci. 69:1254-1257 (1980).

Communication 16

KINETICS AND ANTIARRHYTHMIC EFFECT OF DIHYDROQUINIDINE

M.B. Regazzi, M. Chimienti,[1] A. Salerno[1] and
R. Rondanelli

Department of Pharmacology and
[1]Division of Cardiology
University Hospital S. Matteo
Pavia, Italy

Relatively little information is available on the absorption, distribution and elimination of dihydroquinidine, a compound known more as an impurity in commercially available quinidine preparations than as a drug itself. Conflicting results have been reported on the antiarrhythmic activity in animals and man of dihydroquinidine compared to quinidine. Different rates and extents of absorption have been reported for the available dihydroquinidine salts (1,2). We investigated the absolute bioavailability of conventional tablets of 150 mg and of sustained release capsules of 250 mg dihydroquinidine chloride in 12 patients with heart disease. Each patient received, at 3-day intervals, 300 mg (two tablets) dihydroquinidine chloride as conventional tablets, 500 mg (two capsules) dihydroquinidine as sustained release capsules, and 300 mg dihydroquinidine gluconate solution by constant intravenous infusion over a 25-minute period according to a randomized 3-way cross-over design. During the bioavailability study, the plasma and urine samples were assayed by the Cramer-Isaksson method.

After administration of 300 mg dihydroquinidine chloride as tablets, a mean peak plasma concentration of 0.74 mg/L (CV = 45.4%) was obtained at about 5 hours. Oral administration of 500 mg dihydroquinidine chloride sustained release capsules produced mean peak plasma concentrations of 0.55 mg/L (CV = 50.3%) about 7 hours later. The conventional tablets provided greater and less variable absorption of dihydroquinidine than the sustained release capsules: F = 0.89 (CV = 10.5%) and F = 0.52 (CV = 29.3%), respectively. Dihydroquinidine chloride as conventional tablets is more poorly

459

absorbed than conventional tablets of quinidine sulfate (1).
Following intravenous infusion of 300 mg dihydroquinidine gluconate
over 25 minutes, the disposition of dihydroquinidine can be described by a two-compartment pharmacokinetic model as previously
reported by Ueda et al. (2). However, the 24-hour time point was
above the fitted curve and that results in a longer half-life of
elimination ($t_{1/2}$ = 10.8 hr, CV = 43.8%). The urinary excretion
rate decayed with a half-life of 12.2 hr (CV = 26.2%). Whether
this longer half-life, apparent with our sampling schedule of 24
hours but not with the sampling schedule of 12 hours used by Ueda
et al. (2), is due to a longer exponential phase or to a decrease

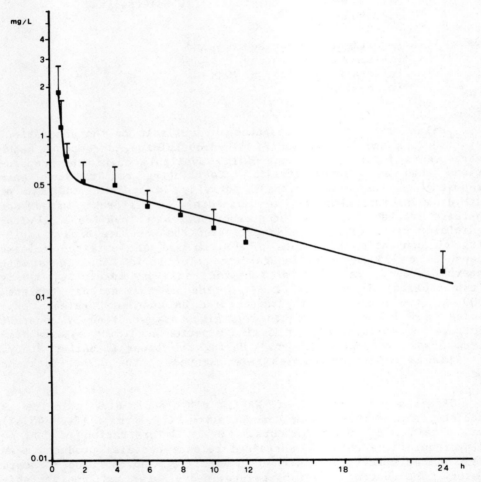

Figure 1. Mean (± SD) plasma dihydroquinidine concentration for 10
patients after i.v. infusion over a period of 25 minutes
with 300 mg of dihydroquinidine gluconate.

in metabolic activity during the night should be investigated.
Moreover, as reported for quinidine, a shoulder was frequently
observed in the plasma concentration curve after the distribution
phase, possibly due to enterohepatic cycling of dihydroquinidine
(3). The clearance of dihydroquinidine, 0.28 L/hr/kg (CV = 20.3%),
is of the same order of magnitude as that previously estimated by
Ueda et al. (2).

A discrepancy exists between the value of the volume of
distribution (V) obtained in our study (V = 4.67 L/kg, CV = 28%)
and the value calculated by Ueda et al. (2) (V = 2.7 L/kg, CV =
61.8%), reflecting, partially, the dependence of V on the terminal
disposition constant in fitting the data to the model equation
employed (Fig. 1). However, the absence in this study of a quinidine control group and the possible contribution of metabolites to
the estimate of dihydroquinidine plasma concentrations prevents
assessment of the possible contribution of a larger volume of
distribution to the reportedly more powerful action of dihydroquinidine when compared to quinidine.

In the second part of our studies we investigated the effect
of dihydroquinidine chloride (as conventional tablets) on ventricular ectopy (PVC) in 7 patients (six male, one female) aged 46 ± 17
yr. The double-blind cross-over protocol included control 24-hour
Holter monitoring (H) and 2 consecutive 72-hour periods of treatment (DQ and placebo, randomly). On the second and third day of
each period H was carried out. Plasma concentrations of dihydroquinidine were determined by HPLC assay (reversed phase). Compared
to placebo (740 ± 304), dihydroquinidine (144 ± 130, p < 0.01)

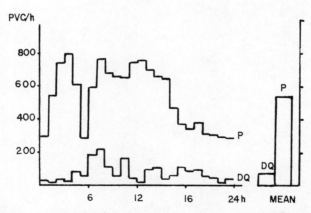

Figure 2. Number of PVC/hr on the third day of treatment with
placebo (P) and with dihydroquinidine (DQ) in patient
P.S. (DQ plasma levels: 1.31 mg/L and 1.05 mg/L, 2.5 hr
and 8 hr, respectively, after the morning dose.)

significantly reduced the mean PVC/hr, and six patients (86%) had more than a 70% decrease in PVC on dihydroquinidine (Fig. 2). The mean dihydroquinidine plasma concentrations were 1.39 ± 0.32 (SD) mg/L and 0.91 ± 0.35 mg/L at 2.5 hours and 8 hours, respectively, after administration of the morning dose of dihydroquinidine chloride tablets (300 mg every 8 hours) on the third day of therapy. The mean plasma concentration at 2.5 hours after the morning dose on the second day was 16% lower than the corresponding value on the third day. The clinical efficacy of dihydroquinidine in significantly reducing PVCs at a dose of 300 mg every 8 hours, and the lower rate of absorption of dihydroquinidine chloride with less fluctuation in plasma concentrations during multiple dosing make this molecule clinically interesting not only as an impurity of quinidine but as a potential medicinal agent itself.

REFERENCES

1. D.M. Hailey, A.R. Lea, D.M. Coles, P.E. Heaume and W.J. Smith, Absorption of quinidine and dihydroquinidine in humans, Eur. J. Clin. Pharmacol. 21:195–199 (1981).
2. C.T. Ueda, B.J. Williamson and B.S. Dzindzio, Disposition kinetics of dihydroquinidine following quinidine administration, Res. Commun. Chem. Pathol. Pharmacol. 14:215–224 (1976).
3. T.W. Guentert, P.E. Coates, R.A. Upton, D.L. Combs and S. Riegelman, Determination of quinidine and its major metabolites by high-performance liquid chromatography, J. Chromatogr. 162:59–70 (1979).

Communication 17

QUINIDINE-N-OXIDE: STRUCTURE AND PHARMACOKINETICS OF A NEW QUINIDINE METABOLITE

T.W. Guentert

School of Pharmacy
University of Basel
Basel, Switzerland

The effects of quinidine after oral doses cannot be explained by the presence of unchanged drug alone. Several pharmacologically active metabolites have been identified (1) but it remains to be established which of these or other as yet unknown metabolites contribute significantly to the clinical effects of quinidine.

We have observed a previously unreported major metabolite during single and multiple dose studies. This metabolite was isolated, identified and synthesized. Furthermore, its pharmacokinetic properties were evaluated in dogs and its binding properties to human serum proteins were determined.

ISOLATION AND SYNTHESIS

The new metabolite was isolated from 10.5 liters of human urine by extraction into dichloromethane under alkaline conditions and back-extraction into dilute sulfuric acid. After addition of ammonium hydroxide to the aqueous phase, basic compounds were again extracted with dichloromethane. Preparative thin layer chromatography (TLC), further purification by high pressure liquid chromatography (HPLC), and crystallization from hexane/ethyl acetate/methanol yielded 2 mg of white crystals with a melting point of 152-156°C.

Oxidation of quinidine with dilute hydrogen peroxide in acetone or with m-chloroperbenzoic acid in dichloromethane yielded a compound that was identical to the isolated metabolite as judged

463

from its ^{1}H-NMR spectrum, MS, melting point properties and chromatographic behavior (TLC, HPLC).

CHARACTERIZATION

^{13}C-NMR studies indicated 20 carbon atoms in the isolated metabolite. The highest mass in EI-MS studies was seen at m/e 340 and therefore a molecular formula of $C_{20}H_{40}N_2O_3$ was proposed. The MS fragmentation pattern, ^{1}H- and ^{13}C-NMR spectra agreed with the structure of quinidine-N-oxide with the additional oxygen in the quinuclidine ring. Final proof for this structure came from an x-ray diffraction analysis of synthetic quinidine-N-oxide ethanolate.

PHARMACOKINETIC BEHAVIOR IN DOGS

A dose of 32 mg/kg quinidine-N-oxide in 60 ml of a sterile solution containing 5% dextrose and 10% ethanol was administered to three male beagle dogs by intravenous infusion for 80 minutes. To maintain water balance in the animals during the experiment, a slow infusion of saline at a rate of 0.52 ml/min was begun at the end of drug administration and maintained for the first 10 hours. Drug concentrations in collected plasma and urine samples were determined using reversed phase HPLC techniques (2).

Quinidine-N-oxide concentrations in plasma followed multi-compartment characteristics. The clearance of quinidine-N-oxide (4.1 ± 0.74 ml/min/kg; mean ± SD) was comparable to that for quinidine in the same dogs (5.4 ± 3.2 ml/min/kg) or in humans (4.9 ± 1.6 ml/min/kg, (3)). Probably due to increased polarity, the volume of distribution for the metabolite (V_{ss} = 1.2 ± 0.22 L/kg) was smaller than that observed for quinidine (dogs: V_{ss} = 5.0 ± 0.91 L/kg; humans: V_{ss} = 2.3 ± 0.70 L/kg). This difference was reflected in a shorter terminal half-life for quinidine-N-oxide than for quinidine in the dogs (4.8 ± 1.6 hr versus 13.2 ± 0.63 hr).

Quinidine-N-oxide was eliminated mostly unchanged via the kidneys; 75-80% of the dose administered was recovered from urine. The renal elimination pathway was, however, concentration-dependent with saturation at higher plasma concentrations. Michaelis-Menten constants of 18.05 mg/L for K_m and 0.73 mg/min for V_{max} were estimated.

PROTEIN BINDING CHARACTERISTICS

In contrast to other quinidine metabolites, the N-oxide is bound to human serum proteins to a larger extent than is the parent drug. In five healthy volunteers between the ages of 35-62 years only 3-4% of the total N-oxide concentration in serum was unbound. As can be seen from the two examples listed in Table I, the binding was independent of the spiked concentration in the range of 70-2000 ng/ml. Interindividual variability of the binding values in the volunteers examined was very small. This might, however, be due to the restrictions imposed on the volunteers (no drug ingestion for 14 days before the study; blood collection in the morning after a light breakfast without beverages containing caffeine). A greater variability might be expected in patients.

The average binding of quinidine-N-oxide in clinical samples collected from patients with arrhythmias controlled by quinidine was not different from that found in spiked serum of normal volunteers. However, a larger span of free fractions was observed (Table I). The percent unbound values for the metabolite ranged from 2% to 7% in samples collected after multiple quinidine doses (1-2 g/day) with metabolite concentrations between 270 and 500 ng/ml. Similar binding values (fraction unbound: 3%) were observed in spiked serum from 3 cirrhotics studied. Protein binding was also determined in spiked serum samples taken from four patients following a heart attack and preceding therapy. The unbound metabolite fraction in these samples (2%) was not different from the values in the normal volunteers.

Table I. Binding of quinidine-N-oxide to human serum proteins.

Healthy Volunteers			Patients on Quinidine Therapy[a]	
Added concentration of quinidine N-oxide (ng/ml)	% unbound subject 1	subject 2	Concentration of quinidine-N-oxide (ng/ml)	% unbound
67	4.5	4.7	268	2.2
167	3.7	3.6	280	4.7
333	3.5	3.5	404	6.5
667	3.8	3.3	435	2.7
1333	4.5	3.9	502	6.7
2000	5.5	4.9		

[a]Clinical samples from 4 different subjects.

REFERENCES

1. N.H.G. Holford, P.E. Coates, T.W. Guentert, S. Riegelman and
    L.B. Sheiner, The effect of quinidine and its metabolites on
    the electrocardiogram and systolic time intervals: Concentra-
    tion-effect relationships, Br. J. Clin. Pharmacol. 11:187-195
    (1981).
2. T.W. Guentert, A. Rakhit, R.A. Upton and S. Riegelman, An
    integrated approach to measurements of quinidine and metabo-
    lites in biological fluids, J. Chromatogr. 183:514-518 (1980).
3. T.W. Guentert, N.H.G. Holford, P.E. Coates, R.A. Upton and S.
    Riegelman, Quinidine pharmacokinetics in man: Choice of a
    disposition model and absolute bioavailability studies, J.
    Pharmacokin. Biopharm. 7:315-330 (1979).

Communication 18

PHENOBARBITAL INDUCTION OF QUINIDINE PLASMA PROTEIN BINDING IN DOGS AND ITS EFFECT ON QUINIDINE DISPOSITION

A. Rakhit,[1] N.H.G. Holford[2] and D.J. Effeney[3]

[1] Drug Metabolism
CIBA-GEIGY Corporation
Ardsley, New York

[2] Department of Pharmacology and
Clinical Pharmacology
University of Auckland Medical School
Auckland, New Zealand

[3] Department of Surgery
VA Medical Center
San Francisco, California

Major known metabolites of quinidine (Q), a drug which is primarily eliminated by the nonrenal route, are similar in humans and dogs. Jaillon et al. (1) reported a decrease in clearance and volume of distribution of Q in dogs treated with phenytoin. The present study was undertaken to investigate a) whether phenobarbital (PB), like phenytoin, affects the disposition of Q in dogs, b) the mechanism of such changes in Q disposition and c) the metabolic pathways which are PB inducible. In this report, however, we will discuss only the changes in Q disposition.

METHODS

Chronic portacaval transposition and biliary cannulation were performed in each of two mongrel dogs (2). In this preparation forelimb infusion is similar to normal intravenous administration, while hindlimb infusion administers drug directly into the portal vein. The physical condition and blood chemistry of each dog were normal before and after PB treatment. The study period was divided into five phases:

467

Phase I. Quinidine gluconate in 0.9% saline was administered i.v. via the right forelimb vein for 1 hour to reach a plasma concentration of about 4.0 mg/L. This was followed by a slower rate infusion for the next 9 hours to maintain an apparent steady-state plasma concentration of 4.0 mg/L. Blood, urine and bile samples were taken at scheduled intervals during the entire infusion period. Blood sampling was continued post-infusion for a total of 50 hours.

Phase II. Two weeks later the infusion was repeated via the hindlimb (direct portal infusion) following the same schedule as in Phase I.

Phase III. One week after the end of Phase II, oral administration of phenobarbital USP tablets (10 mg/kg/day) was initiated and was continued until the end of the study.

Phases IV and V. After 2 weeks of PB administration, the forelimb i.v. administration and hindlimb infusion of Q were repeated as in Phases I and II, respectively.

Q and its metabolites in plasma, urine and bile were measured by an HPLC procedure (3). The extent of protein binding was determined using equilibrium dialysis on the 8 and 10 hour plasma samples, when the apparent steady-state concentration of Q was achieved.

RESULTS AND DISCUSSION

Changes in the plasma concentration-time course of Q before and after PB treatment are depicted in Figure 1 for dog A after an i.v. infusion. The plasma Q concentration at the end of the first hour infusion was 4.0 and 12.0 mg/L during the control and PB phases, respectively. The terminal half-life of Q decreased from a mean value of 15.6 ± 4.2 (SD) hours to a mean value of 6.2 ± 1.6 hours after PB administration (n = 4).

A comparison of systemic and portal infusion experiments showed that the liver extraction ratio for Q in dogs was very low, since the ratio of clearance values was not statistically different from one (1.08 ± 0.15, n = 4). Therefore, for practical purposes the portal and intravenous infusions have been treated as duplicate experiments in each animal. The higher plasma Q concentrations in the early part of the infusion after PB indicate a decrease in the volume of distribution for Q as a result of PB treatment. The V_{ss} decreased from a control value of 153.6 ± 20.5 L to 53.9 ± 6.1 L after PB treatment (n = 4). The volume of distribution of the central compartment (V_1) derived from a two-compartment model decreased from 37.5 ± 15.3 L to 3.4 ± 0.4 L (n = 4) after PB

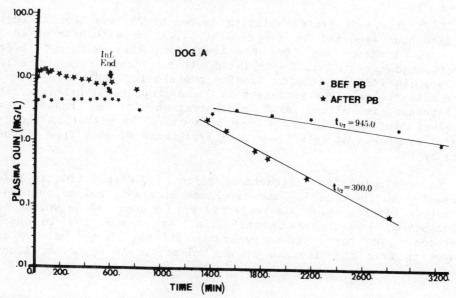

Figure 1. Plasma quinidine concentrations in dog A before and after phenobarbital (PB) treatment.

treatment. The total clearance of Q calculated from the area under the plasma concentration versus time curve was affected negligibly by PB administration (control: 6.6 ± 2.1 L/hr; PB treatment: 5.6 ± 0.8 L/hr, n = 4). The renal clearance of Q, however, decreased significantly from 1.00 ± 0.16 L/hr to 0.31 ± 0.15 L/hr (n = 4).

When plasma protein binding was measured, a marked decrease (61%) in the free fraction of Q in plasma was observed (control: 0.12 ± 0.02; PB treatment: 0.05 ± 0.01, n = 4). This increase in protein binding by PB treatment appears to be the key factor for changes in Q disposition. The steady-state volume of distribution and renal clearance for unbound Q in contrast to total Q were unaltered after PB treatment, while there was a large increase in unbound nonrenal clearance (control: 50.5 ± 23.6 L/hr; PB treatment: 124.5 ± 38.0 L/hr, n = 4). Since Q was not excreted in the bile, this increase in unbound nonrenal clearance reflects an increase in the unbound metabolic clearance of Q.

An important observation is that although the plasma Q concentration at the end of the 10 hour infusion increased from 4 to 8 mg/L, the free concentration did not increase. If unbound drug is responsible for therapeutic and also toxic effects of Q, such an increase in total drug concentration would not require a reduction of dose or discontinuance of drug.

An increase in protein binding caused by PB treatment in dogs has also been reported for propranolol (4). The mechanism of such increased binding due to PB treatment has not yet been investigated. It is speculated that changes in α_1-acid glycoprotein (AAGP), a major binding protein for basic drugs, may be responsible for such increases in Q and propranolol binding. If an increase in plasma AAGP concentration is the reason for increased binding, this could have been caused by either an induction of synthesis of this protein or by release of AAGP from tissue sites by PB.

In conclusion, PB pretreatment affected Q disposition in dogs by causing an increase in unbound plasma clearance and an increase in protein binding which was reflected by: a decrease in volume of distribution, a decrease in half-life, and a decrease in renal clearance. The total plasma clearance did not change because of changes in free fraction and unbound clearance in opposite directions.

REFERENCES

1. P. Jaillon and R.E. Kates, Phenytoin induced changes in quinidine and 3-hydroxyquinidine pharmacokinetics in conscious dogs, J. Pharmacol. Exp. Ther. 213:33-37 (1980).
2. D.J. Effeney, S.M. Pond, M-W. Lo, B. Silber and S. Riegelman, A technique to study hepatic and intestinal drug metabolism separately in the dog, J. Pharmacol. Exp. Ther. 221:507-511 (1982).
3. A. Rakhit, M. Kunitani, N.H.G. Holford and S. Riegelman, Improved liquid-chromatographic assay of quinidine and its metabolites in biological fluids, Clin. Chem. 28:1505-1509 (1982).
4. F.P. Abramson, S.A. Bai and V.T. Vu, The induction of plasma protein binding of propranolol by phenobarbital in dogs, Fed. Proc. 39:850 (1980).

Communication 19

COVALENT BINDING OF QUINIDINE

K. Maloney, W. Sadée and N. Castagnoli

School of Pharmacy
University of California
San Francisco, California

Quinidine, an antiarrhythmic agent, is known to cause a number of immunologically mediated side effects. One of these, a kind of granulomatous hepatitis, occurs in about 5 percent of the patient population. It is believed that the problem is not caused by the drug itself but rather by a reactive intermediate covalently binding to a protein. Previous investigations have been able to account for only about 50 percent of a quinidine dose in terms of the parent drug and known metabolites. One of these metabolites is the 10,11-diol. The formation of diols is known to proceed via epoxides. Epoxides are known to covalently bind to tissue macromolecules. This study was undertaken to determine if quinidine, after metabolic activation, could covalently bind to proteins and thus possibly cause these side effects.

Covalent binding was studied using the 100,000 x g microsomal pellet from rat liver. Male Sprague-Dawley rats were induced by intraperitoneal injection of 80 mg/kg of sodium phenobarbital for 4 days. On the 5th day, the rats were decapitated and the livers perfused in situ with ice cold 1.15% KCl. The livers were homogenized in KCl solution using a Dounce tissue grinder, the homogenate centrifuged at 10,000 x g for 20 minutes at 4°C, and the resulting supernatant was centrifuged at 100,000 x g for 1 hour at 4°C. The microsomal pellet was then homogenized in potassium/sodium phosphate buffer (pH 7.4) and diluted to a protein concentration of 2 mg/ml.

Incubations were performed with 3 ml of homogenate, 1mM NADPH/0.5 ml buffer, 92 μg of quinidine sulfate, or 112 μg of dihydroquinidine chloride/0.5 ml buffer and, where applicable, 10^{-4} M SKF 525A or metyrapone, 5.5×10^{-5} M trichloropropane oxide

(TCPO) and 5.6 x 10⁻⁴ M N-acetyl cysteine. Incubations were carried out for 1 hour at 37°C and NADPH was added at 0, 20 and 40 minutes. For the gel filtration experiments, 920 µg of quinidine sulfate was incubated for 3 hours with 5.5 x 10⁻⁴ M TCPO and the NADPH (3 mM final concentration) was added in portions over the 3 hours.

Incubations (except in the case of the gel filtration experiments) were stopped with 5 ml of CH_3CN. In the gel filtration studies, the microsomal pellets were repeatedly washed with aqueous buffer, again subjected to ultracentrifugation, solubilized with SDS and dialyzed overnight. After addition of CH_3CN, the samples were vortexed for 5 minutes, centrifuged at 1500 rpm, decanted and subsequently washed with CH_3CN, MeOH and 0.1 N $HClO_4$. After each washing and the first precipitation with CH_3CN, the pellets were homogenized in buffer and subjected to fluorometric analysis. Fluorescence was measured in a Perkin Elmer fluorescence spectrophotometer, at an excitation wavelength of 330 nm and an emission wavelength of 385 nm. The samples for gel filtration were placed on a Bio-Rad Bio-Gel TSK-125 HPLC column with a sodium sulfate/sodium phosphate buffer. The results are presented in Figure 1.

In the blank pellet homogenates, the residual fluorescence corresponded to 1 µg of quinidine equivalent per sample. When NADPH or quinidine was added alone, the fluorescence did not increase. However, when quinidine and NADPH were added together the fluorescence increased to 8 µg of quinidine equivalents. In the presence of SKF 525A, metyrapone and N-acetyl cysteine, the fluorescence did not exceed the blank values. In the presence of TCPO, the residual fluorescence increased to 14 µg. In the case of dihydroquinidine, there was no significant amount of residual fluorescence associated with the microsomal pellet under any experimental conditions (see Fig. 1).

In all of the gel filtration samples there is a fluorescent peak with a molecular weight of approximately 50,000 or greater. In the samples with quinidine, NADPH and TCPO together, however, the area under the peak is 10 to 15 times that of the control samples with either quinidine or NADPH alone (see Fig. 1).

These results provide strong experimental evidence that quinidine covalently binds after metabolic activation. Cytochrome P-450 may be responsible for such activation since SKF 525A and metyrapone, potent cytochrome P-450 inhibitors, decrease the covalent binding. Moreover, the increase of quinidine binding with the addition of TCPO, a potent epoxide hydrase inhibitor, and the decreased binding with N-acetyl cysteine support the hypothesis that covalent binding proceeds via an epoxide intermediate. Finally, the fact that dihydroquinidine does not seem to bind

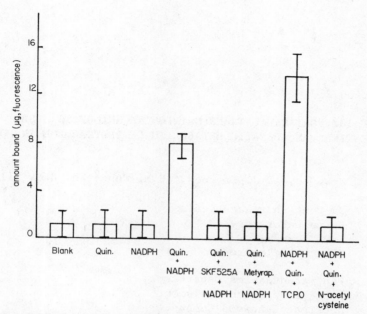

Figure 1. Binding of quinidine to microsomal proteins; the blank contains microsomal protein.

demonstrates that quinidine is probably binding via an intermediate after metabolic activation of the C-10,11 double bond. In conclusion, covalent binding of quinidine to tissue macromolecules may account for the unknown fraction of the drug in the body and moreover may be ultimately responsible for the immunological side effects.

Communication 20

THE USE OF THE PORTACAVAL TRANSPOSITION TECHNIQUE TO STUDY GASTROINTESTINAL AND HEPATIC METABOLISM OF PROPRANOLOL IN DOGS

M-W. Lo,[1] D.J. Effeney,[2] S.M. Pond[2] and B.M. Silber[2]

[1] Du Pont Pharmaceuticals
Stine Laboratory
P.O. Box 30
Newark, Delaware

[2] Pharmacodynamics Department
Medical Research Division
American Cyanamid Company
Pearl River, New York

One of the drugs used extensively to validate the "well-stirred" perfusion model of hepatic drug clearance is propranolol. However, two of the basic assumptions of the model may not be met by propranolol. These are: 1) the liver is the only eliminating organ, and 2) the intrinsic clearance of propranolol is independent of drug concentration entering the liver, and therefore, metabolism is not capacity limited. To test, in vivo, whether or not these assumptions hold when a high first-pass drug such as propranolol is considered, we studied dogs before and after portacaval transposition.

Portacaval transposition is a surgical technique that allows investigators to study gastrointestinal (GI) and hepatic metabolism of drugs in each organ separately in healthy animals (1). The surgery involves an end-to-end transposition of the inferior vena cava and the portal vein. After portacaval transposition, an orally administered drug passes through the GI tract and then enters the systemic circulation directly, bypassing metabolism in the liver after drug absorption. The same drug given by a forelimb vein is like a conventional intravenous (i.v.) dose. When the drug is administered via a hindlimb vein it enters the liver directly. In essence, the dog provides a model in which to perform chronic direct infusions of drug into the intestine or liver.

Due to the altered vasculature in dogs after portacaval transposition, the bioavailability of an oral dose obtained after surgery is the fraction of drug escaping GI metabolism, as shown by Equation (1) (assuming complete absorption):

$$F = \frac{AUC_{oral}}{AUC_{iv,forelimb}} \times \frac{Dose_{iv, forelimb}}{Dose_{oral}} \tag{1}$$

where F is the fraction escaping GI metabolism and AUC is the area under the blood concentration-time curve from zero time to infinity.

The detection of capacity limited metabolism during single or multiple dose studies may be very difficult if only the concentration-time curves of unchanged drug are examined, particularly if first-order and capacity limited metabolic pathways coexist. However, analysis of the excretion rates of metabolites easily provides the information on the kinetics of metabolism via a metabolic pathway.

After portacaval transposition, whether or not a particular metabolite (M_1) of propranolol has a constant intrinsic clearance of formation (CL_f) can be tested by infusing drug into the liver via a hindlimb vein and measuring the total excretion rate of M_1 into bile and urine. At steady state:

$$(\text{Total excretion rate of } M_1)_{ss} = CL_{f,M_1} \cdot C_{b,prop,ss} \tag{2}$$

where $C_{b,prop,ss}$ is the blood concentration of propranolol at steady state. Plotting the total excretion rate of M_1 at steady state versus $C_{b,prop,ss}$ should yield a straight line if CL_{f,M_1} is constant and independent of concentration. If a hyperbola results, the clearance term is not constant and should be expressed in Michaelis-Menten kinetic terms, V_{maxf,M_1} amd K_{mf,M_1}.

We followed three major metabolic pathways of propranolol: O-glucuronidation to propranolol-O-glucuronide (PG), ring oxidation to 4-hydroxypropranolol (4-OH-P) and subsequent conjugation to the glucuronide (4-OH-PG) and N-dealkylation to N-desisopropylpropranolol and subsequent conversion to propranolol glycol glucuronide (GLY-G) and α-naphthoxylactic acid (NLA). These metabolites were collected in bile and urine at steady state. The excretion rates were determined and plotted against the blood concentration of propranolol at steady state according to Equation (2). Since NLA and GLY-G both arise from dealkylation, their excretion rates were summed.

EXPERIMENTAL

Five dogs were given 20 mg propranolol orally and 5 mg fore-limb i.v. doses before and after transposition surgery to study the contribution of GI metabolism. Plasma was analyzed for unchanged propranolol only.

To examine the kinetics of hepatic metabolism of propranolol, three of these dogs (after transposition) were given 4 to 6 hind-limb infusions of propranolol at rates of 1 to 6 mg propranolol per minute for 10 hours to reach steady state. Plasma bile and urine where collected and analyzed for propranolol and four major metabolites, PG, 4-OH-PG, GLY-G and NLA (2). Blood:plasma distribution ratios at various propranolol concentrations were measured in each dog to allow conversion of plasma propranolol concentrations to blood concentrations.

RESULTS AND DISCUSSION

The dogs remained healthy after the operation as judged by appearance, weight, hematologic indices and liver function tests. Systemic bioavailability of the oral dose increased from $8 \pm 8\%$ (mean $\pm$ SD) before transposition to $102 \pm 9\%$ after transposition (3). This shows that propranolol's first-pass metabolism is completely hepatic. The systemic plasma clearance increased from 766 ± 192 ml/min to 976 ± 280 ml/min. The increased clearance reflects the increase in liver blood flow produced by portacaval transposition due to the greater blood flow draining into the inferior vena cava than into the portal vein.

Plots of the steady-state total excretion rates of the metabolites versus steady-state blood concentrations of propranolol in one dog are shown in Figure 1. Results in the two other dogs are similar. Whereas CL_f of PG is constant, the formation clearances are not constant for (NLA + GLY-G) and 4-OH-PG. CL_f for PG ranged from 0.40 to 0.61 L/min. The nonlinear clearances for (NLA + GLY-G) and 4-OH-PG, expressed in V_{maxf} and K_{mf}'s, ranged from 2.1 to 8.8 μmole/min for V_{maxf} and 3.4 to 9.8 μmole/L for K_{mf}.

In summary, portacaval transposition in the dog provides a valuable tool in pharmacokinetic studies because it allows the investigator to separate the GI and hepatic contributions to first-pass metabolism. Studies in these dogs have allowed examination of the kinetics of hepatic metabolism of propranolol. The results demonstrate that the elimination is nonlinear because of capacity limitation in the metabolic pathways that results in the formation of NLA + GLY-G and 4-OH-PG. The well-stirred model for hepatic clearance of propranolol would be appropriate if capacity limited metabolism is incorporated.

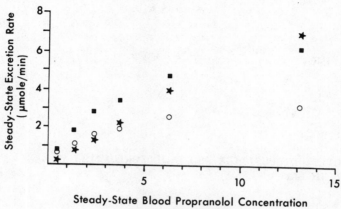

Figure 1. Plots of the steady-state total (bile + urine) excretion rates of propranolol metabolites versus steady-state blood propranolol concentrations in one dog after portacaval transposition. Key: propranolol-O-glucuronide (stars); α-naphthoxylactic acid plus propranolol glycol glucuronide (squares); 4-hydroxypropranolol glucuronide (circles).

REFERENCES

1. D.J. Effeney, S.M. Pond, M-W. Lo, B.M. Silber and S. Riegelman, A technique to study hepatic and intestinal drug metabolism separately in the dog, J. Pharmacol. Exp. Ther. 221:507-511 (1982).
2. M-W. Lo and S. Riegelman, Determination of propranolol and its major metabolites in plasma and urine by HPLC without solvent extraction, J. Chromatogr. 183:213-220 (1980).
3. M-W. Lo, D.J. Effeney, S.M. Pond, B.M. Silber and S. Riegelman, Lack of gastrointestinal metabolism of propranolol in dogs after portacaval transposition, J. Pharmacol. Exp. Ther. 221:512-515 (1982).

Communication 21

STEREOSELECTIVE DISPOSITION AND GLUCURONIDATION OF PROPRANOLOL IN MAN

B.M. Silber[1] and N.H.G. Holford[2]

[1] Pharmacodynamics Department
Medical Research Division
American Cyanamid Company
Pearl River, New York

[2] Department of Pharmacology and
Clinical Pharmacology
Auckland Medical School
Auckland, New Zealand

Previous pharmacokinetic studies on propranolol based their conclusions on total [S(-) plus R(+)] propranolol concentrations. The purpose of this study was to investigate, over a wide range of doses in humans, possible differences in the disposition of S(-) and R(+)-propranolol and in the formation of their glucuronide conjugates following oral doses of the racemate. After oral dosing to steady state, the disposition of S(-) and R(+)-propranolol and their corresponding glucuronide conjugates was studied in four healthy adults using doses from 40 to 320 mg of the racemate per day. Concentrations of S(-) and R(+)-propranolol and those of their corresponding glucuronide conjugates in plasma were determined using a previously reported technique (1). Because concentrations of propranolol were near the sensitivity limit of the stereospecific assay with doses of 40 and 80 mg per day, enantiomer and glucuronide conjugate concentrations were determined only at steady-state dosing rates of 160, 240 and 320 mg per day. Concentrations of S(-)-propranolol and its glucuronide conjugate were always higher than those for R(+)-propranolol and its glucuronide conjugate in all subjects at all dosing rates. Representative data from one subject are depicted in Figure 1. The ratio of steady-state concentrations of S(-)/R(+)-propranolol during the 13th dosing interval was 2.45 ± 1.12 (mean $\pm$ SD) at 160, 1.78 ± 0.60 at 240, and 1.51 ± 0.05 at 320 mg per day. The ratio of the

478

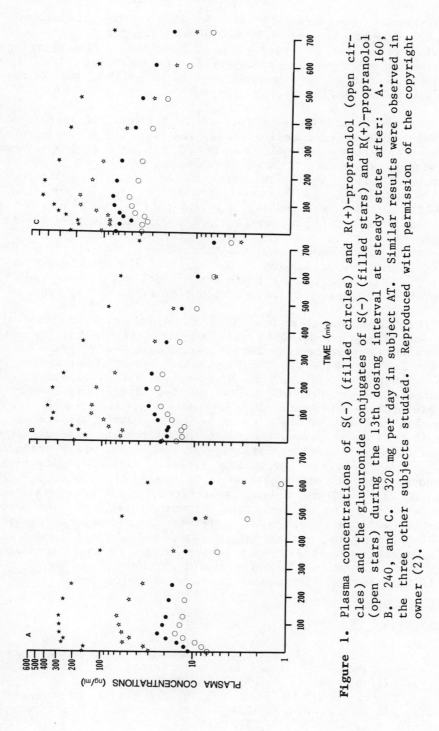

Figure 1. Plasma concentrations of S(-) (filled circles) and R(+)-propranolol (open circles) and the glucuronide conjugates of S(-) (filled stars) and R(+)-propranolol (open stars) during the 13th dosing interval at steady state after: A. 160, B. 240, and C. 320 mg per day in subject AT. Similar results were observed in the three other subjects studied. Reproduced with permission of the copyright owner (2).

steady-state concentrations of the glucuronide conjugates of S(-)/R(+)-propranolol was 4.74 ± 0.96 at 160, 3.64 ± 0.41 at 240, and 2.93 ± 0.17 at 320 mg per day. There was a disproportionate increase in the average steady-state concentration of S(-) and R(+)-propranolol in each subject as the daily dose was increased from 160 to 320 mg.

The intrinsic clearance (CL_{int}) of S(-) and R(+)-propranolol was determined at each dosing rate. The CL_{int} of S(-)-propranolol was always found to be lower than the CL_{int} of the R(+)-enantiomer. On average, there was a 52 ± 7% decrease in the CL_{int} of S(-)-propranolol and a 65 ± 22% decrease in the CL_{int} of R(+)-propranolol when the dose was increased from 160 to 320 mg per day. The half-life of S(-)-propranolol was 1.5-fold longer than for the R(+)-enantiomer at 160 mg per day (p < 0.05) and 1.6-fold longer at 320 mg per day (p < 0.05). Also, the half-life of the S(-)-propranolol glucuronide was 1.4-fold longer than for the R(+)-enantiomer at 160 mg per day (p < 0.05) and 1.3-fold longer at 320 mg per day (p < 0.05). The half-life of both enantiomers and their glucuronide conjugates increased with increasing dosing rate.

The formation clearance (CL_f) of glucuronide conjugates of S(-) and R(+)-propranolol in all four subjects was best described as a saturable process. The CL_f estimated by V'_{max}/K_m for the glucuronide conjugate of S(-)-propranolol ranged from 496 to 1831 ml/min, whereas the formation clearance for the conjugate of R(+)-propranolol ranged from 202 to 447 ml/min. Therefore, the CL_f for the glucuronide conjugate of S(-)-propranolol was from 2.1 to 4.9 times higher than the CL_f for the R(+)-enantiomer. The results of this investigation demonstrate that the disposition and glucuronidation of S(-) and R(+)-propranolol are not equal after oral doses of the racemic mixture in healthy adults. Since S(-)-propranolol is about 100-fold more potent as a beta adrenergic blocking agent than is the R(+)-enantiomer, administration of the drug as a racemic mixture, in essence, involves administration of two pharmacological entities, each with different pharmacokinetic behavior. Therefore, we propose that future pharmacokinetic and pharmacodynamic studies involving propranolol be focused on the pharmacologically more important S(-)-propranolol enantiomer rather than on total [S(-) plus R(+)] concentrations of the drug.

REFERENCES

1. B. Silber and S. Riegelman, Stereospecific assay for (-)- and (+)-propranolol in human and dog plasma, J. Pharmacol. Exp. Ther. 215:643-648 (1980).
2. B. Silber, N.H.G. Holford and S. Riegelman, Stereoselective disposition and glucuronidation of propranolol in humans, J. Pharm. Sci. 71:699-704 (1982).

Communication 22

EFFECT OF RENAL AND HEPATIC INSUFFICIENCY ON THE PHARMACOKINETICS OF BETAXOLOL, A NEW ADRENERGIC β-BLOCKER

J.F. Thiercelin,[1] G. Bianchetti,[1] P. Padovani,[1]
P.L. Morselli,[1] D. Fries,[2] J.M. Costa,[3] J. Paccalin,[3]
J.L. Bouchet[4] and C. Martin-Dupont[4]

[1] LERS-Synthelabo, Paris, France
[2] Hôpital Paul Brousse, Villejuif, France,
[3] Hôpital Saint André, Bordeaux, France
[4] Hôpital Pellegrin-Tondu, Bordeaux, France

The disposition of betaxolol (B), a new cardioselective β-blocker with proven antihypertensive activity, was studied following a single 20 mg oral dose in:

1. Eight patients with chronic renal insufficiency and a creatinine clearance between 5 and 50 ml/min (Group I).

2. Twelve patients needing periodic hemodialysis (Group II).

3. Six patients treated by continuous ambulatory peritoneal dialysis (Group III).

4. Six patients with hepatic cirrhosis proven by liver biopsy but with no liver shunt or ascites (Group IV).

5. Eight healthy volunteers, matched for age as controls.

The last two groups also received a 20 mg i.v. dose of betaxolol.

The mean (± SD) age of each group was 40.8 ± 19.0, 53.9 ± 12.8, 61.0 ± 16.4, 56.1 ± 13.2 and 50.6 ± 4.5 years, respectively. Blood, urine and dialysate were collected up to 48 hours for patients under dialysis and for up to 72 hours for other subjects. Concentrations of unchanged drug were measured by a specific and sensitive GLC method.

The pharmacokinetic results of the studies are summarized in Table I. As might be expected from the minor contribution of the kidneys to the overall elimination of B (15 < fe < 20%), not many changes were observed in Group I versus controls. In the most seriously impaired patients (Groups II and III), however, the total body clearances were decreased by 30 to 40% and terminal half-lives were prolonged by 60 to 100%.

The volume of distribution was significantly increased in Group II although large variations in this parameter were observed. It is also interesting to note that the dialysance of the drug is rather low irrespective of the type of dialysis used, showing that the procedure is not likely to change significantly the overall elimination of B from the body. These data indicate that in these dialyzed patients the daily dose of B should be reduced from 20 to 10 mg.

The pharmacokinetic profiles of B in cirrhotic patients were not significantly different from the controls as seen in Table I. Only the volume of distribution was significantly increased. It is therefore apparent that even a serious impairment of liver function does not significantly alter the overall disposition of betaxolol and therefore no dosage adjustment seems needed.

Table I. Pharmacokinetic parameters of betaxolol in different populations (mean ± standard deviation).

	Controls Healthy Subjects	Group I Chronic Renal Impairment	Group II Hemo-dialysis	Group III Peritoneal Dialysis	Group IV Cirrhosis
N =	8	8	12	6	6
$t_{1/2}$ (hr)	16.4 ± 5.1	21 ± 6	34 ± 10	27 ± 7	22.3 ± 5.4
CL_T (ml/hr/kg)	220 ± 60	230 ± 110	150 ± 30	130 ± 20	250 ± 70
CL_R (ml/hr/kg)	42 ± 23	15 ± 6	0	1.5 ± 1.0	30 ± 5
V_d (L/kg)	5.5 ± 1.4	6.8 ± 2.5	7.5 ± 2.1	5.0 ± 1.0	7.9 ± 1.7
CL_D (ml/min)	-	-	14 ± 14	11 ± 2	-
t_{max} (hr)	5.2 ± 1.4	4.8 ± 2.8	3.5 ± 3.5	3.7 ± 2.7	3.7 ± 0.7
C_{max} (ng/ml)	43 ± 11	43 ± 14	56 ± 14	61 ± 17	45 ± 15
$AUC_{0\to\infty}$ (ng/ml x hr)	1030	1350	2050	2065	1292
F %	76 ± 20	-	-	-	92 ± 20

The results of this study are consistent with the properties of the drug. It is a basic, lipophilic substance, mainly eliminated by metabolism although not rapidly cleared by the liver.

Due to its particular pharmacokinetic features (long half-life, small first-pass effect, low renal excretion, limited binding to plasma proteins (55%), formation of metabolites with low activity) and the above reported results, clinical use of B seems less complicated than that of many existing beta-blockers.

Communication 23

A SELECTIVE HPLC ASSAY FOR SIMULTANEOUS QUANTITATION OF FOURTEEN METHYLXANTHINES AND METHYLURIC ACIDS IN URINE

D.D-S. Tang-Liu,[1] J.H.G. Jonkman,[2]
K. Muir[3] and M. Kunitani[4]

[1] Drug Metabolism Pharmacokinetics
Drug Discovery Research
Allergan Pharmaceuticals
Irvine, California

[2] Laboratory for Pharmaceutical and Analytical Chemistry
State University
Groningen, The Netherlands

[3] School of Pharmacy
University of Southern California
Los Angeles, California

[4] Cetus Corporation
Berkeley, California

Until recently, the pharmacokinetics and metabolism of caffeine, theophylline and their metabolites were not well defined, although caffeine is widely ingested in foods and beverages and theophylline plays an important role in the treatment of asthma. To study the disposition kinetics of theophylline, caffeine and their metabolites, a reliable method to accurately quantify methyl-xanthines and methyluric acids is a prerequisite. We have developed a sensitive and selective HPLC-UV assay to quantify fourteen xanthines and uric acids in urine. This method involves a combination of normal and ion pair liquid-to-liquid extraction (1), with subsequent quantitation by reversed phase ion pair gradient elution. The method has proved to have sufficient sensitivity and selectivity for pharmacokinetic studies.

The compounds of interest, listed in Table I, can be categorized into two groups; the xanthines (pKa~8.5) and the uric acids

484

(pKa~5.5). Because of the large differences in physico-chemical properties of these compounds, selection of a simple organic extraction solvent providing high extraction efficiencies for both compounds was not possible. With the addition of an ion pairing agent (tetrabutylammonium hydrogen sulfate), the extraction of the more polar substituted uric acids was much enhanced. A solvent mixture of ethyl acetate, chloroform and isopropanol (45:45:10) was chosen so that the unionized xanthines were also efficiently extracted by normal liquid-to-liquid partition. Extraction was further enhanced by adding high concentrations of ammonium sulfate to the aqueous phase to produce a salting-out effect. The optimum pH value was 6.0. The extraction efficiencies are given in Table I.

To obtain sufficient retention and resolution of the polar methyluric acids, addition of tetrabutylammonium counter ions to the mobile phase was essential. The two mobile phases used in the gradient system contained the same concentrations of salts (10 mM sodium acetate and 5 mM tetrabutylammonium hydrogen sulfate). Solvent system A was water at pH 4.9 and solvent system B was 50% methanol with an apparent pH of 4.8. The two mobile phases were mixed according to a five step gradient program (2) in order to obtain maximal resolution among methylxanthines and methyluric acid ion pairs. The methanol composition in the mobile phase varied from 0 to 22.5%, and the flow rate from 1.25 to 1.5 ml/min with a run time of 60 minutes for each sample. The use of an exhaustively silylated column (Altex Ultrasphere ODS, 5μ, 250 x 4.6 mm), together with a replaceable precolumn, maintained column performance over a period of approximately one year during the injection of several thousand samples. The high efficiency column, together with a fast time constant detector, allowed for the resolution of rapidly eluting peaks. The detection wavelength was set at 280 nm to optimize the absorbance of both methylxanthines and methyluric acids (λ_{max} = 270 nm and 290 nm, respectively). Although both xanthines and uric acids have significant absorbance at 254 nm, much less interference was observed at 280 nm.

To ensure reproducible chromatography, the column was water-jacketed at a constant temperature (25°C) and the chromatographic system was automated. A WISP 710A Auto-Sampler (Waters Assoc., Milford, MA) was used to inject samples and to initiate an Altex Model 420 solvent-controller (Altex, Berkeley, CA) every 60 minutes. An integrator (SP4100, Spectra Physics, Santa Clara, CA), supplemented with customized calibration and peak width monitoring programs, was used for data reduction. The reproducible elution pattern and the high degree of peak resolution aided in quantitation of low concentrations of methylxanthines and methyluric acids. This assay has subsequently been shown to be sufficiently selective for pharmacokinetic studies.

Table I. The pK_a values, extraction efficiencies and retention times of the xanthines and uric acids.

	pK_a	Extraction Efficiency[a] (%)	Retention Time[b] (min)
Xanthines			
xanthine (X)	1.3, 9.9	--	--
1-methylxanthine (1-MX)[d]	7.7, 12.0	95.5 ± 5.6	11.56
3-methylxanthine (3-MX)[d]	8.1, 11.3	96.8 ± 5.4	8.90
7-methylxanthine (7-MX)[c]	8.3	78.1 ± 9.3	7.91
1,3-dimethylxanthine (1,3-MX; theophylline)[c]	8.8	100.1 ± 3.2	22.61
1,7-dimethylxanthine (1,7-MX; paraxanthine)[c]	8.7	97.7 ± 4.4	20.14
3,7-dimethylxanthine (3,7-MX; theobromine)[c]	9.9	96.2 ± 4.3	13.33
1,3,7-trimethylxanthine (1,3,7-MX; caffeine)[e]	14.0	101.5 ± 6.5	29.60
Uric Acids			
uric acid (U)	5.5	--	--
1-methyluric acid (1-MU)[d]	5.5	92.1 ± 9.9	15.41
3-methyluric acid (3-MU)	6.2, 11.4	80.3 ± 10.1	6.85
7-methyluric acid (7-MU)[c]	5.5, 10.9	81.3 ± 7.7	14.84
1,3-dimethyluric acid (1,3-MU)[d]	--	98.9 ± 3.2	18.35
1,7-dimethyluric acid (1,7-MU)[c]	5.7, 10.9	87.5 ± 4.8	27.19
3,7-dimethyluric acid (3,7-MU)	--	76.7 ± 10.3	14.00
1,3,7-trimethyluric acid (1,3,7-MU)[c]	--	91.8 ± 3.7	28.55

[a] n = 7, mean ± SD.
[b] n = 26.
[c] Metabolite of caffeine.
[d] Metabolite of theophylline and caffeine.
[e] Metabolite of theophylline.

REFERENCES

1. K.T. Muir, J.H.G. Jonkman, D.D-S. Tang, M. Kunitani and S. Riegelman, Simultaneous determination of theophylline and its major metabolites in urine by reversed-phase ion-pair high performance liquid chromatography, J. Chromatogr. 221:85-95 (1980).
2. D.D-S. Tang-Liu and S. Riegelman, An automated HPLC assay for simultaneous quantitation of methylated xanthines and uric acids in urine, J. Chromatogr. Sci. 20:155-159 (1982).

Communication 24

A COMPOSITE VIEW OF THEOPHYLLINE ELIMINATION IN MAN

D. D-S. Tang-Liu[1] and R.L. Williams[2]

[1] Drug Metabolism Pharmacokinetics
Drug Discovery Research
Allergan Pharmaceuticals
Irvine, California

[2] Division of Clinical Pharmacology
Schools of Medicine and Pharmacy
University of California
San Francisco, California

Theophylline has played a major role in the treatment of asthma for many years. Therapy with theophylline has often been associated with reports of serious toxicity and sometimes with fatalities. The plasma concentrations producing efficacy are close to those producing adverse effects. Individualization of the dosing regimen is recommended because of the narrow therapeutic concentration range and the large variation in the elimination half-life of theophylline.

We became interested in this drug because of evidence suggesting dose-dependent disposition of the drug, such as a convex decline in the plasma concentration with time in intoxication cases (1,2) and a disproportionate relationship between steady-state concentrations in serum and dosing rate in children (3). Despite numerous studies, the disposition kinetics of theophylline and its metabolities have remained essentially unexplored. In the past three years, we have performed a series of experiments to elucidate the kinetics of theophylline and its metabolites in healthy volunteers.

Theophylline undergoes ring oxidation to 1,3-dimethyluric acid (40%), oxidative demethylation to 3-methylxanthine (16%) and 1-methylxanthine, which is subsequently oxidized to 1-methyluric acid (20%), and methylation to caffeine (6%) as shown in Figure 1 (4,5).

Because the clearance of caffeine is much higher than that of theophylline, and because only a small portion of theophylline is converted to caffeine, plasma concentrations of caffeine are usually below the limit of detection after single doses of theophylline in adults (5). Caffeine is extensively metabolized after its formation from theophylline and is converted to diverse metabolites. The urinary excretion of these theophylline-derived caffeine degradation products, which can be measured after caffeine administration but not after theophylline dosing, accounts for the incomplete urinary recovery of theophylline and its metabolites after intravenous administration of the drug (4).

Up to 80% of a theophylline dose is eliminated by capacity limited metabolism to 3-methylxanthine, 1-methyluric acid and 1,3-dimethyluric acid (4). The Km values estimated for these three

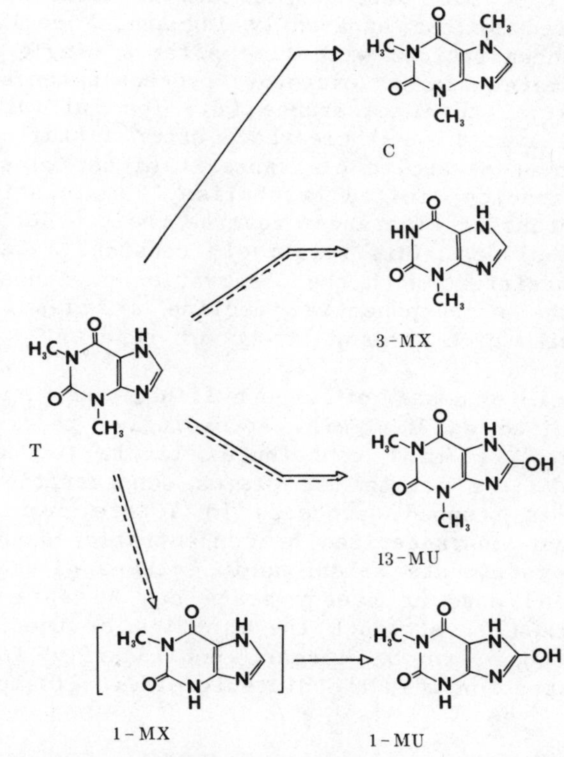

Figure 1. Proposed metabolic pathways of theophylline (capacity limited (broken line) and linear (solid line). T = theophylline, 3-MX = 3-methylxanthine, 13-MU = 1,3-dimethyluric acid, 1-MX = 1-methylxanthine, 1-MU = 1-methyluric acid and C = caffeine. Reprinted from (4) with permission from the C.V. Mosby Co.

pathways are below or within the therapeutic concentration range of theophylline, indicating that the metabolism of theophylline is partially saturated after therapeutic doses. Formation of 1,3-dimethyluric acid is the pathway with the highest Km and Vmax values, that is, the one with the lowest affinity and highest capacity among the three major metabolic pathways of theophylline.

About 13% of a theophylline dose is excreted renally. Theophylline undergoes passive reabsorption in the renal tubule and its renal clearance is highly urine flow-dependent (6). Because theophylline produces diuresis, its renal clearance may initially account for more than 70% of the time-averaged total clearance after a single dose. The diuretic effect diminishes with time and theophylline renal clearance decreases rapidly as urine flow decreases.

The disposition of theophylline demonstrates time, concentration and urine flow rate-dependencies and is much more complicated than is indicated by the apparently log-linear decline of plasma theophylline concentrations with time after a single dose. Compensation between metabolic and excretory processes tends to produce a relatively constant total clearance (7). The initial distribution phase and the elevated renal clearance after a single dose compensate for the lower metabolic clearance at higher plasma concentrations due to capacity limited metabolism. The relative magnitudes of renal and metabolic clearances reverse their order as the plasma concentration declines. This relatively constant value for overall clearance is consistent with the observation of linear kinetics as reflected by the monoexponential decline of plasma theophylline concentration with time in many literature reports.

After multiple doses of theophylline, the urine output is normally maintained at 1 ml/min. Accordingly, renal clearance of the drug (about 4 ml/min) contributes little to total clearance (less than 10%). The decline of plasma concentration, after drug administration is stopped, proceeds in a more pronounced convex-descending manner characterized by concentration-dependent metabolism. A disproportionate relationship between plasma theophylline concentration and dose at steady state can be observed in normal healthy subjects (7). Although the kinetics of theophylline after single doses appear to be linear, nonlinearity is unmasked on chronic administration when the diuretic effect dissipates.

REFERENCES

1. G.J. Kadlec, C.H. Jarboe, S.J. Pollard and J.L. Sublett, Acute theophylline intoxication. Biphasic first-order elimination kinetics in a child, Ann. Allergy 41:337-338 (1978).

2. J.W. Jenne, T.W. Chick, B.A. Miller and R.D. Strickland, Apparent theophylline half-life fluctuations during treatment of acute left ventricular failure, Am. J. Hosp. Pharm. 34:408-409 (1977).

3. E. Sarrazin, L. Hendeles, M. Weinberger, K. Muir and S. Riegelman, Dose-dependent kinetics for theophylline: Observations among ambulatory asthmatic children, J. Pediat. 97:825-828 (1980).

4. D.D-S. Tang-Liu, R.L. Williams and S. Riegelman, Nonlinear theophylline elimination, Clin. Pharmacol. Ther. 31:358-369 (1982).

5. D.D-S. Tang-Liu and S. Riegelman, Metabolism of theophylline to caffeine in adults, Res. Commun. Chem. Path. Pharmacol. 34:371-380 (1981).

6. D.D-S. Tang-Liu, T.N. Tozer and S. Riegelman, Urine flow dependence of theophylline renal chearance, J. Pharmacokin. Biopharm. 10:351-364 (1982).

7. D.D-S. Tang-Liu, "Theophylline Elimination in Man," Ph.D. dissertation, University of California, San Francisco (1981).

Communication 25

THE INFLUENCE OF FOOD ON THE BIOAVAILABILITY OF A SUSTAINED RELEASE THEOPHYLLINE FORMULATION

Lloyd N. Sansom

School of Pharmacy
South Australian Institute of Technology
Adelaide, South Australia

Chronic theophylline therapy is now well established as effective treatment in the management of reversible airway disease. Pharmacodynamic studies have shown that while significant improvement in pulmonary function can be achieved with serum theophylline concentrations between 7 and 20 mg/L, serious toxic effects occur at concentrations exceeding 20-30 mg/L (1). The need to maintain serum concentrations within this narrow range means that a knowledge of the pharmacokinetics of theophylline is essential for proper patient management. Sustained release preparations of theophylline can offer the dual benefit of improved patient compliance and reduction in the interdose fluctuations of serum theophylline concentrations.

The guidelines recommended by regulatory agencies for the bioavailability testing of sustained release theophylline products require both single and multiple dose studies to be performed. The recommendation is for single dose studies to be conducted following an overnight fast of at least 12 hours prior to dosing with a further 2-4 hour fasting period after dosing.

This study examines the influence of food on the absorption of theophylline from an experimental sustained release product (KC capsules). The product was formulated as coated pellets of theophylline packaged into gelatin capsules.

METHODS

Eight healthy adult volunteers (6 male, 2 female, nonsmokers, 24 to 35 years of age and weighing from 52 to 80 kg) participated in the study. In the first study period, each subject received 250 mg theophylline as a rapidly dissolving tablet (2 x Nuelin® tablets) following an overnight fast. No food or drink was allowed for 2 hours after dosing. Data from this study were used to estimate pharmacokinetic parameters for each subject to determine if excessive serum concentrations would be reached following the administration of the sustained release product, which contained a larger amount of theophylline. For 3 further study periods, subjects were randomly assigned to the following treatments: (a) 250 mg theophylline (2 x Nuelin®) following an overnight fast of at least 12 hours; (b) 600 mg theophylline in slow releasing pellets (2 x KC capsules, 300 mg) following an overnight fast of at least 12 hours* and (c) 600 mg theophylline in slow releasing pellets (2 x KC capsules, 300 mg) following a standard breakfast*. Each dose was taken at 8 a.m. with 200 ml of water, with 7 days separating each study period. The breakfast consisted of orange juice, breakfast cereal with milk, 2 eggs, 1 piece of bacon and 2 pieces of toast. The volunteers received 21-32 kcal/kg, with 29% of the calories being obtained from protein, 32% from fat and 39% from carbohydrate. Subjects refrained from caffeine containing food and beverages for 36 hours prior to each study and for the duration of each sampling period.

Blood samples (200 µL) were obtained by finger prick just prior to the dose, and 0.5, 1, 2, 3, 4, 5, 6, 7, 8 and 9 hours after the administration of Nuelin® Tablets, and at the following additional times when the sustained release product was taken: 10, 12, 15, 24, 26, 28 and 30 hours. Serum was separated by centrifugation and kept frozen until assayed. The theophylline concentration in serum was determined by a high pressure liquid chromatography assay able to distinguish theophylline from its metabolites. Bioavailability was determined from the area under the serum concentration time curve (AUC) corrected for the dose administered. The area from zero to infinity was calculated using a combination of linear and logarithmic trapezoid estimation together with an extrapolation technique (2). In view of the difficulty of estimating the elimination rate constant from some of the serum profiles following administration of the sustained release preparation due to continued absorption, the extrapolation was performed using the average elimination rate constant obtained from the 2 administrations of Nuelin® 125 tablets.

---

*One subject had a very low theophylline clearance and received 300 mg theophylline; (1 x KC capsule, 300 mg).

RESULTS

Table I shows the results for the mean bioavailability, peak serum concentration and the time at which peak concentrations occurred (t_{peak}). The test product (KC capsules) given in the fasting state had good bioavailability, based on AUC measurements, when compared to the standard (104 ± 14%). There was a significant difference between the time to peak for the standard (1.5 hours) and the test product (8.8 hours). The significantly lower peak concentration is probably the result of the slower absorption and indicates that the test product is behaving as a sustained release formulation. The length of time during which the serum theophylline concentrations are maintained within 75% of the peak concentration (13.9 hours) further indicates the sustained release characteristics of this formulation. The bioavailability of the test product given with the standard breakfast (33 ± 10%) was significantly lower compared to both the reference and test products given in the fasting state. Significantly lower peak serum concentrations were observed (15 mg/L/g dose) when the test product was given in the nonfasting state. The t_{peak} was not prolonged (6.8 ± 1.5 hours), nor was the length of time that serum concentrations exceeded 75% of the peak level significantly

Table I. Absorption characteristics of test product versus standard.[a]

	Standard[b]	KC (Fasting)	KC (Non-fasting)
Bioavailability (%) (AUC_{test}/AUC_{std})[c]	--	104.2 ± 14.3	33.1 ± 10.4[e]
Peak time (hr)	1.5 ± 0.8	8.8 ± 1.3[d]	6.8 ± 1.5[d]
Peak concentration (mg/L/g dose)	28.7 ± 5.9	12.5 ± 2.8[d]	5.0 ± 2.1[d,e]
Hours with > 75% of peak level	3.1 ± 1.8	13.9 ± 3.5[d]	13.3 ± 5.1[d]

[a]Data are presented as the mean ± SD, N = 8.
[b]Average of 2 separate doses.
[c]Corrected for differences in dose administered.
[d]Significantly different from the standard (p < 0.05).
[e]Significantly different from the fasting state (p < 0.05).

different for the test product in the fasting and nonfasting states. This suggests that food had no significant influence on the relative absorption rate of the bioavailable portion of theophylline from the sustained release test product.

DISCUSSION

The influence of food on the bioavailability of many drugs has been investigated (3) but information on the effect of food on drug release from sustained release products is generally lacking. Food may influence the absorption of orally administered drugs due to a specific interaction between the drug and a food component, an effect on gastrointestinal physiology (motility, stomach emptying rate), a physical impairment of absorption, or an effect on the dissolution of the drug. Welling (4) has shown that the extent of theophylline absorption from a conventional tablet dosage form was unaffected when administered with various types of meals and thus it is unlikely that the reduction in bioavailability of KC capsules when taken in the nonfasting state is due to either a specific interaction of theophylline with a food component or to a physical barrier to the absorption process. Asker et al. (5) examined the influence of pepsin, pancreatin and ox bile on the dissolution behaviour of prolonged release granules of sulfanilamide. These workers showed that the various agents can influence the dissolution depending upon the nature of the dissolution retarding agent. Because of the complexity of sustained release formulations compared to conventional solid dosage forms, it is possible that specific interactions with the retardant or a physical barrier to the dissolution process are responsible for decreased bioavailability of KC capsules when administered with food.

Bogentoft and Sjogren (6) have suggested that an examination of the effect of food on drug absorption should always be included in any documentation of a controlled release dosage form. This study supports their contention and shows that while a preparation can be manufactured showing good bioavailability and release profile in the fasting state, this is no guarantee that either the extent of absorption or the absorption profile will not change when the formulation is administered with food. Since in the absence of any specific label statement to the contrary, the clinical use of most oral sustained release dosage forms involves administration at, or in close proximity to meal times, it is suggested that the guidelines for the bioavailability testing of sustained release products may be improved with the inclusion of a requirement for single dose studies in the presence of food.

REFERENCES

1. R.I. Ogilvie, Clinical pharmacokinetics of theophylline, Clin. Pharmacokin. 3:267-293 (1978).
2. R.A. Upton, J.F. Thiercelin, T.W. Guentert, L. Sansom, J.R. Powell, P.E. Coates and S. Riegelman, Evaluation of the absorption from some commercial sustained release theophylline products, J. Pharmacokin. Biopharm. 8:131-149 (1980).
3. P.G. Welling, Influence of food and diet on gastrointestinal drug absorption: A review, J. Pharmacokin. Biopharm. 5:291-334 (1977).
4. P.G. Welling, L.L. Lyons, W.A. Craig and G.A. Trochta, Influence of diet and fluid on bioavailability of theophylline, Clin. Pharmacol. Ther. 17:475-480 (1975).
5. A.F. Asker, A.M. Motawi and M.M. Abdel Khalek, A study of some factors affecting the in vitro release of drug from prolonged release granulations, Pharmazie 26:904-905 (1981).
6. C. Bogentoft and J. Sjogren, Controlled release from dosage forms, in: "Towards Better Safety of Drugs and Pharmaceutical Products," D.D. Breimer, ed., Elsevier/North Holland Biomedical Press, Amsterdam (1980), pp. 229-246.

Communication 26

PHARMACOKINETICS OF THE VASODILATORS HYDRALAZINE AND ENDRALAZINE

P.A. Reece, I. Cozamanis and R. Zacest

Department of Clinical Pharmacology
The Queen Elizabeth Hospital
Adelaide, South Australia

Hydralazine (1-hydrazinophthalazine, HP) and a new vasodilator, endralazine (6-benzoyl-3-hydrazino-5,6,7,8-tetrahydropyrido-[4,3-c] pyridazine, E) have similar chemical and pharmacological properties (see Fig. 1). Both are effective antihypertensives when used together with β-adrenoceptor blocking drugs. Recently E was proposed as an important alternative to minoxidil, especially for the treatment of refractory hypertension in women, since it lacks the hypertrichosis side effects of minoxidil (1).

Although E and HP undergo similar routes of metabolism, the relative importance of acetylation, hydrazone formation and hydroxylation in the clearance of E have not been determined. Similarly, the extent of differences in the metabolism of E in slow and fast acetylators has not been reported. Using a specific high performance liquid chromatographic-fluorescence assay recently reported for E (2), a placebo controlled, integrated pharmaco-kinetic-pharmacodynamic study of 5 and 10 mg single oral doses of E was undertaken in 17 healthy, fasting male volunteers (8 slow,

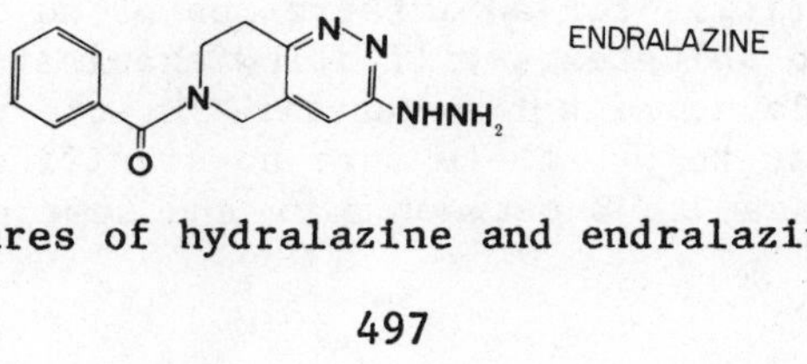

Figure 1. Structures of hydralazine and endralazine.

497

7 heterozygous fast and 2 homozygous fast acetylators). Intravenous E was not available at the time of these studies. The results were compared with those from a previous pharmacokinetic study of single oral and intravenous doses of HP in 10 healthy volunteers (5 slow, 4 heterozygous fast and 1 homozygous fast acetylator) (3).

E had a much longer terminal half-life (mean ± SD = 4.30 ± 1.08 hr) than did HP (27.3 ± 5.4 min, oral dose). However, like HP, there was no difference in the terminal half-life of E between slow and fast acetylators. In human plasma in vitro, E again had a longer half-life (3.80 hr at 37°C) than HP (11 min). This difference was attributed to different rates of reaction of the drugs with endogenous α-keto acids, particularly pyruvic acid, and was confirmed in the case of HP by simultaneously monitoring the formation of hydralazine pyruvic acid hydrazone (HPPAH).

Only a slightly larger area under the plasma concentration-time curve (AUC$_0^\infty$) was observed for E in slow versus fast acetylators; 22.3% larger (p < 0.05) for the 5 mg dose and 12.4% larger (p > 0.05) for the 10 mg dose. For HP, however, the dose-corrected AUC$_0^\infty$ was 148% larger and bioavailability 119% higher (p < 0.001) in the slow versus fast acetylators. Although clearances were unknown, only low plasma concentrations of the acetylated metabolite of E (methyltriazoloendralazine) were observed compared with relatively high concentrations of the equivalent HP metabolite (3-methyl-s -triazolo[3,4-a]phthalazine). For both drugs, highly significant differences between AUC$_0^\infty$'s of the acetylation metabolites were observed between slow and fast acetylators.

There was no evidence of nonlinearity in the pharmacokinetics of E at the two doses studied. That is, the ratio of AUC$_0^\infty$'s was 2.02 ± 0.23 for the 10 to 5 mg doses and the mean terminal half-life was 4.30 ± 1.08 hours for the 5 mg dose and 4.25 ± 1.09 hours for the 10 mg dose. Published results suggesting a nonlinear increase in the AUC$_0^\infty$ of HP with increasing dose will require re-evaluation using the specific assays now available.

Highly significant correlations (p < 0.001) between plasma concentrations of E and decreases in diastolic blood pressure (r = 0.8), decreased peripheral vascular resistance (r = 0.72), and increases in cardiac index (r = 0.9) and in heart rate (r = 0.74) were observed from 2 to 10 hours after a dose. Such analyses were not possible for HP since plasma concentrations of the drug became undetectable 3 to 4 hours after dosing. Recent approval by Australian health authorities for administration of an intravenous formulation of HPPAH to volunteers will allow examination of the role of this quantitatively important metabolite in the prolonged activity of HP. In contrast to HP, there were no significant differences in hemodynamic responses to E between slow and fast acetylators.

In conclusion, E was found to be a more potent vasodilator than HP and, in contrast to HP, only small differences in the metabolism and hemodynamic effects of E were observed between slow and fast acetylators. The acetylator phenotype independence of its metabolism may make E simpler to use clinically than HP.

REFERENCES

1.   J. Kindler, W.M. Glockner, G. Sieberth, K.A. Meurer, A. Konrads and H. Feldkamp, Antihypertensive properties of endralazine, a pyridopyridazine compound in the treatment of refractory hypertension in comparison to minoxidil, Proceedings of the 8th Scientific Meeting of the International Society of Hypertension, Milan (1981).
2.   P.A. Reece, I. Cozamanis and R. Zacest, Sensitive high-performance liquid chromatographic assay for endralazine and two of its metabolites in human plasma, J. Chromatogr. 225:151-160 (1981).
3.   P.A. Reece, I. Cozamanis and R. Zacest, Kinetics of hydralazine and its main metabolites in slow and fast acetylators, Clin. Pharmacol. Ther. 28:769-778 (1980).

Communication 27

FORMATION OF MONO- AND DINITRATE METABOLITES OF NITROGLYCERIN FOLLOWING INCUBATION WITH HUMAN BLOOD

Patrick K. Noonan

Department of Pharmacy
University of California
San Francisco, California

Nitroglycerin (GTN) is rapidly metabolized in humans; reported clearance values are much greater than liver blood flow. Therefore, other body sites, including blood, may be responsible for GTN metabolism. Lee (1) demonstrated the conversion of GTN to 1,2- and 1,3-glyceryldinitrates (1,2-GDN and 1,3-GDN) after incubation with blood, but at GTN concentrations (1 mg/ml) that would not be observed in humans. He was not able to detect the formation of glycerylmononitrates (GMN's). Armstrong et al. (2) demonstrated the disappearance of physiologically relevant concentrations of GTN following incubation with blood. Even though these workers did not measure the appearance of metabolites, they assumed that the loss of GTN was due to metabolism. More recently, Wu et al. (3,4) attempted to measure the formation of metabolites (GDN's) following incubation of GTN with human erythrocytes. These investigators noted that even though levels of GTN decreased with time, the metabolites could not be detected. They concluded that the reaction of GTN with blood was not enzymatic but that the loss was physical in nature. The work described here was designed to elucidate the mechanisms by which GTN might be lost (that is, either a physical or metabolic loss) after incubation with blood.

Tritium labeled GTN (^{3}H-GTN) was incubated (37°C) with fresh human blood, pooled plasma and buffer (pH 7.4). Aliquots of blood, plasma or buffer were withdrawn from the flasks over time. Concentrations of ^{3}H-GTN and ^{3}H-metabolites were determined by selective extractions and normal phase HPLC. Pentane and ether were chosen as extraction solvents because of their respective partitioning properties. GTN is preferentially extracted into pentane relative to the drug's more polar metabolites. In pentane, 75% of GTN is

500

extracted but only 9% of the GDN's and less than 1% of the GMN's will be extracted under the conditions utilized (single extraction, 10:1 organic solvent:biologic fluid, 2 minutes contact time). In contrast, 100% of the GDN's and 60% of the GMN's will partition into an ether extraction. Thus, GTN and metabolite levels may be approximated by the tritium content in the pentane and ether extracts, respectively.

The concentrations of radiolabeled compounds (equivalent to GTN) in the pentane and ether extracts as a function of incubation time in blood are shown in Figure 1A. Concentrations of GTN and metabolites, after normalizing for GTN and metabolite extraction efficiencies, are shown in Figure 1B. The disappearance of GTN may

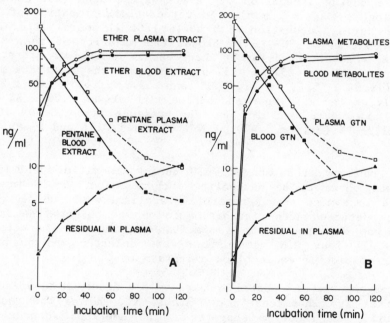

Figure 1. In vitro metabolism of ^{3}H–GTN to ^{3}H–metabolites by human blood at 37°C. Figures show the loss of ^{3}H–GTN measured in both plasma (open squares) and blood (filled squares) and the accumulation of ^{3}H–metabolites (open circles = plasma, filled circles = blood) with time. Bottom curves show the residual concentration of radioactivity in plasma (triangles) after extractions. The concentration of radioactive material (as GTN) found in the extracts is shown in A. This data was normalized for GTN and metabolite extraction efficiencies to show concentrations of ^{3}H–GTN and ^{3}H–metabolites (B).

be followed in both plasma and whole blood and is apparently a pseudo-first-order process. The apparent loss of linearity at the later time points, when GTN concentrations are low with respect to metabolite concentrations, may be caused by the partitioning of GDN's into pentane (since pentane can extract approximately 9% of the GDN's). Under these conditions (very low GTN and high GDN concentrations), the pentane extract may no longer be specific for GTN. The curves at the bottom of Figure 1 show the relationship between the amount of GTN related material not extracted from plasma and the time of incubation. Since only 60% of the GMN's are extracted by ether, this curve may reflect the accumulation of GMN's in plasma. The amount of radioactivity remaining in extracted whole blood was not determined.

After incubation with blood, the decline in ^{3}H-GTN was first-order with half-lives ranging from 22 to 32 minutes (Fig. 1). The half-life during incubation of ^{3}H-GTN with plasma (not shown) was 8-fold longer (202 ± 5 min). No detectable degradation of ^{3}H-GTN occurred during incubation with buffer for 21 hours. After a two-hour incubation of ^{3}H-GTN in blood, the majority of the ^{3}H-label (99 ± 9%) was accounted for by the presence of the mononitrate (4.7 ± 1.4% of 1-GMN and 23.0 ± 4.3% of 2-GMN) and the dinitrate metabolites (19.3 ± 5.7% of 1,3-GDN and 52.9 ± 6.9% of 1,2-GDN). Similarly, after a 21-hour incubation with plasma, 100 ± 8% of the ^{3}H-label was accounted for by the presence of: 1,3-GDN (62.5 ± 5.4%); 1,2-GDN (31.5 ± 5.4%); 1-GMN (3.1 ± 1.0%); and 2-GMN (2.9 ± 3.2%).

In summary, the loss of GTN during in vitro incubation in blood was shown to be metabolic. Incubation of ^{3}H-GTN in plasma resulted in a much slower rate of metabolism, while no degradation could be detected after incubation in pH 7.4 buffer. The decrease in GTN was accompanied by a simultaneous increase in metabolite levels. All four GTN metabolites were detected and quantitated after incubation in whole blood and plasma.

Acknowledgements. Supported in part by NIH Grant GM 26691 and by a grant from Key Pharmaceuticals, Miami, Fl. During the course of this work, PKN received support as the American Foundation for Pharmaceutical Education James F. Hoge Memorial Fellow.

REFERENCES

1. N.H. Lee, The metabolism of glyceryl trinitrate by liver and blood from different species, Biochem. Pharmacol. 22:3122-3124 (1973).
2. J.A. Armstrong, S.E. Slaughter, G.S. Marks and P.W. Armstrong, Rapid disappearance of nitroglycerin following incubation with human blood, Can. J. Physiol. Pharmacol. 58:459-462 (1980).

3.   C.C. Wu, T. Sokoloski, M.F. Blanford and A.M. Burkman, Absence of metabolite in the disappearance of nitroglycerin following incubation with red blood cells, Int. J. Pharm. 8:323-329 (1981).

4.   T.D. Sokoloski, C.C. Wu, L.S. Wu and A.M. Burkman, Interaction of nitroglycerin with human blood components, J. Pharm. Sci. 72:335-338 (1983).

Communication 28

A PHARMACODYNAMIC MODEL FOR THIAZINAMIUM IN ASTHMATIC PATIENTS

N.H.G. Holford,[1] P. Clements,[2] P. Collier,[3]
N.G.M. Orie,[4] L. Eudia van Bork[4] and J.H.G. Jonkman[5]

[1]Department of Pharmacology
and Clinical Pharmacology
Auckland Medical School
Auckland, New Zealand

[2]Department of Medicine
University of California
Los Angeles, California

[3]Department of Pharmacy
Queens University
Belfast, Northern Ireland

[4]Departments of Medicine and [5]Pharmacy
Rijkuniversiteit
Groningen, The Netherlands

Thiazinamium is a quaternary ammonium phenothiazine and clinically useful bronchodilator. Its mechanism of action is thought to be mediated by a combination of antimuscarinic and antihistaminic properties and its efficacy in the treatment of bronchoconstriction appears to be superior to epinephrine and aminophylline (1). Although it has been in clinical use for over 25 years, little is known about its pharmacokinetics and pharmaco-dynamics in humans (2,3). A prominent side effect of thiazinamium use is an increase in heart rate presumed to be due to vagal blockade. We have investigated the relationship between plasma thiazinamium concentration and the change in airways obstruction and heart rate to help provide rational dosing guidelines for the treatment of bronchoconstriction.

504

METHODS

Seven male patients with chronic reversible airways obstruction were given 6.25 mg of thiazinamium as a rapid intravenous injection over 1 minute or by intramuscular administration into the lateral thigh. The median (range) age of the subjects was 50 (29-64) years with a forced expiratory volume in 1 second (FEV1) of 1.7 (1.45-3.0) liters which is 52% (36-110%) of the predicted value for normal subjects. Each subject increased his FEV1 more than 0.4 liters in response to i.m. administration of 25 mg of thiazinamium. Plasma thiazinamium concentrations were measured by gas-liquid chromatography after ion pair extraction (2). Parameter estimation was performed using MKMODEL (4), a computer modeling program available on the PROPHET system (5).

RESULTS

A three-compartment model with bolus input using weights of the reciprocal of the measured concentration squared was marginally better than a two-compartment model in describing the plasma concentrations following i.v. administration. A two-compartment model with constant rate input during absorption was superior to first-order input using weights of the reciprocal of the measured concentration to describe the plasma concentrations following i.m. administration.

Plots of both FEV1 and heart rate responses as a function of plasma concentrations exhibited anti-clockwise hysteresis after i.m. dosing (Fig. 1A), suggesting that the effect site is located in a compartment other than plasma. A combined pharmacokinetic-pharmacodynamic model (6) was used to estimate the time course and magnitude of effect site concentrations (Fig. 1B). An Emax pharmacodynamic model was used with a baseline parameter and the effect site equilibration rate constant estimated from the observed effects. The three-compartment model was preferred to describe concentrations after i.v. dosing because it was superior in describing measurements made when concentrations and effects were changing rapidly.

The equilibration half-time for the achievement of FEV1 and heart rate responses was short (10 and 4 minutes, respectively). The maximum predicted response of FEV1 was 90 and 87% of predicted normal (i.v. and i.m). The concentration producing 50% of maximum drug effect (EC50) was 12 (i.v.) and 25 (i.m.) ng/ml. The maximum predicted response of heart rate was 136 (i.v.) and 179 (i.m.) beats per minute. The EC50 for the heart rate response was much higher than for the bronchodilator response, 174 (i.v.) and 242 (i.m.) ng/ml.

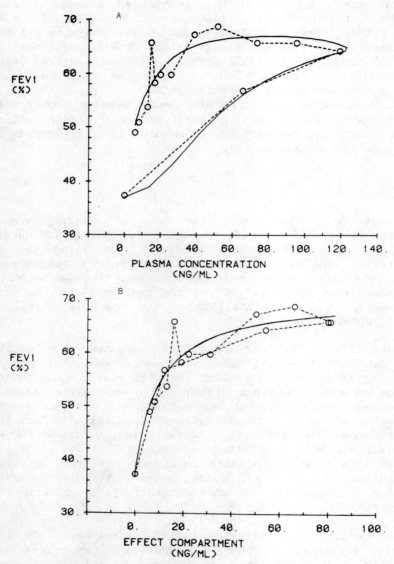

Figure 1. Plot of plasma concentration of thiazinamium versus FEV1
(A) and effect compartment concentration of thiazinamium
versus FEV1 (B).

DISCUSSION

This study of therapeutic (FEV1) and toxic (heart rate) effects of a drug as a function of plasma concentration permits the definition of a target concentration for clinical use. Because the EC50s for the therapeutic and toxic effects are separated by over an order of magnitude, near maximum bronchodilator response will be achieved at concentrations which are still producing substantial increments in heart rate. No benefit can be expected from increasing thiazinamium plasma concentration above 100 ng/ml in a typical patient although potentially hazardous increases in heart rate may occur. It is suggested that dosing with thiazinamium be adjusted to achieve a maximum concentration of 100 ng/ml which is expected to produce 90% of predicted normal FEV1 with a heart rate no greater than 100 beats per minute.

REFERENCES

1. H. Booy-Noord, N.G.M. Orie, H.J. Ten Cate, S. Sloots and D. Bolt, The influence of various drugs on the vital capacity of asthmatics, Int. Arch. Allergy 10:321-341 (1957).
2. J.H.G. Jonkman, J. Wijsbeek, S. Hollenbeek Brouwer-de Boer, R.A. de Zeeuw, L.E. van Bork and N.G.M. Orie, Determination of low concentrations of the quaternary ammonium compound thiazinamium methylsulphate in plasma and urine, J. Pharm. Pharmacol. 27:849-854 (1975).
3. L.E. Van Bork, J.H.G. Jonkman, R.A. de Zeeuw, N.G.M. Orie, R. Peset and K. de Vries, Diagnostisch en therapeutisch gebruik van thiazinamium (Multergan), Ned. T. Geneesk. 121:1196-1202 (1977).
4. N.H.G. Holford, MKMODEL - A mathematical modelling tool for the PROPHET system, "PROPHET Public Procedures Manual," H.M. Perry, ed., Bolt, Beranek and Newman, Boston (1982) 4:125-129.
5. W.F. Raub, The PROPHET system and resource sharing, Fed. Proc. 33:2390 (1976).
6. N.H.G. Holford and L.B. Sheiner, Understanding the dose-effect relationship, Clin. Pharmacokin. 6:429-453 (1981).

Communication 29

PROTEIN BINDING ESTIMATES IN THE PRESENCE OF VOLUME SHIFTS DURING EQUILIBRIUM DIALYSIS

Thomas N. Tozer

Department of Pharmacy
University of California
San Francisco, California

With the advent of translucent acrylic plastic cells, it has become apparent that sizable and variable volume shifts occur across a semipermeable membrane during equilibrium dialysis. These volume shifts, toward the plasma or protein side, influence the estimation of binding parameters and the unbound fraction. A method of correcting for volume shifts is presented using binding data for salicylate and prednisolone. The specific dialysis procedures employed have been described elsewhere (1,2).

The binding of each drug to plasma proteins was determined in separate studies using radiolabeled drug. ^{14}C-Salicylic acid was added to the plasma and ^{3}H-prednisolone was added to the buffer. The concentration of the radiolabel was measured in each sample before dialysis and in the plasma and buffer after dialysis. The total concentration of drug in plasma was determined before dialysis as described elsewhere (1,2). The duration of dialysis was 4 hours for salicylate and 16 hours for prednisolone in the respective studies.

Equations for calculating volume shifts, unbound concentration, bound concentration and unbound fraction were derived using principles of conservation of amount of drug and radiolabel and volume of solvent. Another major principle used was the conservation of amount bound when a volume shift occurs. The relationships are applicable when there is no binding to the dialysis cell or semipermeable membrane. Their derivation has been published (3).

The volume shift, expressed as the change in the volume on the protein side relative to the initial volume, is summarized in the following equations:

Radiolabel added to:	Buffer side (prednisolone)	Plasma side (salicylate)
	$$\dfrac{R\,(DB - DB') - DP'}{DP' - DB'}$$	$$\dfrac{DP - DP' - R \cdot DB'}{DP' - DB'}$$

where R is the initial ratio of buffer to plasma volumes, DB and DP are the initial predialysis concentrations of radiolabel in the buffer or plasma samples, and DB' and DP' are the concentrations of radiolabel on the buffer and plasma sides of the membrane postdialysis. The relationships are applicable to prednisolone and salicylate as neither drug was found to bind to the dialysis cell or the membrane when the radiolabel in buffer was dialyzed against an equal volume of buffer; all the radiolabel remained in solution.

Figures 1 and 2 show the distribution of volume shifts in the two separate studies. The differences in the volume shifts are, in large part, accounted for by the differences in the duration of dialysis. The coefficients of variation of the volume shifts were remarkably similar, about 0.5.

The unbound, C_b' and bound, C_{bnd}^*, concentrations corrected for volume shifts were calculated from the following derived relationships, when the radiolabel was added to the buffer side (prednisolone):

$$C_b' = \frac{(C_p + L \cdot R)}{R} \cdot \frac{DB'}{DB}$$

$$C_{bnd}^* = \frac{(C_p + L \cdot R)(R(DB - DB') - DB')}{DB \cdot R}$$

and when the radiolabel was added to the plasma side (salicylate):

$$C_b' = (C_p + L)\frac{DB'}{DP}$$

$$C_{bnd}^* = \frac{(C_p + L)(DB - DB' - R \cdot DB')}{DP}$$

where C_p is the initial drug concentration on the plasma side, L is the initial concentration of radiolabel and the other terms are as defined above.

The unbound and bound concentrations, with and without correction for a volume shift, were fitted to the following models:

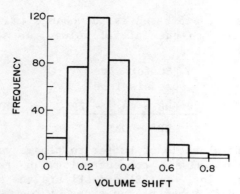

Figure 1. Distribution of volume shifts in the prednisolone
studies (N = 388). The average shift was 0.31 ± 0.15
(SD). Volume shift is expressed as the change in volume
on the protein side relative to the initial volume.
Reproduced with permission of the copyright owner (3).

Prednisolone   Salicylate

$$C^*_{bnd} = \frac{CAP_1 \cdot C'_b}{K_1 + C'_b} + S \cdot C'_b \qquad\qquad C^*_{bnd} = \frac{CAP_1 \cdot C'_b}{K_1 + C'_b} + \frac{CAP_2 \cdot C'_b}{K_2 + C'_b}$$

where CAP_1 and CAP_2 are parameters for binding capacities at two
different sets of binding sites, K_1 and K_2 are the respective
dissociation constants, and S is CAP_2/K_2. The estimates of the
binding parameters for prednisolone and salicylate differed from
those obtained without volume shift correction by 10 to 40%.

The fraction unbound, fu, corrected for volume shift, was
calculated from the relationships:

Radiolabel   Buffer side   Plasma side
added to: (prednisolone)   (salicylate)

$$fu = \frac{DB'}{R(DB - DB')} \qquad\qquad fu = \frac{DB'}{DP - R \cdot DB'}$$

The difference in the estimates of the fraction unbound, by correcting for volume shift and by not doing so (the ratio of counts
on the buffer and plasma sides), was approximately equal to the
volume shift. These studies show the importance of correcting for
the net movement of water during equilibrium dialysis and provide a
means for doing so.

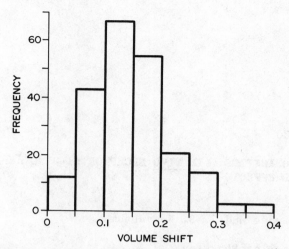

Figure 2. Distribution of volume shifts in the salicylate studies (N = 219). The average shift was 0.15 ± 0.07 (SD).

REFERENCES

1. D.E. Furst, T.N. Tozer and K.L. Melmon, Salicylate clearance, the resultant of protein binding and metabolism, Clin. Pharmacol. Ther. 26:380-389 (1979).
2. J.G. Gambertoglio, F.J. Frey, N.H.G. Holford, J.L. Birnbaum, P.S. Lisak, F. Vincenti, N.J. Feduska, O. Salvatierra and W.J.C. Amend, Prednisone and prednisolone bioavailability in renal transplant patients, Kidney Int. 21:621-626 (1982).
3. T.N. Tozer, J.G. Gambertoglio, D.E. Furst, D.S. Avery and N.H.G. Holford, Volume shifts and protein binding estimates using equilibrium dialysis – application to prednisolone binding in man, J. Pharm. Sci. 72:1442-1446 (1983).

Communication 30

OPIATE PHARMACOKINETICS: IN VIVO RECEPTOR BINDING AND PHARMACOLOGICAL EFFECTS

W. Sadée and J. S. Rosenbaum

School of Pharmacy
University of California
San Francisco, California

The discovery of a specific cerebral opiate receptor in 1973 (reviewed in reference 1) rapidly led to the detection of endogenous peptides as putative neurotransmitters/modulators associated with the opiate receptor (2). However, Martin et al. (3) presented the first pharmacological evidence that the opiate receptor system consists of several subpopulations of distinct receptor sites, and it was subsequently postulated that there are multiple opiate receptors and endogenous ligands (2), including Leu-enkephalin, Met-enkephalin, β-endorphin and dynorphin. In [^{3}H]-ligand binding studies on rodent brain homogenates (4), at least three distinct binding sites were detectable; the μ, δ and κ/σ sites. Despite the rapid advance in opiate molecular pharmacology, several key questions concerning the molecular mechanisms remain unsolved. We are studying the problem with regard to which receptor subsites mediate the different pharmacological effects of the opiates. Effects include analgesia, dependence, tolerance and many other behavioral and peripheral changes that are seemingly unrelated to each other.

The experimental approach uses newly developed in vivo receptor binding assays that can determine the receptor occupancy by various opiates in the intact rat and therefore allow one to directly correlate in vivo receptor binding with the effect under study. Briefly, a radioactive opiate tracer is subcutaneously injected, the animals are sacrificed at suitable times, and the fraction of brain [^{3}H] activity that is specifically bound to the membranous fraction of brain homogenates is measured by a rapid filtration technique (5). The pharmacokinetics and metabolism of each tracer must be known in detail to select suitable in vivo receptor assay conditions; fractional occupancy, total number of binding sites, and _in vivo_ off-rates can then be determined with reasonable accuracy.

The objective of the first part of these studies was to determine any differences that might exist between _in vitro_ and _in vivo_ opiate receptor binding, an important problem that has previously not been addressed in a systematic fashion. First, we noted a deviation of the _in vivo_ receptor binding kinetics of opiate antagonists from the law of mass action; the results could be simulated by combining a pharmacokinetic model with a new receptor binding model (receptor microcompartment) (6). Other major differences were noted, including an unexpected disparity between _in vivo_ fractional receptor occupancy and pharmacological effect for agonists but not antagonists (5), and a much lower apparent _in vivo_ binding affinity for agonists relative to antagonists (7). We also observed changes in the binding sensitivity to the effects of metal cations _in vitro_ (8), and a partial loss in the binding sensitivity to the effects of guanyl nucleotides (which are thought to mediate coupling of the receptor to adenylate cyclase) in the _in vitro_ system (unpublished results). These results demonstrate important _in vivo/in vitro_ receptor binding differences and underscore the need to obtain direct _in vivo_ receptor binding-effect comparisons in order to understand receptor subsite functions.

In the second phase of this project, we attempt to develop _in vivo_ labeling techniques that are capable of discriminating between the opiate receptor subtypes, analogous to similar binding studies _in vitro_. However, different tracers and methods are required _in vivo_. We have thus far employed four tritiated opiate tracers: ^{3}H-diprenorphine, an opiate antagonist with equal affinity for the μ, δ and κ/σ binding sites _in vitro_; ^{3}H-etorphine, a potent opiate agonist; ^{3}H-naloxone, a universal opiate antagonist with preference for the μ receptor; and ^{3}H-ethylketocyclazocine, a putative κ-agonist. Specific saturable _in vivo_ binding was established for each tracer; moreover, the bound radioactivity was accounted for (> 90%) as the unchanged drug in each case, thereby excluding possible metabolite interferences. Time of peak binding coincided with time of peak effect, as tested for etorphine (5).

The saturation isotherms of _in vivo_ binding by these four tracers are shown in Figure 1. Because of its rather low _in vivo_ affinity, it was not possible to accurately determine the total _in vivo_ binding site population of ^{3}H-ethylketocyclazocine. However, measurable plateau levels were reached with the other three tracers. There were significant differences in the total number of binding sites that were labeled by ^{3}H-naloxone (~50 pmole/g), ^{3}H-diprenorphine (~25 pmole/g) and ^{3}H-etorphine (15–20 pmole/g brain tissue) over the observed dosage range. This result suggests that each tracer labels a different set of binding site subpopulations. _In vivo_ displacement studies with a series of unlabeled

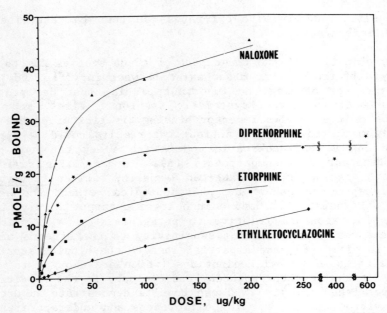

Figure 1. <u>In vivo</u> saturation isotherms of four opiate ligands, plotted against the total injected dose. Tritiated tracers were injected along with increasing amounts of the respective unlabeled drug and results were corrected for specific [³H] activity. Nonspecific binding after high saturating doses was subtracted from all values. Reprinted with permission from Life Sciences 31:1299–1301 (1982), Pergamon Press, Ltd.

opiates revealed that a fraction of the bound ³H-naloxone is associated with an additional binding site population of unknown function, that is not identical to the known μ, δ and κ/σ sites and that is selective for morphinan derivatives. We have recently termed this binding site population the λ site (9). Moreover, by blocking specific receptor subsites with unlabeled opiates, it appears that at least three and possibly four opiate receptor subsites can be distinguished with these tracers (Rosenbaum and Sadée, unpublished data).

As a first application of these differential <u>in vivo</u> labeling techniques, the molecular mechanisms responsible for the bell shaped dose-response curve of buprenorphine were studied. The results demonstrated that buprenorphine saturates one receptor subpopulation when reaching its peak agonistic effects (~0.5 mg/kg), and then saturates another receptor subpopulation at higher doses (up to 10 mg/kg) with a concomitant decline of the agonistic effect (Sadée and Herz, unpublished data). This result, for the first time, provides evidence suggesting the existence of noncompetitive auto-inhibition among the opiate receptor subsites. Certainly, such a finding may reveal an important physiological component (i.e., the interaction of several pain processing pathways) in the striking phenomenon of opiate tolerance.

REFERENCES

1. S.H. Snyder and R. Simantov, The opiate receptor and opioid peptides, J. Neurochem. 28:13-20 (1977).

2. J.A.H. Lord, A.A. Waterfield, J. Hughes and H.W. Kosterlitz, Endogenous opioid peptides: Multiple agonists and receptors, Nature 267:495-499 (1977).

3. W.R. Martin, C.G. Eades, J.A. Thompson, R.E. Huppler and P.E. Gilbert, The effects of morphine- and nalorphine-like drugs in the nondependent and morphine-dependent chronic spinal dog, J. Pharmacol. Exp. Ther. 197:517-532 (1976).

4. K.-J. Chan, E. Hazum and P. Cuatrecasas, Novel opiate binding sites selective for benzomorphan drugs, Proc. Natl. Acad. Sci. USA. 78:4141-4145 (1981).

5. D.C. Perry, J.S. Rosenbaum, M. Kurowski and W. Sadée, [^{3}H]-Etorphine receptor binding in vivo: Small fractional occupancy elicits analgesia, Mol. Pharmacol. 21:272-279 (1982).

6. D.C. Perry, K.B. Mullis, S. Øie and W. Sadée, Opiate antagonist receptor binding in vivo: Evidence for a new receptor binding model, Brain Res. 199:49-61 (1980).

7. M. Kurowski, J.S. Rosenbaum, D.C. Perry and W. Sadée, [^{3}H]-Etorphine and [^{3}H]-diprenorphine receptor binding in vitro and in vivo: Differential effects of Na$^+$ and GPP(NH)P, Brain Res. 249:345-352 (1982).

8. W. Sadée, A. Pfeiffer and A. Herz, Opiate receptor: Multiple effects of metal ions, J. Neurochem. 36:659-667 (1982).

9. J. Grevel and W. Sadée, An opiate binding site in the rat brain is highly selective for 4,5-epoxymorphinans, Science 221:1198-1201 (1983).

Communication 31

CEFOPERAZONE PHARMACOKINETICS IN HEALTHY CHINESE VOLUNTEERS

Russel Rhei-Long Chen

School of Pharmacy
National Taiwan University
Taipei, Taiwan, Republic of China

Cefoperazone is a new third generation broad spectrum cephalosporin with antibacterial activities encompassing gram negative microorganisms including Pseudomonas aeruginosa (1). Pharmacokinetic studies on this antibiotic have been carried out by several groups but only one of these studies was performed on Orientals, namely Japanese volunteers (2-4). The current study was designed to elucidate the kinetic profile of this drug in Chinese subjects to meet the needs of clinical practice in our geographical area.

Four healthy volunteers were given an intramuscular injection of 1 g cefoperazone and intravenous infusions of 1 g and 2 g of cefoperazone over a one-hour period. Blood samples were drawn at 0, 0.5, 1, 2, 3, 4, 6 and 8 hours after each dose. Urine samples were collected at 0-1, 1-2, 2-4, 4-8 and 8-12 hours after each i.m. injection and at 0-1, 1-2, 2-4, 4-6, 6-8, 8-10 and 10-12 hours after each i.v. infusion. The plasma and urine samples were assayed microbiologically with Micrococcus lutea ATCC 9341 as the test organism.

Plasma cefoperazone concentrations after drug administration, percent urinary recovery and some calculated pharmacokinetic parameters are shown in Table I. The biological half-life after i.m. injection was 2.69 ± 0.21 hours. This is longer than the half-life estimates obtained from i.v. infusions (1.80 ± 0.06 hr for 1 g, 1.90 ± 0.08 hr for 2 g). The two half-life estimates from i.v. infusions are not statistically different ($p > 0.05$). The cumulative urinary excretion following i.m. injection ($14.2 \pm 1.1\%$) was less than after i.v. infusion ($22.3 \pm 1.7\%$ for 1 g, $25.2 \pm 0.5\%$ for 2 g). The biological half-life after the i.v. infusions and

516

Table I. Plasma cefoperazone concentrations (µg/ml) and some derived pharmacokinetic parameters.[a]

Time	Intramuscular	Intravenous Infusion[b]	
	1 g	1 g	2 g
0.5	34.3 ± 12.0	79.3 ± 14.9	184.8 ± 12.0
1	77.8 ± 13.6	148.6 ± 22.2	252.2 ± 28.9
2	52.8 ± 10.8	90.8 ± 11.6	181.5 ± 20.0
3	39.8 ± 12.1	49.9 ± 10.4	121.4 ± 10.6
4	33.0 ± 11.0	31.9 ± 7.6	87.8 ± 11.7
6	20.4 ± 4.9	17.5 ± 3.0	40.8 ± 2.6
8	11.7 ± 1.7		
$t_{1/2}$(hr)	2.69 ± 0.21	1.80 ± 0.06	1.90 ± 0.08
V (L)	--	5.11 ± 1.18	5.40 ± 0.63
CL (ml/min)	--	32.7 ± 6.3	32.8 ± 3.0
CL_R (ml/min)	10.1 ± 2.9	8.4 ± 2.7	8.7 ± 2.2
% Urinary recovery 0-12 hr	14.2 ± 1.1	22.3 ± 1.7	25.2 ± 0.5
AUC (µg • hr/ml)	263 ± 57	306 ± 35	636 ± 0.83

[a] Mean ± SD; N = 4.
[b] Over a one-hour period.

the urinary excretion data are similar to previously reported data (2-4).

There was no significant difference between the mean volume of distribution values and the mean total body clearance values calculated from the two sets of i.v. infusion data (p > 0.05). Volumes of distribution were calculated according to a one-compartment model and were 5.11 ± 1.18 L for the 1 g infusion and 5.40 ± 0.63 L for the 2 g infusion. Total body clearances were 32.7 ± 6.3 ml/min and 32.8 ± 3.0 ml/min after 1 g and 2 g infusions, respectively. These clearance and volume data are similar to those obtained from Japanese volunteers (2) but lower than those from Western groups (3,4).

Renal clearances following cefoperazone i.v. infusions in the present study (8.4 ± 2.7 ml/min for 1 g, 8.7 ± 2.2 ml/min for 2 g) were lower than previously reported values (2-4). No significant difference between the two data sets in the present work was observed (p > 0.05).

REFERENCES

1. A.M. Hinkle, B.M. Le Blanc and G.P. Bodey, In vitro evaluation of cefoperazone, Antimicrob. Agents Chemother. 17:423-427 (1980).
2. A. Saito, M. Ohmori, K. Shiba, T. Yamji and H. Ihara, Clinical studies on T-1551, Investigator Reference Manual, Toyama Chemical Company and Pfizer International, Inc. (1979).
3. W.A. Craig, Single dose pharmacokinetics of cefoperazone following intravenous administration, Clin. Ther. 3(Special Issue):46-49 (1980).
4. L. Balant, P. Dayer, M. Rudhardt, A.F. Allaz and J. Fabre, Cefoperazone: Pharmacokinetics in humans with normal and impaired renal function and pharmacokinetics in rats, Clin. Ther. 3 (Special Issue):50-59 (1980).

APPENDIX - SCIENTIFIC BIBLIOGRAPHY

SIDNEY RIEGELMAN

1. S. Riegelman, J.V. Swintosky and L.W. Busse, Colloids, emulsions and suspensions, in: "American Pharmacy," (Vol. II), R.A. Lyman, ed., J.B. Lippincott Co., Philadelphia (1947), ch. 3.
2. J.V. Swintosky, S. Riegelman, T. Higuchi and L.W. Busse, Studies on pharmaceutical powders and the state of subdivision. I. The application of low-temperature nitrogen adsorption isotherms to the determination of surface area, J. Am. Pharm. Assoc., Sci. Ed. 38:210-215 (1949).
3. J.V. Swintosky, S. Riegelman, T. Higuchi and L.W. Busse, Studies on pharmaceutical powders and the state of subdivision. II. Surface area measurements of some pharmaceutical powders by the low-temperature nitrogen adsorption isotherm technique, J. Am. Pharm. Assoc., Sci. Ed. 38:308-313 (1949).
4. J.V. Swintosky, S. Riegelman, T. Higuchi and L.W. Busse, Studies on pharmaceutical powders and the state of subdivision. III. An evaluation of pharmaceutical dispensing techniques employed to increase the specific surface area of powders, J. Am. Pharm. Assoc., Sci. Ed. 38:378-381 (1949).
5. S. Riegelman, J.V. Swintosky, T. Higuchi and L.W. Busse, Studies on pharmaceutical powders and the state of subdivision. IV. The application of spray-drying techniques to pharmaceutical powders, J. Am. Pharm. Assoc., Sci. Ed. 39:444-450 (1950).
6. R. Pratt, J. Dufrenoy, P.P.T. Sah, J. Oneto, D.C. Brodie, S. Riegelman and V.L. Pickering, Vitamin K_5 as an antimicrobial medicament and preservative, J. Am. Pharm. Assoc., Sci. Ed. 39:127-134 (1950).
7. S.J. Dean, D.C. Brodie, E. Brochmann-Hanssen and S. Riegelman, The preparation of belladonna and stramonium tinctures through the use of colloid mill, J. Am. Pharm. Assoc., Sci. Ed. 42:88-90 (1953).
8. N.A. Allawala and S. Riegelman, The release of antimicrobial agents from solutions of surface-active agents, J. Am. Pharm. Assoc., Sci. Ed. 42:267-275 (1953).
9. N.A. Allawala and S. Riegelman, The properties of iodine in solutions of surface-active agents, J. Am. Pharm. Assoc., Sci. Ed. 42:396-401 (1953).
10. N.A. Allawala and S. Riegelman, Phenol coefficients and the Ferguson principle, J. Am. Pharm. Assoc., Sci. Ed. 43:93-97 (1954).
11. S. Riegelman, D.G. Vaughan, Jr. and M. Okumoto, Evaluation of the sporicidal activity of Post's sterilizing solution, A.M.A. Arch. Ophthalmol. 53:847-851 (1955).
12. S. Riegelman, D.G. Vaughan, Jr. and M. Okumoto, Rate of sterilization as a factor in the selection of ophthalmic solutions, A.M.A. Arch. Ophthalmol. 54:725-732 (1955).

13. S. Riegelman, D.C. Vaughan, Jr. and M. Okumoto, Compounding ophthalmic solutions, J. Am. Pharm. Assoc., Pract. Ed. 16:742-746 (1955).

14. S. Riegelman, Suppositories, in: "American Pharmacy," (4th Edition), R.A. Lyman and J.B. Sprowls, eds., J.B. Lippincott Co., Philadelphia (1955), ch. 18, pp. 347-360.

15. S. Riegelman, D.G. Vaughan, Jr. and M. Okumoto, Antibacterial agents in Pseudomonas aeruginosa contaminated ophthalmic solutions, J. Am. Pharm. Assoc., Sci. Ed. 45:93-98 (1956).

16. S. Riegelman and W.J. Crowell, The kinetics of rectal absorption. I. Preliminary investigations into the absorption rate process, J. Am. Pharm. Assoc., Sci. Ed. 47:115-122 (1958).

17. S. Riegelman and W.J. Crowell, The kinetics of rectal absorption. II. The absorption of anions, J. Am. Pharm. Assoc., Sci. Ed. 47:123-127 (1958).

18. S. Riegelman and W.J. Crowell, The kinetics of rectal absorption. III. The absorption of undissociated molecules, J. Am. Pharm. Assoc., Sci. Ed. 47:127-133 (1958).

19. S. Riegelman and D.G. Vaughan, Jr., A rational basis for the preparation of ophthalmic solutions. I., J. Am. Pharm. Assoc., Pract. Ed. 19:474-477 (1958). Also: Survey of Ophthalmology 3:471-492 (1958).

20. S. Riegelman and D.G. Vaughan, Jr., A rational basis for the preparation of ophthalmic solutions. II., J. Am. Pharm. Assoc., Pract. Ed. 19:537-540 (1958). Also: Survey of Ophthalmology 3:471-492 (1958).

21. S. Riegelman and D.G. Vaughan, Jr., A rational basis for the preparation of ophthalmic solutions. III., J. Am. Pharm. Assoc., Pract. Ed. 19:665-668 (1958). Also: Survey of Ophthalmology 3:471-492 (1958).

22. S. Riegelman, N.A. Allawala, M.K. Hrenoff and L.A. Strait, The ultraviolet absorption spectrum as a criterion of the type of solubilization, J. Colloid Sci. 13:208-217 (1958).

23. D.G. Vaughan, Jr. and S. Riegelman, New irrigating device especially useful for anterior chamber irrigation, Am. J. Ophthalmol. 47:34-35 (1959).

24. S. Riegelman, Ear, nose and throat, in: "Husa's Pharmaceutical Dispensing," (5th Edition), E.W. Martin, ed., Mack Publishing Co., Easton, PA (1959), pp. 245-290.

25. S. Riegelman, Suppositories, in: "American Pharmacy," (5th Edition), J.B. Sprowls, ed., J.B. Lippincott Co., Philadelphia (1960), ch. 19, pp. 347-366.

26. S. Riegelman, The effect of surfactants on drug stability. I., J. Am. Pharm. Assoc., Sci. Ed. 49:339-343 (1960).

27. S. Riegelman and R.P. Penna, Effect of vehicle components on the absorption characteristics of sun screen compounds, J. Soc. Cosmet. Chem. 11:280-291 (1960).

28. D. Vaughan, R. Shaffer and S. Riegelman, A new stabilized form of epinephrine for the treatment of open-angle glaucoma, A.M.A. Arch. Ophthalmol. 66:232-235 (1961).

29. E. Nelson and S. Riegelman, Gastrointestinal irritation by salicylate and route of administration, Gastroenterology 41:644-645 (1961).

30. S. Riegelman, L.A. Strait and E.Z. Fischer, Acid dissociation constants of phenylalkanolamines, J. Pharm. Sci. 51:129-133 (1962).

31. S. Riegelman, A critical re-evaluation of factors affecting emulsion stability. I. The hydrophilic-lipophilic balance postulate. Am. Perfum. 77:31-33 (1962).

32. S. Riegelman and E.Z. Fischer, Stabilization of epinephrine against sulfite attack, J. Pharm. Sci. 51:206-210 (1962).

33. S. Riegelman and E.Z. Fischer, Effect of boric acid and bisulfite on the rate of oxidation of epinephrine, J. Pharm. Sci. 51:210-213 (1962).

34. S. Riegelman, New data on determining emulsion stability, Am. Perfum. Cosmet. 1:59-62 (1962).

35. D.G. Vaughn, Jr. and S. Riegelman, The preparation of ophthalmic solutions, in: "Ocular Pharmacology and Therapeutics and the Problems of Medical Management," S. Kimura and E. Goodner, eds., F.A. Davis, Co., Philadelphia (1963), pp.129-135.

36. M.E. Corwin, V. Coleman, S. Riegelman, M. Okumoto, E. Jawetz and P. Thygeson, Effect of IUDR and amethopterin on experimental herpes simplex keratitis, Invest. Ophthalmol. 2:578-583 (1963).

37. L.J. Fischer and S. Riegelman, Absorption and distribution of griseofulvin in rabbits, J. Pharm. Sci. 54:1571-1575 (1965).

38. S.A. Kaplan, S. Riegelman and K.H. Lee, Effects of potential inhibitors on metabolism of griseofulvin in vitro. J. Pharm. Sci. 55:14-18 (1966).

39. S. Riegelman and D.L. Sorby, EENT preparations, in: "Husa's Pharmaceutical Dispensing" (6th Edition), E.W. Martin, ed., Mack Publishing Co., Easton, PA (1966), ch. 16, pp. 311-358.

40. O.N. Rambo, F.F. Zboralske, P.A. Harris, S. Riegelman and A.R. Margulis, Toxicity studies on tannic acid administered by enema. I. Effects of enema-administered tannic acid on the colon and liver of rats, Am. J. Roentgenol., Rad. Ther. Nucl. Med. 96:488–497 (1966).

41. P.A. Harris, F.F. Zboralske, O.N. Rambo, A.R. Margulis and S. Riegelman, Toxicity studies on tannic acid administered by enema. II. The colonic absorption and intraperitoneal toxicity of tannic acid and its hydrolytic products in rats, Am. J. Roentgenol., Rad. Ther. Nucl. Med. 96:498–504 (1966).

42. F.F. Zboralske, P.A. Harris, S. Riegelman, O.N. Rambo and A.R. Margulis, Toxicity studies on tannic acid administered by enema. III. Studies on the retention of enemas in humans. IV. Review and conclusions, Am. J. Roentgenol., Rad. Ther. Nucl. Med. 96:505–509 (1966).

43. L.J. Fischer and S. Riegelman, Quantitative determination of griseofulvin and griseofulvin-4'-alcohol in plasma by fluorimetry on thin layer chromatograms, J. Chromatogr. 21:268–274 (1966).

44. L.J. Fischer and S. Riegelman, Absorption and activity of some derivatives of griseofulvin, J. Pharm. Sci. 56:469–476 (1967).

45. P.A. Harris and S. Riegelman, Acetylsalicylic acid hydrolysis in human blood and plasma. I. Methodology and in vitro studies, J. Pharm. Sci. 56:713–716 (1967).

46. M. Rowland and S. Riegelman, Determination of acetylsalicylic acid and salicylic acid in plasma, J. Pharm. Sci. 56:717–720 (1967).

47. M. Rowland, S. Riegelman, P.A. Harris, S.D. Sholkoff and E.J. Eyring, Kinetics of acetylsalicylic acid disposition in man, Nature 215:413–414 (1967).

48. S.D. Sholkoff, E.J. Eyring, M. Rowland and S. Riegelman, Plasma and synovial fluid concentrations of acetylsalicylic acid in patients with rheumatoid arthritis, Arthritis Rheum. 10:348–351 (1967).

49. M. Rowland and S. Riegelman, Use of carbon disulfide as a solvent for the silylation of submicrogram amounts of carboxylic acids, Anal. Biochem. 20:463–465 (1967).

50. S. Riegelman, J.C.K. Loo, and M. Rowland, Shortcomings in pharmacokinetic analysis by conceiving the body to exhibit properties of a single compartment, J. Pharm. Sci. 57:117–123 (1968).

51. S. Riegelman, J.C.K. Loo and M. Rowland, Concept of a volume of distribution and possible errors in evaluation of this parameter, J. Pharm. Sci. 57:128–133 (1968).

52. F.F. Zboralske, F.R. Margolin, O.N. Rambo and S. Riegelman, Experimental oral hepatography in rats, Invest. Radiol. 3:35–43 (1968).

53. J.C.K. Loo and S. Riegelman, New method for calculating the intrinsic absorption rate of drugs, J. Pharm. Sci. 57:918–928 (1968).

54. M. Rowland, S. Riegelman and W.L. Epstein, Absorption kinetics of griseofulvin in man, J. Pharm. Sci. 57:984–989 (1968).

55. M. Rowland and S. Riegelman, Pharmacokinetics of acetylsalicylic acid and salicylic acid after intravenous administration in man, J. Pharm. Sci. 57:1313–1319 (1968).

56. P.A. Harris and S. Riegelman, Influence of the route of administration on the area under the plasma concentration-time curve, J. Pharm. Sci. 58:71–75 (1969).

57. P.A. Harris and S. Riegelman, Metabolism of griseofulvin in dogs, J. Pharm. Sci. 58:93–96 (1969).

58. S. Riegelman, Clinical evaluation of the effect of formulation variables on therapeutic performance of drugs, Drug Informat. Bull. 1:59–67 (1969).

59. W.L. Chiou, S. Riegelman and J.R. Amberg, Complications in using rabbits for the study of oral drug absorption, Chem. Pharm. Bull. 17:2170–2173 (1969).

60. W.L. Chiou and S. Riegelman, Disposition kinetics of griseofulvin in dogs, J. Pharm. Sci. 58:1500–1504 (1969).

61. W.L. Chiou and S. Riegelman, Preparation and dissolution characteristics of several fast-release solid dispersions of griseofulvin, J. Pharm. Sci. 58:1505–1510 (1969).

62. J.C.K. Loo and S. Riegelman, Assessment of pharmacokinetic constants from postinfusion blood curves obtained after i.v. infusion, J. Pharm. Sci. 59:53–55 (1970).

63. W.H. Barr and S. Riegelman, Intestinal drug absorption and metabolism. I. Comparison of methods and models to study physiological factors of in vitro and in vivo intestinal absorption, J. Pharm. Sci. 59:154–163 (1970).

64. W.H. Barr and S. Riegelman, Intestinal drug absorption and metabolism. II. Kinetic aspects of intestinal glucuronide conjugation, J. Pharm. Sci. 59:164–168

(1970).

65.   M. Rowland, L.Z. Benet and S. Riegelman, Two-compartment model for a drug and its
       metabolite: Application to acetylsalicylic acid pharmacokinetics, J. Pharm. Sci.
       59:364-367 (1970).

66.   J.E. Tingstad and S. Riegelman, Dissolution rate studies. I. Design and
       evaluation of a continuous flow apparatus, J. Pharm. Sci. 59:692-696 (1970).

67.   W.L. Chiou and S. Riegelman, Oral absorption of griseofulvin in dogs: Increased
       absorption via solid dispersion in polyethylene glycol 6000, J. Pharm. Sci.
       59:937-942 (1970).

68.   S. Riegelman, M. Rowland and W. L. Epstein, Griseofulvin-phenobarbital
       interaction in man, J. Am. Med. Assoc. 213:426-431 (1970).

69.   W. Sadée S. Riegelman and L.F. Johnson, On the mechanism of steroid fluorescence
       in sulfuric acid.   Part I.   The formation of trienones, Steroids 17:595-606
       (1971).

70.   S. Riegelman, The kinetic disposition of aspirin in humans, in: "Aspirin,
       Platelets and Stroke," W.S. Fields and W.K. Hass, eds., W.H. Green, Inc., St.
       Louis (1971) ch. 10, pp. 105-114.

71.   W.L. Chiou and S. Riegelman, Pharmaceutical applications of solid dispersion
       systems, J. Pharm. Sci. 60:1281-1302 (1971).

72.   W.L. Chiou and S. Riegelman, Absorption characteristics of solid dispersed and
       micronized griseofulvin in man, J. Pharm. Sci. 60:1376-1380 (1971).

73.   W.L. Chiou and S. Riegelman, Increased dissolution rates of water-insoluble
       cardiac glycosides and steroids via solid dispersion in polyethylene glycol 6000,
       J. Pharm. Sci. 60:1569-1571 (1971).

74.   K. Asghar and S. Riegelman, Ocular absorption of catecholamines, Arch. Int.
       Pharmacodyn. Ther. 194:18-38 (1971).

75.   M. Rowland, S. Riegelman, P.A. Harris and S.D. Sholkoff, Absorption kinetics of
       aspirin in man following oral administration of an aqueous solution, J. Pharm.
       Sci. 61:379-385 (1972).

76.   V.P. Shah, S. Riegelman and W.L. Epstein, Determination of griseofulvin in skin,
       plasma and sweat, J. Pharm. Sci. 61:634-636 (1972).

77.   W. Sadee, M. Dagcioglu and S. Riegelman, Fluorometric microassay for
       spironolactone and its metabolites in biological fluids, J. Pharm. Sci. 61:1126-
       1129 (1972).

78.   W. Sadee, S. Riegelman and S.C. Jones, Plasma levels of spirolactones in the dog,
       J. Pharm. Sci. 61:1129-1132 (1972).

79.   W. Sadee, S. Riegelman and S.C. Jones, Disposition of tritium-labeled
       spirolactones in the dog, J. Pharm. Sci. 61:1132-1135 (1972).

80.   W.L. Epstein, V.P. Shah and S. Riegelman, Griseofulvin levels in stratum
       corneum.   Study after oral administration in man, Arch. Dermatol. 106:344-348
       (1972).

81.   S.H. Wan and S. Riegelman, Renal contribution to overall metabolism of drugs.
       I.   Conversion of benzoic acid to hippuric acid, J. Pharm. Sci. 61:1278-1284
       (1972).

82.   S.H. Wan and S. Riegelman, Renal contribution to overall metabolism of drugs.
       II.   Biotransformation of salicylic acid to salicyluric acid, J. Pharm. Sci.
       61:1284-1287 (1972).

83.   S.H. Wan, B. von Lehmann and S. Riegelman, Renal contribution to overall
       metabolism of drugs.   III.   Metabolism of p-aminobenzoic acid, J. Pharm. Sci.
       61:1288-1292 (1972).

84.   E.J. Mroszczak and S. Riegelman, Rapid spectrofluorometric assay for total bile
       salts in bile, Clin. Chem. 18:987-991 (1972).

85.   S. Riegelman, Physiological and pharmacokinetic complexities in bioavailability
       testing, Pharmacology 8:118-141 (1972).

86.   S. Riegelman, M. Rowland and L.Z. Benet. Use of isotopes in bioavailability
       testing, J. Pharmacokin. Biopharm. 1:83-87 (1973).

87.   D. Schuppan, S. Riegelman, B. von Lehmann, A. Pilbrandt and C. Becker,
       Preliminary pharmacokinetic studies of propylthiouracil in humans, J.
       Pharmacokin. Biopharm. 1:307-318 (1973).

88.   B. von Lehmann, S.H. Wan, S. Riegelman and C. Becker, Renal contribution to
       overall metabolism of drugs.   IV.   Biotransformation of salicylic acid to
       salicyluric acid in man, J. Pharm. Sci. 62:1483-1486 (1973).

89.   S. Riegelman and M. Rowland, Effect of route of administration on drug
       disposition, J. Pharmacokin. Biopharm. 1:419-434 (1973).

90.   M. Rowland and S. Riegelman, Determination of 6-demethyl-griseofulvin in urine,

J. Pharm. Sci. 62:2030-2032 (1973).

91. H.G. Boxenbaum, S. Riegelman and R.M. Elashoff, Statistical estimations in pharmacokinetics, J. Pharmacokin. Biopharm. 2:123-148 (1974).

92. L. Plon and S. Riegelman, Are there risks in long-term, low-dose tetracycline therapy of acne vulgaris? J. Am. Med. Assoc. 228:900 (1974).

93. H.G. Boxenbaum, G.S. Jodhka, A.C. Ferguson, S. Riegelman and T.R. MacGregor, The influence of bacterial gut hydrolysis on the fate of orally administered isonicotinuric acid in man, J. Pharmacokin. Biopharm. 2:211-237 (1974).

94. V.P. Shah, W.L. Epstein and S. Riegelman, Role of sweat in accumulation of orally administered griseofulvin in skin, J. Clin. Invest. 53:1673-1678 (1974).

95. V.P. Shah, S. Riegelman and W.L. Epstein, Griseofulvin, absorption, metabolism and excretion, in: "The Diagnosis and Treatment of Fungal Infections," H.M. Robinson, Jr., ed., (1974), ch. 24, pp. 315-353.

96. M. Weinberger and S. Riegelman, Rational use of theophylline for bronchodilatation, N. Engl. J. Med. 291:151-153 (1974).

97. H.G. Boxenbaum and S. Riegelman, Determination of isoniazid and metabolites in biological fluids, J. Pharm. Sci. 63:1191-1197 (1974).

98. S. Riegelman and M. Rowland, Effect of route of administration on drug disposition, in: "Pharmacology and Pharmacokinetics," T. Teorell, R.L. Dedrick and P.G. Condliffe, eds., Plenum Press, New York (1974) pp. 87-107.

99. V.P. Shah and S. Riegelman, GLC determination of theophylline in biological fluids, J. Pharm. Sci. 63:1283-1285 (1974).

100. V.P. Shah, S.M. Wallace and S. Riegelman, Microultrafiltration technique for drug-protein binding determination in plasma, J. Pharm. Sci. 63:1364-1367 (1974).

101. S. Riegelman, Pharmacokinetic factors affecting epidermal penetration and percutaneous absorption, Clin. Pharmacol. Ther. 16:873-883 (1974).

102. S. Riegelman, Disposition factors as determinants of drug activity, in: "Pharmacokinetics, Drug Metabolism and Drug Interactions," (Vol. III), F.G. McMahon, ed., Futura Publishing Co., Mt. Kisco, NY (1974) ch. 3, pp.25-50.

103. J.A. Nelson, A.E. Staubus and S. Riegelman, Saturation kinetics of iopanoate in the dog, Invest. Radiol. 10:371-377 (1975).

104. W.L. Epstein, V.P. Shah and S. Riegelman, Dermatopharmacology of griseofulvin, CUTIS 15:271-275 (1975).

105. E.J. Mroszczak and S. Riegelman, Disposition of diethylstilbestrol in the rhesus monkey, J. Pharmacokin. Biopharm. 3:303-327 (1975).

106. W.L. Epstein, V.P. Shah, H.E. Jones and S. Riegelman, Topically applied griseofulvin in prevention and treatment of Trichophyton mentagrophytes, Arch. Dermatol. 111:1293-1297 (1975).

107. H.G. Boxenbaum and S. Riegelman, Pharmacokinetics of isoniazid and some metabolites in man, J. Pharmacokin. Biopharm. 4:287-325 (1976).

108. S.K. Lin, A.A. Moss and S. Riegelman, Saturation kinetics of iodipamide, Invest. Radiol. 12:175-179 (1977).

109. J.R. Powell, J.F. Thiercelin, S. Vozeh, L. Sansom and S. Riegelman, The influence of cigarette smoking and sex on theophylline disposition, Am. Rev. Respir. Dis. 116:17-23 (1977).

110. S.M. Wallace, V.P. Shah and S. Riegelman, GLC analysis of acetazolamide in blood, plasma, and saliva following oral administration to normal subjects, J. Pharm. Sci. 66:527-530 (1977).

111. S.M. Wallace and S. Riegelman, Uptake of acetazolamide by human erythrocytes in vitro, J. Pharm. Sci. 66:729-731 (1977).

112. E. Martin, T.N. Tozer, L.B. Sheiner and S. Riegelman, The clinical pharmacokinetics of phenytoin, J. Pharmacokin. Biopharm. 5:579-596 (1977).

113. S.M. Wallace, V.P. Shah, W.L. Epstein, J. Greenberg and S. Riegelman, Topically applied antifungal agents. Percutaneous penetration and prophylactic activity against Trichophyton mentagrophytes infection, Arch. Dermatol. 113:1539-1542 (1977).

114. S.K. Lin, A.A. Moss and S. Riegelman, Iodipamide kinetics: Capacity-limited biliary excretion with simultaneous pseudo-first-order renal excretion, J. Pharm. Sci. 66:1670-1674 (1977).

115. E.J. Mroszczak and S. Riegelman, Biliary excretion of diethylstilbestrol in the rhesus monkey, J. Pharmacokin. Biopharm. 6:339-354 (1978).

116. J.R. Powell, S. Vozeh, P. Hopewell, J. Costello, L.B. Sheiner and S. Riegelman, Theophylline disposition in acutely ill hospitalized patients. The effect of smoking, heart failure, severe airway obstruction, and pneumonia, Am. Rev. Resp. Dis. 118:229-238 (1978).

117. S. Vozeh, R.A. Upton, S. Riegelman, L.B. Sheiner and J.R. Powell, Bronchodilator therapy, N. Engl. J. Med. 298:220 (1978).

118. S.M. Wallace, V.P. Shah, S. Riegelman and W.L. Epstein, Electron capture gas chromatographic assay for miconazole and clotrimazole in skin samples, Anal. Letters 11:461-468 (1978).

119. S.K. Lin, A.A. Moss, R. Motson and S. Riegelman, Pharmacokinetics of iodoxamic acid in rhesus monkey: Biliary excretion, plasma protein binding and enterohepatic circulation, J. Pharm. Sci. 67:930-934 (1978).

120. T.W. Guentert and S. Riegelman, Specificity of quinidine determination methods, Clin. Chem. 24:2065-2066 (1978).

121. S. Vozeh, J.R. Powell, S. Riegelman, J. Costello, L.B. Sheiner and P. Hopewell, Changes in theophylline clearance during acute illness, J. Amer. Med. Assoc. 240:1882-1884 (1978).

122. T.W. Guentert, P.E. Coates, R.A. Upton, D.L. Combs and S. Riegelman, Determination of quinidine and its major metabolites by high-performance liquid chromatography, J. Chromatogr. 162:59-70 (1979).

123. M.R. Bonora, T.W. Guentert, R.A. Upton and S. Riegelman, Determination of quinidine and metabolites in urine by reverse-phase high-pressure liquid chromatography, Clin. Chimica Acta 91:277-284 (1979).

124. A.A. Moss, S.K. Lin, E.R. Margules, R.W. Motson and S. Riegelman, Pharmacokinetics of iopanoic acid in the rhesus monkey: Biliary excretion plasma protein binding and biotransformation, Invest. Radiol. 14:171-176 (1979).

125. L.B. Sheiner, R.A. Upton, J.-F. Thiercelin and S. Riegelman, Bioavailability studies and drug design as influenced by variation in drug disposition, in: "Biologic Availability of Medicines", Pharmaceutical and Chemical Manufacturers Association of South Africa, Pretoria (1979) pp. 43-50.

126. T.W. Guentert, R.A. Upton, N.H.G. Holford and S. Riegelman, Divergence in pharmacokinetic parameters of quinidine obtained by specific and nonspecific assay methods, J. Pharmacokin. Biopharm. 7:303-311 (1979).

127. T.W. Guentert, M.G. Wientjes, R.A. Upton, D.L. Combs and S. Riegelman, Evaluation of a modified high-performance liquid chromatography assay for acebutolol and its major metabolite, J. Chromatogr. 163:373-382 (1979).

128. S.K. Lin, A.A. Moss and S. Riegelman, Kinetics of drug-drug interactions: Biliary excretion of iodoxamic acid and iopanoic acid in the rhesus monkey, J. Pharm. Sci. 68:1430-1433 (1979).

129. T.W. Guentert, N.H.G. Holford, P.E. Coates, R.A. Upton and S. Riegelman, Quinidine pharmacokinetics in man: Choice of a disposition model and absolute bioavailability studies, J. Pharmacokin. Biopharm. 7:315-330 (1979).

130. K.T. Muir and S. Riegelman, Curve fitting and modeling in pharmacokinetics, J. Pharmacokin. Biopharm. 7:685-687 (1979).

131. R.A. Upton, J-F. Thiercelin, T.W. Guentert, L. Sansom, J.R. Powell, P.E. Coates and S. Riegelman, Evaluation of the absorption from some commercial sustained release theophylline products, J. Pharmacokin. Biopharm. 8:131-149 (1980).

132. R.A. Upton, J.R. Powell, T.W. Guentert, J-F. Thiercelin, L. Sansom, P.E. Coates and S. Riegelman, Evaluation of the absorption from some commercial enteric release theophylline products, J. Pharmacokin. Biopharm. 8:151-164 (1980).

133. R.A. Upton, J.N. Buskin, T.W. Guentert, R.L. Williams and S. Riegelman, A convenient and sensitive high pressure liquid chromatography assay for ketoprofen, naproxen and other allied drugs in plasma or urine, J. Chromatogr. 190:119-128 (1980).

134. R.A. Upton, L. Sansom, T.W. Guentert, J.R. Powell, J-F. Thiercelin, V.P. Shah, P.E. Coates and S. Riegelman, Evaluation of the absorption from 15 commercial theophylline products indicating deficiencies in currently applied bioavailability criteria, J. Pharmacokin. Biopharm. 8:229-242 (1980).

135. B. Silber, M-W. Lo and S. Riegelman, The influence of heparin administration on the plasma protein binding and disposition of propranolol, Res. Commun. Chem. Pathol. Pharmacol. 27:419-429 (1980).

136. T.W. Guentert, R.A. Upton, N.H.G. Holford, A. Bostrom and S. Riegelman, Gastrointestinal absorption of quinidine from some solutions and commercial tablets, J. Pharmacokin. Biopharm. 8:243-255 (1980).

137. M-W. Lo and S. Riegelman, Determination of propranolol and its major metabolites in plasma and urine by HPLC without solvent extraction, J. Chromatogr. 183:213-220 (1980).

138. E. Sarrazin, L. Hendeles, M. Weinberger, K. Muir and S. Riegelman, Dose-dependent kinetics of theophylline: observations among ambulatory asthmatic children, J.

Pediatrics 97:825-828 (1980).

139. K. Muir, J.H.G. Jonkman, D. Tang, M. Kunitani and S. Riegelman, Simultaneous determination of theophylline and its major metabolites in urine by reversed-phase ion-pair high performance liquid chromatography, J. Chromatogr. 221:85-95 (1980).

140. T.W. Guentert, A. Rakhit, R.A. Upton and S. Riegelman, An integrated approach to measurements of quinidine and metabolites in biological fluids, J. Chromatogr. 183:514-518 (1980).

141. S. Vozeh, J.R. Powell, G.C. Cupit, S. Riegelman and L.B. Sheiner, Influence of allopurinol on theophylline disposition in adults, Clin. Pharmacol. Ther. 27:194-197 (1980).

142. S. Riegelman and J.W. Jenne, Controlled release theophylline, Chest 78:250-251 (1980).

143. B. Silber and S. Riegelman, Stereospecific assay for (-)- and (+)-propranolol in human and dog plasma, J. Pharmacol. Exp. Ther. 215:643-648 (1980).

144. R.A. Upton, J.N. Buskin, R.L. Williams, N.H.G. Holford and S. Riegelman, Negligible excretion of unchanged ketoprofen, naproxen and probenecid in urine, J. Pharm. Sci. 69:1254-1257 (1980).

145. S. Riegelman, K. Muir and R.A. Upton, Factors affecting the pharmacokinetics of theophylline, Eur. J. Resp. Dis., Suppl. 61:67-82 (1980).

146. S. Riegelman and P. Collier, The application of statistical moment theory to the evaluation of in vivo dissolution time and absorption time, J. Pharmacokin. Biopharm. 8:509-534 (1980).

147. S. Riegelman, L.B. Sheiner and S.L. Beal, Population based approach to pharmacokinetics and bioavailability studies in patients, in: "Pharmacokinetics, a 25 Year Old Discipline," E. Gladtke and G. Heimann, eds., G. Fischer Verlag, Stuttgart (1980) pp. 83-95.

148. R.A. Upton, S. Riegelman and L.B. Sheiner, Bioavailability assessment as influenced by variation in drug disposition, in: "Drug Absorption and Disposition: Statistical Considerations," K.S. Albert, ed., American Pharmaceutical Association, Washington (1980) pp. 77-85.

149. S. Riegelman and R.A. Upton, In vitro and in vivo bioavailability correlation, in: "Drug Absorption," L.F. Prescott and W.S. Nimmo, eds., ADIS Press, New York (1981) pp. 297-312.

150. T.N. Tozer, D.D-S. Tang-Liu and S. Riegelman, Linear versus nonlinear pharmacokinetics, in: "Topics in Pharmaceutical Sciences," D.D. Breimer and P. Speiser, eds., Elsevier/North Holland Biomedical Press, Amsterdam (1981) pp. 3-17.

151. N.H.G. Holford, P.E. Coates, T.W. Guentert, S. Riegelman and L.B. Sheiner, The effect of quinidine and its metabolites on the electrocardiogram and systolic time intervals: concentration-effect relationships, Br. J. Clin. Pharmacol. 11:187-195 (1981).

152. J.H.G. Jonkman, D. Tang, R.A. Upton and S. Riegelman, Measurement of excretion characteristics of theophylline and its major metabolites, Eur. J. Clin. Pharmacol. 20:435-441 (1981).

153. R.A. Upton, R.L. Williams, T.W. Guentert, J.N. Buskin and S. Riegelman, Ketoprofen pharmacokinetics and bioavailability based on an improved, sensitive and specific assay, Eur. J. Clin. Pharmacol. 20:127-133 (1981).

154. M.G. Kunitani, D.A. Johnson, R.A. Upton and S. Riegelman, Convenient and sensitive high-performance liquid chromatography assay for cimetidine in plasma or urine, J. Chromatogr. 224:156-161 (1981).

155. B. Silber, B.A. Mico, P.R. Ortiz de Montellano, D.M. Dols and S. Riegelman, In vivo effects of the cytochrome P-450 suicide substrate 2-isopropyl-4-pentenamide (allylisopropylacetamide) on the disposition and metabolic pattern of propranolol, J. Pharmacol. Exp. Ther. 219:125-133 (1981).

156. R.A. Prince, D.S. Wing, M.M. Weinberger, L.S. Hendeles and S. Riegelman, Effect of erythromycin on theophylline kinetics, J. Allergy Clin. Immunol. 68:427-431 (1981).

157. L. Sansom, J.R. Powell and S. Riegelman, Bioavailability of aminophylline suppositories - clinical implications, Proc. First Eur. Congr. Biopharm. Pharmacokin. 1:389-398 (1981).

158. D.D-S. Tang-Liu and S. Riegelman, Metabolism of theophylline to caffeine in adults, Res. Commun. Chem. Path. Pharmacol. 34:371-380 (1981).

159. J.H.G. Jonkman, K.T. Muir, D-S. Tang and S. Riegelman, Selective quantitative determination of methylxanthines and methyluric acids in urine, in:

"Theophylline and other Methylxanthines," N. Rietbrock, B.G. Woodcock and A. H. Staib, eds., F. Vieweg & Sohn, Braunschweig/Wiesbaden, (1982) pp. 169-174.

160. R.A. Upton, J-F. Thiercelin, T.W. Guentert, S.M. Wallace, J.R. Powell, L. Sansom and S. Riegelman, Intra-individual variability in theophylline pharmacokinetics: Statistical verification in 39 of 60 healthy young adults, J. Pharmacokin. Biopharm. 10:123-134 (1982).

161. R.A. Upton, J-F. Thiercelin, J.K. Moore and S. Riegelman, A method for estimating within-individual variability in clearance and in volume of distribution from standard bioavailability studies, J. Pharmacokin. Biopharm. 10:135-146 (1982).

162. D.D-S. Tang-Liu and S. Riegelman, An automated HPLC assay for simultaneous quantitation of methylated xanthines and uric acids in urine, J. Chromatogr. Sci. 20:155-159 (1982).

163. D.D-S. Tang-Liu, T.N. Tozer and S. Riegelman, Urine flow-dependence of theophylline renal clearance in man. J. Pharmacokin. Biopharm. 10:351-364 (1982).

164. D.D-S. Tang-Liu, R.L. Williams and S. Riegelman, Nonlinear theophylline elimination, Clin. Pharmacol. Ther. 31:358-369 (1982).

165. M-W. Lo, B. Silber and S. Riegelman, An automated HPLC method for the assay of propranolol and its basic metabolites in plasma and urine, J. Chromatogr. Sci. 20:126-131 (1982).

166. D.J. Effeney, S.M. Pond, M-W. Lo, B.M. Silber and S. Riegelman, A technique to study hepatic and intestinal drug metabolism separately in the dog, J. Pharmacol. Exp. Ther. 221:507-511 (1982).

167. M-W. Lo, D.J. Effeney, S.M. Pond, B.M. Silber and S. Riegelman, Lack of gastrointestinal metabolism of propranolol in dogs after portacaval transposition, J. Pharmacol. Exp. Ther. 221:512-515 (1982).

168. T.W. Guentert, J.J. Daly and S. Riegelman, Isolation, characterization and synthesis of a new quinidine metabolite, Eur. J. Drug Metab. Pharmacokin. 7:31-38 (1982).

169. J.R. Powell, R. Okada, K.A. Conrad, T.W. Guentert and S. Riegelman, Altered quinidine disposition in a patient with chronic active hepatitis, Postgrad. Med. J. 58:82-84 (1982).

170. B.M. Silber, N.H.G. Holford and S. Riegelman, Stereoselective disposition and glucuronidation of propranolol in humans, J. Pharm. Sci. 71:699-704 (1982).

171. A. Rakhit, M. Kunitani, N.H.G. Holford and S. Riegelman, Improved liquid-chromatographic assay of quinidine and its metabolites in biological fluids, Clin. Chem. 28:1505-1509 (1982).

172. R.L. Williams, R.A. Upton, R.J. Seidehamel and S. Riegelman, Multiple-dose bioavailability of a sustained release theophylline product, Curr. Ther. Res. 31:45-55 (1982).

173. B.M. Silber, N.H.G. Holford and S. Riegelman, Dose-dependent elimination of propranolol and its major metabolites in humans, J. Pharm. Sci. 72:725-732 (1983).

174. D. D-S. Tang-Liu, T.N. Tozer and S. Riegelman, Dependence of renal clearance on urine flow: A mathematical model and its application. J. Pharm. Sci. 72:154-158 (1983).

175. P.S. Collier and S. Riegelman, Estimation of absolute bioavailability assuming steady-state apparent volume of distribution remains constant. J. Pharmacokin. Biopharm. 11:205-214 (1983).

176. P.K. Noonan, I. Kanfer, S. Riegelman and L.Z. Benet, Determination of picogram nitroglycerin plasma concentrations using capillary GC with on-column injection. J. Pharm. Sci., in press (1984).

527